IMMUNOLOGY AND IMMUNOPATHOLOGY OF THE HUMAN FOETAL-MATERNAL INTERACTION

"The history of man for the nine months preceding his birth would, probably, be far more interesting and contain events of greater moment than all the three-score and ten years that follow it."

Samuel Taylor Coleridge

IMMUNOLOGY AND IMMUNOPATHOLOGY OF THE HUMAN FOETAL-MATERNAL INTERACTION

Y. W. Loke M.A., M.D.

Lecturer, Division of Experimental and Cellular Pathology, Department of Pathology, University of Cambridge, England

Fellow and Director of Studies in Medicine, King's College, Cambridge, England

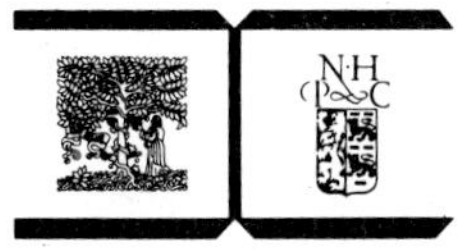

1978

Elsevier/North-Holland Biomedical Press
Amsterdam • New York • Oxford

Cover photo Paul Curtis

Published by:
Elsevier/North-Holland Biomedical Press
335, Jan van Galenstraat, P.O. Box 211
Amsterdam, The Netherlands

Sole distributors for the U.S.A. and Canada:
Elsevier/North-Holland Inc.
52 Vanderbilt Avenue
New York, N.Y. 10017

Library of Congress Cataloging in Publication Data

Loke, Y W
Immunology and immunopathology of the human foetal-maternal interaction.

Bibliography: p.
Includes indexes.
1. Pregnancy—Immunological aspects.
2. Maternal-fetal exchange. 3. Pregnancy, Complications of—Immunological aspects. I. Title.
[DNLM: 1. Maternal—Fetal exchange. 2. Fetus—Immunology. 3. Placenta—Immunology. 4. Antibody formation—In pregnancy. 5. Immunity—In pregnancy. QW553 L836i]
RG557.L65 618.3 78-8634
ISBN 0-444-80055-7

With 13 illustrations

PRINTED IN THE NETHERLANDS

Preface

The immunological aspects of human reproduction constitute a comparatively new field of study and only within the last few years sufficient human data have accumulated to permit a meaningful discussion against the background of animal studies on which most of the present concepts are based. It is also a subject which spans a wide variety of disciplines so that available information tends to be scattered among different scientific publications. The aim of the present monograph is to provide, conveniently within one volume, a comprehensive account of the subject together with an extensive review of the literature, in the hope that it will serve the need of all those human biologists who wish to obtain an overview of this fascinating aspect of reproduction as applied to our own species.

My own interest in this field began from a study of cancer as exemplified by trophoblast neoplasms when it soon became apparent that, until more was known about the immunobiology of normal trophoblast, little could be gained by studying its abnormal counterpart. Much of the earlier work was done in collaboration with many colleagues, experts in immunology, tissue typing and cell culture, to all of whom I am greatly indebted for introducing me to experimental methods. In particular, I would like to mention Dr. Robert Borland with whom I worked for many years on the in vitro study of human trophoblast. The biochemical studies of trophoblast cell surface incorporated in this volume are by Dr. Anthony Whyte. I thank him for this valuable contribution and also for his help in the preparation of the manuscript. I would like to record my deep gratitude to Professor

Kendal Dixon who has been a guide and mentor from my undergraduate days right up to the present moment. Many others have assisted me with my work and have acted as sources of constructive ideas as well as providers of valuable material. To all of them I express my thanks.

I am also indebted to those authors and publishers who have kindly given permission to reproduce published material. Full reference to these can be found in relation to the appropriate diagrams and tables. I am happy to have the opportunity to record the financial support which I have received from the Cancer Research Campaign, The Lalor Foundation and The American Friends of Cambridge University.

Finally, I dedicate this book to my family who were most helpful, encouraging and interested throughout with what I was doing. I hope the final product will serve as evidence that all my efforts have not entirely been in vain.

Y. W. LOKE
Autumn 1978

Contents

1

Introduction

Ever since the initial recognition that transplant rejection is mediated by an immunological mechanism due to genetically determined antigenic disparity between graft and recipient, the successful development of the mammalian conceptus in utero is a paradox which has continued to intrigue biologists from a wide variety of disciplines. The conceptus possesses a mixture of antigens inherited from both maternal and paternal sources so that, in an outbred population like man, it is analogous to an allograft implanted in the uterus. Many clinical observations have been recorded and a great deal of experimental work has been done to elucidate the problem and, although new facts continue regularly to emerge, the solution remains tantalisingly beyond reach.

Expanding knowledge in basic immunology has dictated a reappraisal of the immunological processes involved in human reproduction. The concept of the allergic reaction as an 'all or none' phenomenon, that, once mounted will progress relentlessly until the destruction of the foreign cells, is no longer tenable. Instead, like all physiological processes, it is subjected to homeostatic control with complex ways of regulation, so that antigens, antibodies, or both in combination with each other, can lead to switching-off of the allergic reaction. These immunoregulatory mechanisms are thought to influence tumour-host interactions and they may also be responsible for the survival of parasites in immunocompetent hosts. In the context of human reproduction, the demonstration of paternally derived antigens on foetal tissues and the presence of effective maternal immune response, therefore, need no longer be considered as incompatible to the success of the foetus as an allograft. Indeed, a functional immune response may even be an essential factor for a successful foetal-maternal relationship, since placentation has generally evolved in those species with a highly developed immunological system. In addition, there are many other non-specific factors like placental hormones and other proteins which have been shown to play an important regulatory role so much so that pregnancy sera have become a rich source for the isolation of natural immunosuppressive substances.

There may be occasions when this immunological equilibrium is disrupted, leading either to a consistent failure of the alien conceptus to survive or to an over-successful degree of implantation. The former may be exemplified by cases of habitual abortion or sterility, while choriocarcinoma may be a manifestation of the latter. There are other diseases of pregnancy, like toxaemia, the aetiology of which may have a similar immunological basis.

Although the human placenta divides the foetal and maternal circulations, it does not form an absolute barrier. Some serum proteins as well as cells can traverse in either direction, so that there is a constant exchange of these elements between the foetus and mother throughout pregnancy. This can be undoubtedly beneficial to the foetus, like the passive transfer of humoral immunity but, in many instances, the transplacental transmission of maternal antibodies can lead to grave consequences. The production of erythroblastosis foetalis by maternal iso-antibodies is well recognised. Recent demonstration that some auto-allergic diseases may also be transmitted to the foetus by maternal auto-antibodies has provided further examples, and also afforded an insight into the pathogenesis of these diseases. The transfer of maternal immunocompetent cells to the foetus will similarly be expected to be potentially harmful. Indeed, the development of graft-versus-host disease has occasionally been reported in man but the rarity with which this occurs attests to the early maturation of immunocompetence in the human foetus. Most of these maternal cells are probably rapidly destroyed, for the human foetus has been shown to posses a useful range of immunological defense mechanisms very early on in gestation.

Maternal influence on the foetus does not end with birth, for there is increasing evidence that the transfer of passive immunity continues via milk. Although the main immunoprotective role is within the neonatal intestine against enteropathogens, the possibility of the adoptive transfer of systemic immunity by this route should not be entirely dismissed.

Recognition of the immunological nature of human gestation has prompted many attempts at devising a method for the artificial interruption of pregnancy based on maternal sensitisation. Earlier studies have suffered from a lack of an appropriate trophoblast-specific antigen. There is hope that this obstacle may now be circumvented by immunising with the placental hormone HCG. Detailed studies on the structure of this molecule have shown that one portion of the amino-acid sequence is specific to the hormone with no cross-reactivity with other endogenous hormones.

There have been many reviews on various immunological aspects of mammalian reproduction (Anderson 1972; Borland 1975; Edwards and Coombs 1975; Beer and Billingham 1976). The present monograph is intended to deal specifically with the human foetal-maternal interaction. The anatomy and physiology of the human placenta differ greatly from those of animal species, and even those animals with a similar haemochorial placentation are not directly comparable. Furthermore, some pregnancy-associated conditions like trophoblast neoplasms appear to be unique in man. Thus, while those animal studies which have resulted in important concepts are included, most of the discussion is based directly on human in vivo and in vitro data.

2

Immunological status of the human foetus and placenta

2.1 Antigenicity of human embryonic tissue

It was Little, in 1924, who postulated that the embryo developed its antigenic individuality relatively late, and it has been widely believed that this antigenic immaturity could play an important part in the survival of the foetus during pregnancy. Current opinion, however, has moved away from this concept because subsequent investigations have shown that antigens are expressed by early human embryonic tissue.

In a series of transplantation studies, Goldstein and Baxter (1958) found that skin grafts from 17—33 weeks gestation age human foetuses transplanted to allogeneic hosts were all rejected within an average time of 12.6 days. Even implants of skin from foetuses of less than 16 weeks gestation age to subcutaneous sites of allogeneic hosts were found to become necrotic and surrounded by mononuclear cell infiltration, indicating that foetal skin at an early stage of development can evoke an active homograft rejection response.

In vitro studies have further confirmed the presence of antigens on early embryonic tissue. By means of a mixed agglutination technique Högman (1959) demonstrated the presence of 'A' and 'B' blood group antigens on cultured cells derived from various organs of foetuses ranging from 3—6 months gestation age. Although positive reactions were seen with cells cultured from most organs, the number of cells per culture actually reacting with indicator red cells varied in different organs, suggesting that there could be a differential expression of 'A' and 'B' antigens by different organs at a particular stage of development. Cells cultured from foetal kidney were the most reactive. Szulman (1964), in an immunofluorescent localisation of ABH antigens on tissue sections, reported that these antigens were demonstrable on the surface of epithelial cells from most foetal tissues as early as 6 weeks gestation age. Paradoxically, there seemed to be a gradual loss of these epithelial cell surface antigens as the tissue matured, so that by the 12th week of gestation age these antigens became increasingly difficult to demonstrate in many organs. It was postulated that the widespread presence of these antigens on the surface of very young epithelial cells could contribute to the molecular profile of the cell wall and thereby played a part in cell to cell contact and differentiation.

Blood group antigens have also been detected on foetal red cells (Constandoulkis and Kay 1962). However, foetal erythrocytes appear to exhibit a quantitative as well as qualitative difference in the expression of these antigens when compared to adult erythrocytes. Foetal group 'A' and group 'B' erythrocytes were found to absorb less anti-A and anti-B antibody, respectively, than the corresponding adult cells in spite of the relatively large size of foetal cells. This could be due to fewer antigenic sites on foetal red cells. In addition, A1 antigens were entirely lacking on foetal erythrocytes. All foetal group 'A' red cells were phenotypically A2. The change to an adult antigenic profile probably takes place after birth through some mechanisms similar to that for transformation from foetal to adult-type haemoglobin. Rhesus antigens have been demonstrated on red cells of a 10 mm foetus estimated to be equivalent to 38 days gestation age (Bergström et al. 1967).

Cells of the erythromyeloid series obtained from lymph node, spleen and bone marrow of foetuses from 10—26 weeks gestation age can be typed for the presence of HL-A antigens (Ceppellini et al. 1971). These antigens have also been demonstrated on other foetal tissues. Seigler and Metzgar (1970), using a mixed agglutination method (perhaps a more accurate description would be a mixed antiglobulin reaction), incubated monolayer cultures of foetal cells with antisera defining a broad spectrum of HL-A specificities. Human red blood cells sensitised with chimpanzee anti-human red blood cell antibody were used as indicator cells with a goat anti-human globulin as the link. They found that positive reactions occurred with foetal cells from 6 weeks gestation age. There was a suggestion that these antigens were present in a greater concentration on cells from some organs than from others, a situation which was similar to that found for the distribution of ABH antigens on foetal tissue.

Water-soluble substances bearing HL-A2, 5,7,8,9 specificities could be extracted by low frequency sonification from spleen, lung, liver, and kidney tissues of 3—5½ months old embryos, these substances being able to inhibit allo-antisera in a pattern consistent with the phenotype of the antigen donor (Pellegrino et al. 1970). Again there appeared to be differences in the expression of these HL-A antigens during the course of development in different organs. No HL-A antigens were eluted from foetal lung specimens until 5½ months gestation age. The foetal kidney had the most soluble HL-A antigens at a very early stage of development. Soluble antigens extracted from 5,000 foetal kidney cells yielded a 50% inhibition of an anti-HL-A2 serum as compared to 8,000 cultured peripheral lymphocytes, 30,000 adult spleen cells and 75,000 adult kidney cells. A greater ease in solubilisation of foetal antigens compared to adult antigens could be an alternative explanation of these findings.

Cells from thymus, spleen, liver and blood lymphocytes obtained from foetuses as early as at 11 weeks gestation age are all capable of stimulating and responding to adult allogeneic lymphocytes in one-way MLC reactions (Pegrum 1971; Ohama and Kajii 1974).

The conclusion to be drawn from the evidence presented is that antigens are present in immunologically effective concentrations on most tissues of the human embryo from a very early stage of development, with perhaps some variation in the expression of these antigens by different tissues.

2.2. Antigenicity of human trophoblast

In the preceding section, it was concluded that the concept of foetal antigenic immaturity was unlikely to be the explanation for why the foetus was not rejected by the mother. In any case, in human gestation, the foetal and maternal systems are entirely separate and it is the extra-embryonic structure, the placenta, which lies in intimate contact over a considerable surface area with maternal tissue. Therefore, it is the antigenic status of placental trophoblast cells which is particularly relevant to our understanding of the immunological paradox of human pregnancy.

Animal transplantation experiments have shown that when mouse embryos were transferred ectopically to maternal strain hosts previously sensitised to paternal strain antigens, the embryonic grafts were quickly destroyed. In contrast, similar grafts of trophoblast tissue from ectoplacental cones proved somewhat refractory to destruction (Simmons and Russell 1962). This is further confirmed by in vitro studies, where mouse trophoblast cells from 7½ days ectoplacental cones were found to be insusceptible to immune cell lysis, while cells from other components of the conceptus, like the embryonic sac, were killed (Jenkinson and Billington 1974). These findings have led to the suggestion that trophoblast represents a specialised form of embryonic tissue which is either devoid of, or incapable of expressing antigenic specificities on its surface.

It is obvious that in vivo allogeneic transplantation studies cannot readily be performed with human placental tissue, so much of the evidence relating to the antigenicity of human trophoblast is based on investigations using xenogeneic animals or in vitro techniques.

2.2.1 Studies of human trophoblast antigens in animals

Heterologous antisera have been raised in mice (Curzen 1968; Curzen 1970) and in rabbits (Boss 1965) to mitochondrial and microsomal fractions of homogenised human placenta. The antibody was localised to the cytoplasm of trophoblast cells on sections of human placenta by immunofluorescent staining. Cross-reaction with human kidney tissue was observed and it was concluded that the antibody was directed at 'organ-specific' antigens which were shared by trophoblast and kidney cells. Whole placental homogenates, when injected into rabbits, also elicited the formation of antibodies which reacted with certain stromal and intracellular cytotrophoblastic elements but not with syncytiotrophoblast (Jones et al. 1972). The specificity of these antisera is difficult to determine and the biological significance in relation to trophoblast-maternal interaction is not clear, since none of the activity is directed at syncytiotrophoblast cell membrane components.

The cytotoxic property of heterologous antisera raised against a product of human trophoblast cells has also been reported. Currie (1967) found that rabbit antibody to human chorionic gonadotrophin, even at high dilutions, was cytotoxic to cultured human trophoblast cells in vitro in the presence of complement. Normal rabbit serum, however, was also cytotoxic but only at low dilutions. Rabbit sera are notoriously difficult to use as they frequently contain 'natural' antibodies to surface components, possibly carbohydrates, of cultured human cells so that any observed cytotoxic activity must be interpreted with care.

2.2.2. *In vitro demonstration of allo-antigens on human trophoblast cells*

Maternal lymphocytes as well as lymphocytes from unrelated donors were found to be cytotoxic to human trophoblast cells grown in culture (Currie and Bagshawe 1967a). This phenomenon of 'allogeneic inhibition', which was maximal after four days, was interpreted as showing that foreign antigenic groupings were expressed by human trophoblast cells. Essentially similar results were obtained by Douthwaite and Urbach (1971), except that they found that buffy coat leucocytes were cytotoxic to trophoblast cultures but purified lymphocytes were not, indicating that more than one cell type may be needed for the reaction. In a later report, Taylor and Hancock (1975) observed that the cytotoxic reaction was preceded by the lymphocytes transforming into blast cells. Thus, the long period (about four days) of incubation before cytotoxic reaction occurs, the need for the presence of another cell type (? macrophage), the cytotoxicity by both maternal and unrelated lymphocytes, and the blast cell transformation are all features which can be explained on the basis of an in vitro primary immune response analogous to the MLR (mixed lymphocyte reaction) but with trophoblast cells as stimulators. This would imply that human trophoblast cells express antigens belonging to the major histocompatibility complex. In contrast, Fikrig et al. (1967), using trophoblast cells obtained by superficial trypsinisation of intact chorionic villi as stimulators, and peripheral lymphocytes from mother and unrelated donors as responders, found no blastogenic response by the lymphocytes. This negative finding seems more in line with what is known about the MLR. Not all nucleated cells bearing allogeneic antigens can necessarily act as stimulators. Furthermore, although lymphoblasts generated in the MLR may have cytotoxic properties towards some cell types like Chang cells and Burkitt lymphoma cells, they do not usually kill the stimulating lymphocyte population (Ling and Kay 1975). Therefore the killing of trophoblast cells by allogeneic lymphocytes does not appear to fit in with any definite in vitro models of cell-mediated immunity.

Many attempts have been made to demonstrate HL-A antigens on human trophoblast cells, but the results are conflicting. Seigler and Metzgar (1970), using a mixed agglutination assay, found positive reactions for HL-A antigens on foetal tissues from 6 weeks gestation age onwards, but trophoblast syncytium was repeatedly negative. In addition, trophoblast tissue failed to absorb sera with anti-HL-A specificities. Negative findings were also reported by Faulk and Temple (1976) and Faulk et al. (1977). They could not demonstrate HL-A or Ia antigens of β_2 microglobulin in early and full-term placentae when using immunofluorescent staining of cryostat sections and electron microscopic examination of sections stained by the peroxidase antibody technique. Cells of the villous mesenchymal stroma, however, showed positive reactions. Treatment of trophoblast sections with neuraminidase, hyaluronidase, collagenase, or trypsin all failed to unmask any underlying antigenic determinants. The only antisera that stained trophoblasts were those directed against actin, plasminogen and transferrin (Faulk and Johnson 1977). Using preparations of placental villous surface membranes (Snary et al. 1976), and an antibody-binding assay. Goodfellow et al. (1976) reported a very low degree of expression, if at all, of HL-A antigens. In an immunofluorescent study on single or aggregates of trophoblast cells of 8—13 weeks gestation age, Sundqvist et al. (1977) were also unable to demonstrate the presence of HL-A antigens. The only positive findings appear to be those of Loke et al. (1971) who found that cultured cells from trophoblast villi and foetal skin of 12—13 weeks old conceptuses were killed in the presence of a multispecific anti-HL-A serum and complement. A monospecific anti-HL-A2 serum was cytotoxic to one out of three cases treated which was in agreement with the frequency of HL-A2 phenotype of 49% in the Cambridge area. The main drawback about using cultured trophoblast cells is the possible presence of contaminating cells. The human placenta is a composite organ which, on culture, generally yields several cell types (Chung et al. 1969; Loke and Borland 1970). These are derived from syncytiotrophoblast, cytotrophoblast and the fibrous stroma of the villous mesenchyme. Although trophoblast cells predominate during the early stages of a primary culture, they are soon replaced by fibroblastic elements after about the 9th day (Taylor and Hancock 1973).

A similar degree of controversy surrounds evidence for the presence of blood group antigens on human trophoblast cells. Immunofluorescent studies by Thiede et al. (1965) and by Szulman (1972) indicated that human placental villi were deficient in blood group antigens. In contrast, Gross (1966), when using a similar technique, found fluorescent staining of trophoblast sections by a rabbit anti-blood-group 'A' antiserum, the intensity of fluorescence diminishing as the placenta matured. The other positive report was by Loke and Ballard

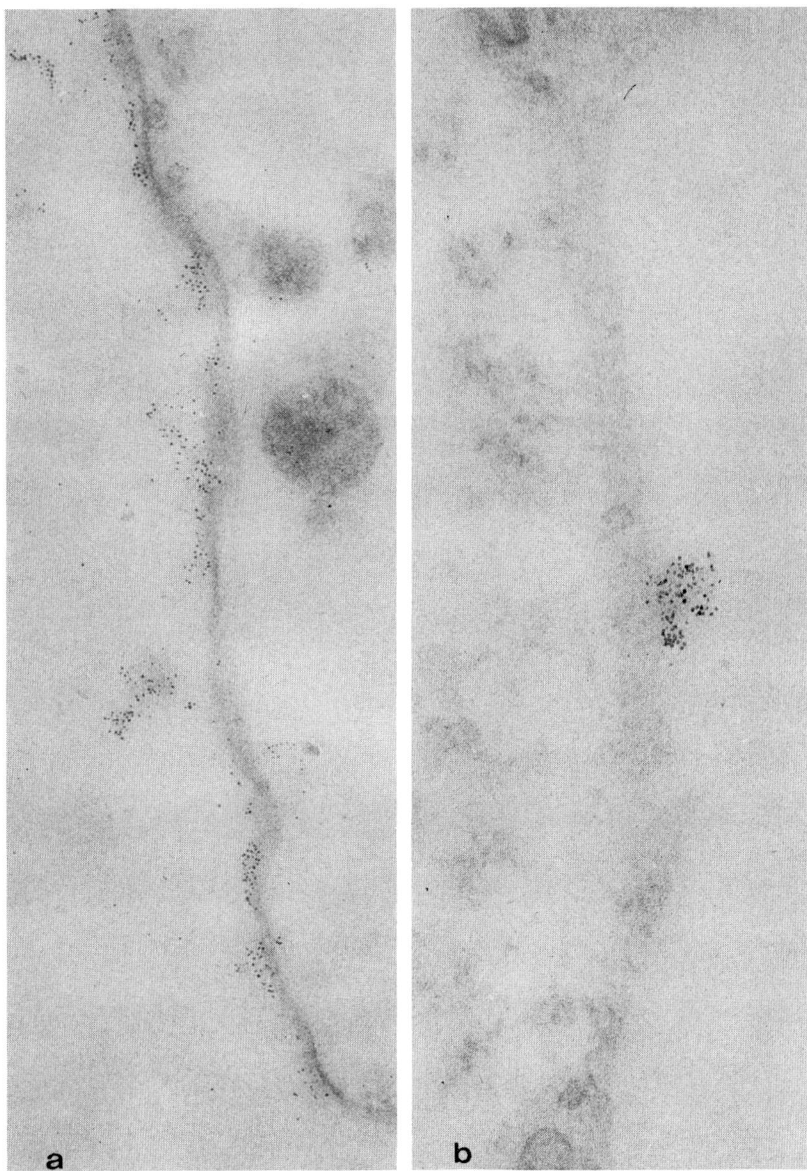

Fig. 2.1 (a) Blood group 'A' foetal skin cell treated with immune anti-A serum and ferritin-labelled anti-human IgG showing labelling over greater part of cell membrane. (b) Blood group 'A' trophoblast cell treated with immune anti-A serum and ferritin-labelled anti-human IgG showing only discrete areas of labelling. From Loke, Y. W. and Ballard, A-C. (1973) *Nature*, 245, 329—330.

(1973). These authors used three methods to detect blood group 'A' antigens on separated skin and trophoblast cells from 12—13 weeks old conceptuses which had been confirmed as belonging to Group 'A' by analysing foetal heart blood. Using a mixed agglutination method with an immune anti-A serum and group 'A' red blood cells as indicator cells, positive reactions were obtained with foetal skin cells but not with trophoblast cells from the same conceptus. Trophoblast cells treated with neuraminidase were equally negative. However, when a mixed antiglobulin method was used by coating trophoblast cells and group 'A' red cells with anti-A serum and cross-linking the two with a rabbit anti-human globulin, then positive rosettes were seen. These results were interpreted as due to antigens on trophoblast cells being so sparse that insufficient antibody was taken up to form stable bridges directly with the indicator red cells until another link was introduced in the form of an antiglobulin, a situation which was analogous to the demonstration of Rh antigens on red cells by the Coombs' test. This interpretation was supported by electron microscopic visualisation of immuno-ferritin labelled antigens occurring as discrete, sparsely distributed patches (Fig. 2.1). However, a subsequent electron microscopic study by Goto et al. (1977) failed to reveal blood group 'A' or 'B' antigens on human placentae taken from all stages of pregnancy even after digestion with neuraminidase, hyaluronidase, chondroitinase, trypsin, pepsin or pronase.

From the preceding review, it can be seen that antigens are certainly more difficult to demonstrate on trophoblast cells than on other foetal cells. The experiments of Loke and Ballard (1973) suggest that this may be due to a relative deficiency of antigens rather than to a total absence. However, in view of the consistently negative findings in whole placental sections, it must be admitted that there is justifiable suspicion that contaminating cells of non-trophoblast origin may have been responsible for the few positive results obtained in experiments using separated or cultured cells from trophoblast villi.

2.2.3 *In vivo immunogenicity of human trophoblast*

As we shall see in a later section, there is evidence that the pregnant mother is frequently sensitised by her developing foetus. The question that arises is to what extent placental cells contribute to the antigenic source for this maternal sensitisation. This question is difficult to answer, for other foetal cells undoubtedly can gain access to the maternal circulation during pregnancy. All that can be said is that placental cells certainly have ample opportunity of sensitising the mother, if indeed they possess immunogenic potential. Syncytiotrophoblast cells have been found frequently in the circulating blood drawn from vessels draining the uterus at various stages of gestation (Douglas et al. 1959). Although rapidly destroyed by proteolytic enzymes in maternal blood, many of these trophoblast cells could be found to lodge in the lungs. Attwood and Park (1961) studied 220 pregnant women and found pulmonary trophoblast embolism in 43.6% of them. In most of these cases, there were only limited amounts of tissue available for study and the authors were of the opinion that the percentage of positive cases might well be much higher if serial sections from different areas of the lungs were studied.

Antibodies to trophoblast cells of their own placentae were found to develop in post partum women (Hulka et al. 1961). A fluorescein-labelled globulin fraction of serum from these women was observed to localise to the cytoplasm of syncytiotrophoblast cells of her own placenta. A subsequent paper reported that other placentae, apart from her own, were also positively stained (Hulka et al. 1963), indicating that the antibody was directed either at some trophoblast-specific antigens or at shared allo-antigens. It is interesting to note from this study that these anti-trophoblast antibodies were not detectable during pregnancy and only appeared around the 4th post partum day. It was suggested that this could be due to a suppression of antibody production during pregnancy, or that the antibodies were absorbed out of the serum by the large placental mass before parturition. This was not confirmed by Burstein and Blumenthal (1969), however. Using a similar technique, they surveyed 824 maternal sera collected at various stages of pregnancy and after delivery and they found anti-trophoblast antibodies to be present in a large number of sera within the first trimester.

Besides the presence of anti-trophoblast antibodies in the sera of pregnant women, there is also evidence for the presence of cell-mediated immunity towards placental antigens. Using macrophage migration inhibition as an in vitro measure of cell-mediated immunity, Youtanannkorn and Matangkasombut (1972) found that leucocytes from post partum women would inhibit the migration of guinea pig peritoneal macrophages in the presence of membranous protein antigens pooled from five placentae. If antigens from only one placenta were used, then only the woman who donated the placenta had leucocytes which reacted. The onset of this cell-mediated immunity appeared to be from the 4th month of gestation onwards, as no inhibition of macrophage migration was found using leucocytes from primiparous women during the first trimester (Youtanannkorn et al. 1974). Furthermore, the concentration of placental antigens required to induce inhibition of macrophage migration gradually became less as pregnancy progressed, which could be indicative of the development of an increasing intensity of cell-mediated immunity. Based on the technique of in vitro cytotoxicity of cultured trophoblast cells by maternal lymphocytes which they have used for the detection of trophoblast antigenicity, Taylor et al. (1975) found that, whereas cultures from trophoblast of 8—24 weeks gestation age were killed by lymphocytes obtained at this stage of pregnancy only after 72 hours incubation, cultures from trophoblast of 32—34 weeks gestation age were killed by lymphocytes from this stage of pregnancy after 24 hours. Since unrelated allogeneic lymphocytes required 72 hours to kill both early and late trophoblast, the shorter period needed by maternal lymphocytes from late pregnancy to kill trophoblast from a similar gestation period was attributed to the development of maternal cell-mediated immune response rather than to any maturation or quantitative differences in antigens between mature and immature trophoblast.

The above studies indicate that pregnant women have humoral as well as cell-mediated immunity which can be shown to be directed at placental antigens in vitro. Does this interaction occur in vivo? Many investigators have examined human placentae for evidence of such an immunological reaction. McCormick et al. (1971) demonstrated, by fluorescent staining, the presence of IgG, βlC, and βlE in areas of fibrinoid necrosis on full term human placentae, which they interpreted as evidence for some sort of immunological reaction having taken place. This was denied by Mφe (1969), who found mainly fibrin and fibrinogen but no γ-globulin in Nitabuch's layer, indicating that this zone did not contain products of an immunological reaction but consisted mainly of platelet-fibrin thrombi. Later fluorescent studies have demonstrated IgG on trophoblast basement membrane of all human placentae (Faulk et al. 1974a). This IgG appeared to be of maternal origin, since it had the same Gm type as the mother, but it was not certain at what placental antigens it was directed. When eluted, this IgG stained the trophoblast basement membrane of homologous placentae but not the basement membrane of lung, thyroid or kidney, suggesting it was directed at some placenta-associated antigens. Other studies on IgG eluted from placental tissue found that the immunoglobulin would agglutinate lymphocytes from different individuals and in some cases were cytotoxic to a panel of 34 donor lymphocytes representing all known HL-A specificities (Bonneau et al. 1973). These eluates also inhibited one-way and two-way MLC reactions. Similar findings of cytotoxic activity against a panel of lymphocytes by placental IgG in subsequent investigations (Doughty and Gelsthorpe 1974; Tongio et al. 1975; Doughty and Gelsthorpe 1976) further confirm that maternal antibody reacts with HL-A determinants on placental cells in vivo.

These observations, however, offer no definitive evidence that the immunological reactions are directed at trophoblast cells. In fact, it seems more likely that other placental cells like those from the villous mesenchyme are involved, for it has been shown that allo-antigens are present on these cells but not on trophoblast (Jeannet et al. 1977). Taken in conjunction with the evidence obtained from in vitro investigations, it does seem that human trophoblast cells are either lacking or deficient in antigenic expression compared to other embryonic tissue. This is in agreement with observations in mice, where it is generally concluded that H-2 antigens are not detectable on peri-implantation trophoblast (Johnson 1975).

If trophoblast cells are indeed devoid of antigens, survival of the allogeneic placenta during pregnancy can be explained purely on the basis of its immunological neutrality. A deficiency of antigens may also be immunologically protective, for it has been demonstrated that when IgG antibody fixes onto cell surface antigens which are sparsely distributed, insufficient antibody 'doublets' are formed to fix complement, thereby transforming a potentially cytotoxic antibody into an enhancing one (Linscott 1970). This is particularly likely to occur in the foetal-maternal interaction, since maternal antibody will have only a limited specificity directed at paternally derived antigens. A similar protective role has been ascribed to 'blocking antibodies' in the survival of antigenic tumour cells in immunocompetent hosts (Hellström and Hellström 1972).

2.3 Special surface properties of human trophoblast cells

Besides a relative deficiency in antigens, there are other surface characteristics which may contribute to trophoblast's immunological inertness.

2.3.1 Surface mucoprotein

Deposits of fibrinoid material at the placental-decidual interface have been described in most haemochorial placentae, including man. This material is probably the result of cellular interaction between the invading trophoblast and maternal decidua (Wynn 1967). To be distinguished from this, there is another kind of fibrinoid-like mucoprotein substance which is intimately associated with the surface of trophoblast cells. Kirby et al. (1964) originated the idea that failure to express antigens by trophoblast cells was due to a covering layer of this fibrinoid material. They studied mouse trophoblast and made the following observations:

(1) Electron microscopic studies showed mouse trophoblast cells to be surrounded by a layer of amorphous, electron-dense material ranging from 0.1 μ to 2 μ thick;

(2) This material stained by PAS and Hale colloidal iron, indicating that it was a mucoprotein which was weakly sulphated but rich in hyaluronic and sialic acids;

(3) Hybrid placentae had more fibrinoid than inbred placentae, indicating that more of this substance was produced with a greater degree of foetal-maternal antigenic disparity;

(4) Extra-uterine trophoblast (e.g. transplanted to kidney capsule) was also surrounded by fibrinoid, indicating that the substance originated from trophoblast rather than from the decidua; and

(5) This trophoblast fibrinoid was very similar to the intercellular matrix of hamster cheek pouch, an organ with well-known antigen barrier qualities.

Similar studies on human trophoblast have also detected a highly sulphated mucoprotein coat around the cells (Bradbury et al. 1969), appearing in the form of a membrane-bound mucoprotein (Bradbury et al. 1970). The chemical composition differs slightly from that of the mouse. The human placental microvilli are covered by a layer of acid mucopolysaccharide which is rich in chondroitin sulphate or hyaluronic acid or both (Tighe et al. 1967), but poor in sialic acid which is abundant in the mouse (Billington 1975).

Attempts to test the concept that this surface coating can mask trophoblast immunogenicity have produced conflicting results. Currie et al. (1968) reported that ectoplacental cones from A_2G mice treated with neuraminidase in vitro would sensitise CBA adults against subsequent skin allograft from A_2G donors, whereas untreated ectoplacental cones did not. It was suggested that the mode of action of neuraminidase was to disrupt the O-glycoside link between sialic acid and its underlying aminosugars, thereby removing the terminal sialic acid group from the covering of sialomucoprotein. Unfortunately, this convincing demonstration of the unmasking of transplantation antigens on mouse trophoblast by neuraminidase has not been confirmed by subsequent investigations, all of which have repeatedly failed to demonstrate mouse trophoblast immunogenicity following enzyme treatment (Simmons et al. 1971; Searle et al. 1975). It is possible that the original experiments by Currie et al. (1968) could have been contaminated by embryonic sac material which is known to be antigenic. The in vitro studies of human trophoblast antigens reviewed in a preceding section were also found not to be affected by prior enzyme treatment. It would seem that, until there is more solid evidence, the antigenic barrier theory cannot, at this point in time, be generally accepted.

Although this mucoprotein coat may not affect the afferent arc of the immunological process by antigenic masking, can it interfere with the efferent arc of the response? Currie and Bagshawe (1967b) have suggested that by virtue of the free carboxyl group on sialic acid, the mucoprotein coat contributes substantially to the negative charge on the trophoblast cell. Since lymphocytes also carry a negative charge, this mutual electrostatic repulsion could interfere with effector lymphocyte cytotoxicity. An alternative mechanism of action is that the oligosaccharide moiety of sialomucin modifies interactions between cells not by any electrostatic effects but by their surface hydration properties (Good 1967). It has been suggested that antigenic tumours may circumvent host immune attack by a similar mechanism. Again, this hypothesis of interfering with effector lymphocytes is not substantiated by experimental evidence, for it has been found that in vitro cultures of mouse trophoblast were insusceptible to immune lymphoid cytolysis even after pre-incubation in various concentrations of neuraminidase (Jenkinson and Billington 1974).

2.3.2 Membrane-associated human chorionic gonadotrophin (HCG)

The possibility that the placental hormone HCG might function as a trophoblast surface immunoprotective layer was suggested by the experiments of Borland et al. (1975), who injected suspensions of viable

Table 2.1 Survival of human foetal cells following transplantation into guinea pig skin.

	Surviving human foetal cells at various times following transplantation				
Cells and treatments	5 days	10 days	15 days	20 days	25 days
Trophoblast	++++	+++++	++++	+++	+++
Trophoblast + HCG	++++	++++++	++++++	++++	++++
Skin	++	++	+	○	○
Skin + HCG	++	++++++	+++++	++++	+++

From Borland, R., Loke, Y. W. and Wilson, D. (1975) In: *Immunobiology of Trophoblast*, Eds.: Edwards, Howe and Johnson. Cambridge University Press, pp. 157–169.

cultured human trophoblast and foetal skin cells intradermally into the backs of guinea pigs. Sections from these injected sites were removed for histological examination at varying intervals. It was found that the survival time of trophoblast cells was much longer than that of foetal skin cells but when foetal skin cells were pre-treated with HCG before inoculation, then their survival time was also prolonged (Table 2.1). The survival time of trophoblast cells was shortened by pre-incubation with neuraminidase but could be restored to that for untreated trophoblast cells by re-incubation with HCG after neuraminidase (Table 2.2).

Table 2.2 Survival of human trophoblast cells following transplantation into guinea pig skin.

	Mean no. of surviving human trophoblast cells following transplantation		
Days post-transplant	Neuraminidase-treated	Controls untreated	Neuraminidase + HCG-treatment
5 days	+	+++	++
10 days	+	++++	+++++
15 days	○	++	+++
20 days	○	+	+++
25 days	○	+	+++

From Borland, R., Loke, Y. W. and Wilson, D. (1975) In: *Immunobiology of Trophoblast*, Eds.: Edwards, Howe and Johnson. Cambridge University Press, pp. 157–169.

To control against any systemic effects of HCG, each guinea pig was injected with different cell suspensions on different areas of its back. Several conclusions may be drawn from these experiments. It seems that HCG can act as a local immunoprotective substance in vivo for both trophoblast and skin cells, suggesting that either there is a non-specific binding due to the substance being 'sticky' or that there are receptors on both skin and trophoblast cells for the hormone. Once on the membrane, the protection lasts for a considerable time. The protection is effective, even in a xenogeneic system. The immunoprotective part of the HCG molecule can be removed by neuraminidase.

HCG, which is a sialoglycoprotein (Bahl 1969), is produced by human trophoblast cells at a rate of about 1.4×10^{-2} IU HCG/day/cell (Braunstein et al. 1973). The hormone can be demonstrated in syncytiotrophoblast cells of the chorionic villi by immunofluorescence (Midgley and Pierce 1962), and by peroxidase immunohisto-enzymologic methods (De Iconicoff and Cedard 1973) on sections of placental tissue, although the specificity of the latter method has since been questioned (Gau and Chard 1976). The distribution of the hormone appears to be predominantly on the maternal surface of the syncytiotrophoblast cells (Naughton et al. 1975), a finding which is confirmed by ultrastructural studies (Dreskin et al. 1970). HCG has also been localised on the surface of cultured human trophoblast cells by immunofluorescence (Loke and Borland 1970) and by a mixed-agglutination technique using trophoblast cells and human group 'O' erythrocytes to which HCG has been chemically coupled via an anti-human erythrocyte antibody as indicator cells, the two being linked by a rabbit anti-HCG antibody (Loke et al. 1972). The positive rosettes obtained by this method suggest that HCG is not only produced by trophoblast but is retained on the surface of the cell. This surface retention has generally been attributed to the 'stickiness' of the hormone due to the molecular structure of the final 30 amino-acid sequence of the carboxyl-terminal end of the β chain (Naughton et al. 1975) but recently Whyte and Loke (unpublished observation) demonstrated that HCG is in fact an integral and major component of the purified plasma membrane of human trophoblast. Such a membrane integration is difficult to explain on the basis of a purely hormonal function because other hormones do not apppear to be similarly integrated into the cell membranes of their secretory cells. It is, therefore, tempting to suggest that this intrinsic nature of HCG on trophoblast plasma membranes may fulfil an immunoprotective function.

The actual mechanism by which it does so is not known. The sialic acid content may interfere with the afferent and efferent arcs of the immunological response in the same way as envisaged for the mucoprotein coat. Incubation of lymphocytes with HCG has been observed to increase their electrophoretic mobility (Wrezlewicz et al. 1977), which is in accord with the postulate that this hormone may increase the negative charge on cell surfaces. The presence of several prolines in the molecule would tend to make it a rather rigid structure and, therefore, stand out in the trophoblast cell surface. It is possible that this could result in steric hindrance, manifested either as poor antigenic expression or interference with maternal effector lymphocytes. McManus et al. (1976) have suggested that HCG is a specific T-cell inhibitory substance which can prevent the maturation of the immune response by interacting with these cells after they have fixed on to paternally derived antigens on the surface of the trophoblast.

The systemic immunosuppressive effects of HCG will be discussed in a later section.

2.3.3 Similarities between trophoblast and neoplastic cells

The invasive behaviour of trophoblast has often been compared to that of malignant tissue. It is, therefore, interesting to note that surface properties, very similar to those of trophoblast cells, are described for malignant cells. The pronase-digested fucose-labelled glycopeptides obtained by mild trypsinisation of neoplastic cells, consistently elute ahead of the corresponding materials from normal cells, this difference being eliminated after treatment with the enzyme neuraminidase (Van Beek et al. 1973). This could be due to an increased content of neuraminidase-sensitive sialic acid on the surface glycoprotein composition of malignant cells which may be analogous to the mucoprotein covering of trophoblast cells. This change in glycoprotein profile appears to accompany all cellular transformation, irrespective of cell type, species, or oncogenic agent responsible, so it could be a universal property of all malignant cells (Van Beek et al. 1975). Using similar methods, Whyte and Loke (unpublished observation) have analysed the surface glycopeptides of human trophoblast cells in comparison with other foetal cells (skin, lung, kidney, heart, and intestine) from the same conceptus. No faster eluting fraction was observed when cells were radiolabelled with L—[1—^{3}H]—fucose and L—[1—^{14}C]—fucose. However, when the experiments were repeated using D—[6—^{3}H]—glucosamine hydrochloride and D—[1—^{14}C]—glucosamine hydrochloride as precursors, trophoblast cells were found to possess a faster eluting fraction (Fig. 2.2). This fraction was observed in both trypsinates and pronase-digested trypsinates. Neuraminidase treatment of the pronase-digested

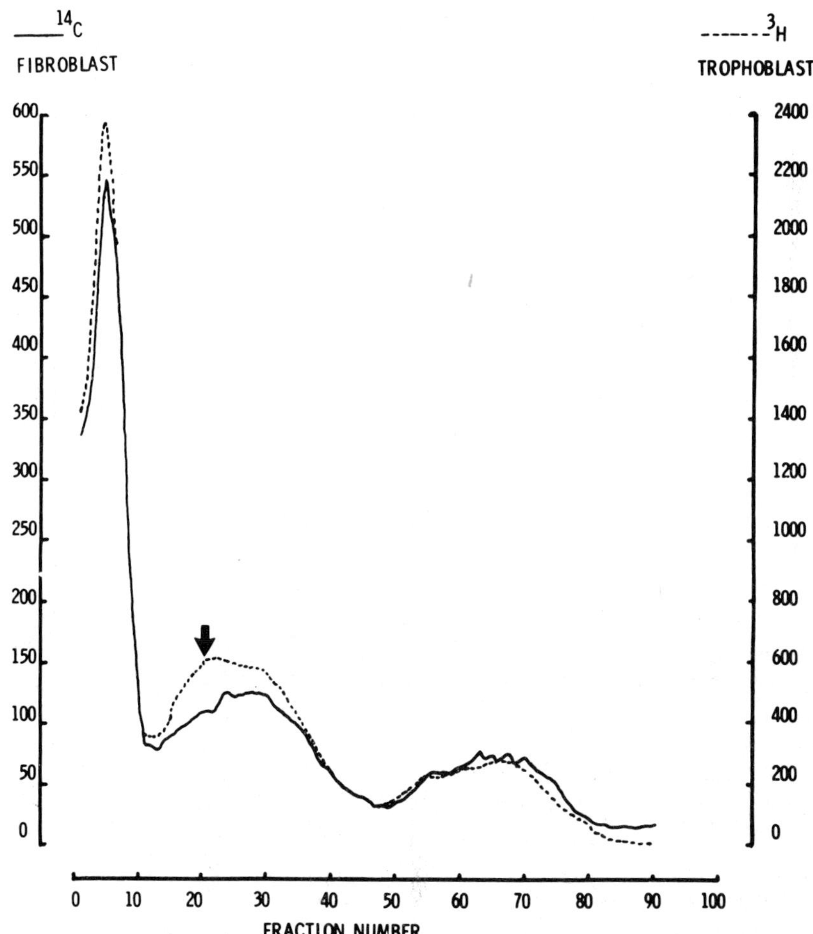

Fig. 2.2 Trophoblast and foetal skin cells incubated with $^{3}H/^{14}C$ glucosamine, treated with trypsin and the trypsinates digested with pronase. Analysis on Sephadex G-50 fine shows a faster eluting fraction in trophoblast (arrow). Activity is expressed as counts/minute. Blue dextran and phenol red were used as high and low molecular weight markers respectively. From Whyte, A. and Loke, Y. W. (Unpublished material).

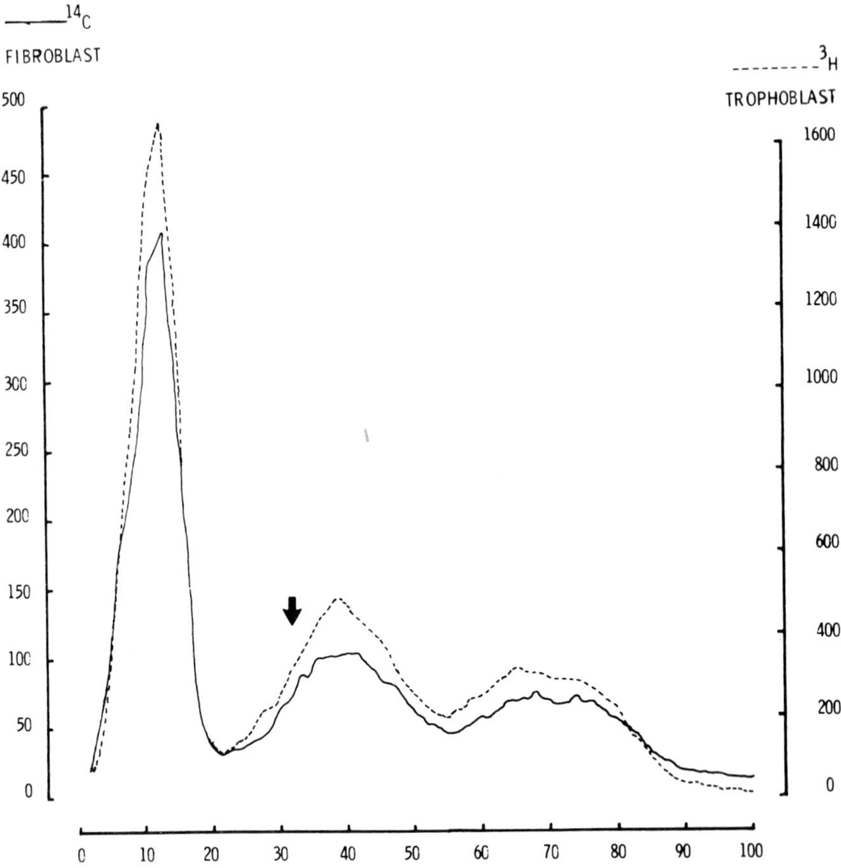

Fig. 2.3 As in Fig. 2.2 except that the pronase digests were further treated with neuraminidase. This caused removal of the faster eluting fraction in trophoblast (arrow) and resulted in co-migration of the trophoblast and fibroblast peaks. From Whyte, A. and Loke, Y. W. (Unpublished material).

trypsinate removed the faster eluting fraction (Fig. 2.3), suggesting that increased sialylation was involved. Thus, trophoblast does appear to exhibit increased glycosylation of certain glycopeptide(s) but this change is not quite the same as that observed in neoplastic cells, in that fucose does not seem to be involved. It does, however, contain glucosamine-derived products including sialic acid. This observation is in agreement with the high levels of sialic acid — 93 nmoles/mg protein

— found in isolated trophoblast plasma membrane (Whyte and Loke, unpublished observation). An increase in glucosamine-derived glycopeptides in implanting mouse blastocysts has also been observed (Pinsker and Mintz 1973), so this surface alteration may be of importance in the process of cellular invasion.

Recent investigations using fluorescein-labelled lectins, have demonstrated the interaction of wheat germ agglutinin (WGA) with human syncytiotrophoblast surface membrane (Whyte, et al., in press). Agglutinating receptors for WGA have been described on some neoplastic cells (Wray and Walborg 1971) which is further evidence for surface resemblance between trophoblast and neoplastic cells.

It is now well documented that frequently there is regression to a foetal phenotype by neoplastic tissue, with the re-expression of embryonic antigens like carcino-embryonic antigen (Gold and Freedman 1965; Terry et al. 1975) and the production of foetal proteins like α-foetoprotein (Abelev 1971; Abelev 1974). The ectopic production of hormones by non-endocrine tumours may be another manifestation of this de-repression (Landon et al. 1974). Of particular relevance to this present review is the frequent synthesis of trophoblast-specific products by tumours of non-trophoblast origin. Stolbach et al. (1969) detected an alkaline phosphatase isoenzyme in the sera of 27 patients with various non-trophoblast malignancies. This isoenzyme was also identified in tumour tissue and in malignant effusion fluids and is biochemically and immunologically indistinguishable from placental alkaline phosphatase. Ectopic production of human chorionic somatomammotrophin (HCS), sometimes also known as human placental lactogen (HPL), has been reported as being present in the sera of 11 out of 128 patients with non-trophoblast tumours and in four of the tumours themselves (Weintraub and Rosen 1971). This hormone has been detected in sections from breast cancers, being positive in 82% of the cases (Horne et al. 1976a). In addition, these authors have detected the pregnancy-specific β_1-glycoprotein in 76% of these breast cancers.

The placental protein, produced ectopically by non-trophoblast tumours, which has been most studied is the hormone human chorionic gonadotrophin (HCG). It is made up of an α- and a β-subunit. The α-subunit resembles that of several other trophic hormones, but the β-subunit shows a certain degree of homology only with the β-subunit of luteinising hormone (LH). Since the availability of specific antisera to the β-subunit of HCG which can discriminate between this hormone and other closely related ones, very sensitive radioimmunoassay

Table 2.3 Presence of detectable immunoreactive HCG in sera of patients with documented tumours.

Type of tumour	No. of patients	No. positive	% positive
Lung	84	6	7.1
Gastrointestinal	323	55	17.0
Gestational trophoblastic disease	49	49	100.0
Haemopoietic	256	7	2.7
Lymphoma	249	5	2.7
Ovarian	28	10	35.7
Testicular	97	59	60.8

With kind permission from Vaitukaitis, J. L. (1974) *Ann. clin. Lab. Sci*, **4**, 276–280.

methods have been developed to detect small quantities of HCG in the circulation. Gailami et al. (1976) reported that 54 out of 320 (17%) patients with non-trophoblastic tumours had modest but measurable levels of HCG in their plasma. As can be seen in Table 2.3, the frequency of ectopic synthesis of HCG appears to vary in different types of cancers (Vaitukaitis 1974). Recently, a case of prostatic carcinoma (Broder et al. 1977) and 17 cases of functioning islet-cell carcinomas (Kahn et al. 1977) associated with HCG production have been added to the rapidly growing list.

Using an enzyme bridge immuno-peroxidase technique, HCG has been localised directly on sections of breast cancers, with 60% of the cases reacting positively (Horne et al. 1976a). Applying a similar method but with an antibody directed specifically at the β-chain of HCG, McManus et al. (1976) demonstrated this hormone on histological sections from 25 non-trophoblast tumours. The hormone was found in the cytoplasm of the tumour cells, and occasionally a discrete band of staining was also seen at the surface of the cells. Only three neoplasms were negative for HCG, but it is possible that extensive necrosis in these tumours might have complicated the interpretations of the staining. It may be concluded, therefore, that the majority of malignant neoplasms of non-trophoblast origin can produce HCG when the tumour tissue is tested directly. It is interesting to note that haptenic coupling of the HCG perhaps with some other surface molecules on the tumour cells may render the hormone immunogenic to the host. Preliminary results with the macrophage electrophoretic mobility test, using lymphocytes from cancer patients and HCG as the antigen, have detected positive responses in 34 out of 44 patients (77%) with various types of cancers (Wass et al. 1977). These results suggest that the ectopic production of HCG and its retention on the surface of tumour cells can be recognised by the host. Monitoring host sensitisation, therefore, could provide an alternative method for the detection of HCG production by tumours.

Ectopic production of HCG has also been detected from cultured cell lines derived from non-trophoblast origin. It was first described by Rabson et al. (1973) from a cell line derived from a bronchogenic carcinoma. The heteroploid HeLa cell line, originally established from a carcinoma of the cervix, has also been reported to produce HCG, in spite of many years of culture (Ghosh and Cox 1976). Recently, HCG has been detected in a new cell line (CaSki), established from a cervical carcinoma which has continued to secrete HCG-β for over 1½ years (Pattillo et al. 1977). These observations point to a relatively stable nature of the de-repression process accompanying neoplasia.

Studies on the ectopic production of HCG have shed some light on the biosynthetic process responsible for assembling the complex HCG heteropolymer molecule. It has been shown that the synthesis of either the α- or the β-subunit of HCG exceeds that of the complete molecule in a bronchogenic carcinoma cell line (Tashjian et al. 1973). Weintraub and Rosen (1973) described a patient with pancreatic carcinoma whose serum and tumour extract contained HCG-β but not HCG-α or complete HCG. These observations of unbalanced synthesis and isolated production would imply that HCG-α and HCG-β are independently transcribed. If this mechanism is applicable to normal trophoblast, it would appear that the formation of HCG is analogous to the formation of antibody where synthesis of the light and heavy chains is independently controlled including translation on separate polyribosomes.

The relationship between developmental gene products and neoplasia is receiving much attention as can be seen from the large number of papers which were presented on this subject in the recent Colloquium on Protides of the Biological Fluids in Brugge in 1976. The ectopic synthesis of placental proteins may be merely one manifestation of this genomic de-repression and has no biological significance apart from providing another tumour marker. However, it is tempting to speculate that the frequent ectopic production of HCG in particular and the presence of this hormone on malignant cell membranes may have an immunoprotective value similar to that postulated for trophoblast cells. In this context, it is pertinent to note that placental gonadotrophin is perhaps the earliest hormone to be produced in ontogeny. An HCG-like gonadotrophin was detected on the surface of pre-implanted mouse embryos as early as the 8 cell stage (Wiley 1974) and the rabbit blastocyst has been shown to contain a gonadotrophin which competes with HCG in binding assays (Haour and Saxena 1974). In human pregnancy, the very early detection of HCG at about the 8th day post ovulation (Wide 1969; Mishell et al. 1974; Saxena et al. 1974) and around the time of implantation (Braunstein et al. 1973), confirms that this hormone is also produced very early in our own species. It is intriguing that de-repression during oncogenesis should so frequently result in the production of this very basic trophoblast-specific hormone. The trophoblast cell-rests theory of cancer which was formulated at the beginning of the century may be due for a revival (Gurchot 1975).

3

Maternal immunocompetence during pregnancy

In the previous chapter, evidence was presented that human trophoblast may be immunologically privileged because of its special cell surface properties. The other side of the story which needs to be considered is whether there is any alteration in maternal immunological reactivity during pregnancy which can contribute to the non-rejection of the foetus.

3.1 Maternal humoral antibody response

The production of anti-Rh antibodies by Rh-negative mothers and the frequent occurrence of anti-HL-A antibodies following pregnancy provide convincing evidence for an intact humoral immune response in pregnant women. However, there have been very few comparative studies of the effect of pregnancy on this response. Recently, Pacsa and Pejtsik (1977) tested the sera from 297 pregnant women for rubella, herpes simplex and toxoplasma antibodies. They found antibody titres to be relatively high at 12—20 weeks, fall to a low level at delivery, but to return to early pregnancy levels 30—45 days post partum. It was postulated that this could be due to pregnancy having a suppressive effect on humoral immunity. Of course, this is but one interpretation of the findings, for it is equally possible that the decreasing antibody titre can be explained by the rapidly growing foetus and placenta absorbing the antibody from the maternal circulation, rather than by any deficit in antibody production. The observation by Tongio and Mayer (1977) that there appears to be a narrowing of lymphocytotoxic antibody specificity at delivery compared to early pregnancy, may be a manifestation of a similar phenomenon. It was found that this narrowing could be very marked, resulting in the total disappearance of all previously detectable lymphocytotoxic antibodies at delivery. Again this effect can be achieved by antibody being sequestered out of the circulation rather than by any suppression by pregnancy.

3.2 Maternal cell-mediated immunity

3.2.1 Inhibition of macrophage migration

The liberation of a macrophage migration inhibition factor (MIF) by sensitised lymphocytes in the presence of specific antigens is generally regarded as a useful in vitro measure of cell-mediated immunity. Rocklin et al. (1973) found that when maternal and her infant's lymphocytes were mixed together in a ratio of 5:1 for 24 hours, the production of MIF against guinea pig macrophages was observed in five out of 10 mothers immediately after delivery. There was no production of MIF when maternal cells were cultured with lymphocytes from unrelated donors. All five mothers positive for MIF production had had three or more babies. These observations suggest the presence of maternal cell-mediated immunity to foetal allo-antigens, and that this sensitisation is more easily detectable in multiparous mothers. Replacing guinea pig macrophages by human leucocytes as a source of migrating cells, Tait et al. (1974) came to very similar conclusions. They found that seven out of 42 pregnant women had positive cell-mediated immunity towards their infant's antigens at the time of birth. There did not seem to be any correlation between a positive cell-mediated immunity as measured by the production of MIF and the presence of lymphocytotoxic antibodies in maternal serum. This dichotomy between maternal humoral and cell-mediated immune response could reflect different modes of sensitisation. The number of cases which responded positively in the preceding two studies was somewhat smaller than that obtained by Youtanannkorn and Matangkasombut (1972), where all 41 post partum mothers were found to have positive cell-mediated immunity. The techniques employed were essentially the same but the source of antigens used were different. Youtanannkorn and Matangkasombut used placental tissue, so it is possible that their experiments were detecting antigens (e.g. trophoblast-specific antigens) which were not present on cord blood lymphocytes.

The production of MIF can be abrogated by maternal serum. This inhibition appears to be specific. Thus, Youtanannkorn and Matangkasombut (1973) found that only autologous plasma blocked maternal leucocyte reactivity to pooled placental antigens but not homologous plasma from unrelated pregnant donors. The inhibition only affected the reactivity to placental antigens and not to PPD. Similar results were obtained by Pence et al. (1975) who also found inhibition by autologous but not homologous maternal serum. In contrast Smith et al. (1972) reported a non-specific depression of maternal lymphocyte reactivity to PPD by autologous serum.

3.2.2 The mixed lymphocyte reaction (MLR)

Unlike the production of MIF which detects the presence of sensitised cells towards specific antigens, the mixed lymphocyte reaction (MLR) is an in vitro measure of the inherent ability of lymphocytes from two genetically non-identical individuals to be stimulated by each other. It is usual to employ a one-way MLR with maternal cells as responders and foetal cells which have been irradiated (and therefore cannot respond) as stimulators but a two-way MLR can also be used if there is no need to distinguish between stimulators and responders.

Maternal lymphocytes have been observed to respond to cord blood lymphocytes from her foetus (Carr et al. 1974) but it seems that this response is perhaps not as marked as that occurring in non-pregnant unrelated controls. Bonnard and Lemos (1972) presented their own results and also summarised the results from other investigators and confirmed that the response by maternal lymphocytes to stimulation by foetal lymphocytes in an unidirectional MLR was consistently low (Table 3.1).

It seems that this lowered response by maternal lymphocytes can extend to allogeneic unrelated cells (Jones and Curzen 1973) and also to rubella virus (Thong et al. 1973), indicating a non-specific depression of maternal MLR during pregnancy, but Lewis et al. (1966) believed that depression of maternal MLR was specific only to husband's cells and not to unrelated cells. Further investigations are necessary to clarify this point.

Besides being poor responders, maternal lymphocytes also appear to be poor stimulators to her own newborn's lymphocytes (Ceppellini

Table 3.1 Unidirectional MLR in various combinations

Stimulators (Mitomycin treated)	Responders	No. of cases	cpm (Mean ± SE)
(a) Unrelated	unrelated	61	15,137 ± 987
(b) Newborn	unrelated	35	16,014 ± 1514
(c) Newborn	father	42	11,350 ± 1259
(d) Newborn	mother	54	6,008 ± 889

With kind permission from Bonnard, G. D. and Lemos, L. (1972) *Transplant. Proc.* 4, 177–180.

1971). This reciprocal hyporeactivity could be a reflection of maternal tolerance due to contact with antigens which have passed in both directions. Husband's lymphocytes, but not those from unrelated adults, also respond poorly to maternal cells (Ceppellini et al. 1971), indicating that whatever factors that could have modulated antigen expression on maternal lymphocytes appear to be specific against those antigens which the mother has encountered during pregnancy. The possibility of maternal tolerance developing during pregnancy is further suggested by the observation that skin grafts exchanged between mother and child in both directions could survive for long periods, sometimes up to 15 months, while grafts exchanged between father and child were all rejected within 20 days (Peer 1958). An interesting finding is that tolerance in the child can be long lasting. There were two cases where mother's skin grafted to her 7- and 12-year-old male children lasted 78 and 253 days respectively.

Like in MIF production, there is some evidence to indicate that the reciprocal hyporeactivity between mother and her newborn in the MLR may also be mediated by serum factors. Maternal serum has been found to depress one-way MLR of her own cells to stimulation by cells from her husband, children and unrelated donors (Gatti et al. 1973). Even MLR between unrelated pairs can be non-specifically inhibited by maternal serum (Curzen et al. 1972). However, not all maternal sera have this inhibitory effect. Revillard et al. (1972) found that maternal sera taken just after delivery inhibited the MLR between her own and husband's lymphocytes and between unrelated pairs in seven instances out of 13. This series was subsequently extended to 45 cases, where inhibition was observed in 16 (Robert et al. 1973). All the sera were from multiparous women. Jenkins and Hancock (1972) found that MLR inhibition was more pronounced with multiparous than with primiparous sera. In a survey of 42 pregnant sera for MLR-inhibiting factors, Jonker et al. (1977) found that half of them would reduce the MLR between cells from the serum donor and her husband to less than 40% of control values, but there did not appear to be any obvious correlation between the frequency of inhibition and parity.

3.2.3 Lymphocyte cytotoxicity

Maternal lymphocytes are capable of killing target placental cells (Currie and Bagshawe 1967a; Douthwaite and Urbach 1971) and foetal cells (Bonnard and Lemos 1972) in vitro. Again, it has been found that the 'blast' transformation and cytotoxicity of maternal lymphocytes on trophoblast cell cultures are entirely inhibited by the addition of autologous serum. This blocking activity appears to be at the level of the target cell rather than the effector lymphocyte, indicating a form of afferent inhibition.

3.2.4 Lymphocyte transformation by phytohaemagglutinin (PHA)

Certain plant mitogens, the best known being phytohaemagglutinin (PHA) can induce lymphocytes to transform into blast cells in the same way as antigenic stimulation. This chiefly affects T-lymphocytes and the degree of transformation has been used as an in vitro measure of T-cell immunocompetence. A large number of conflicting reports on PHA transformation of maternal lymphocytes have appeared in the literature. Some investigators reported that there was no difference in PHA transformation of maternal lymphocytes compared with non-pregnant controls (Comings 1967; Thiede et al. 1968; Watkins 1972; Poskitt et al. 1977). Others thought that maternal lymphocytes showed a progressively increased response to PHA throughout pregnancy together with a greater response at suboptimal doses (Carr and Stites 1972; Carr et al. 1973a). The authors explain these findings by suggesting that the triggering of lymphocytes is a quantitative phenomenon, irrespective of the antigens involved. Thus, maternal lymphocytes which are already exposed to small amounts of foetal antigens will require smaller doses of PHA to generate a response. Maternal lymphocytes have also been found to spontaneously incorporate more radiolabelled thymidine without PHA stimulation than non-pregnant lymphocytes. Again, this could reflect a low level antigenic stimulation during pregnancy. Perhaps there is an actual increase in the number of immunoreactive cells during pregnancy (Petrucco et al. 1976), a situation which is also found in renal transplant patients.

The vast majority of investigators, however, reported a depression of maternal lymphocyte response to PHA (Arala-Chawes and Meirinho 1972; Finn et al. 1972; Leikin 1972; Purtilo et al. 1972; Walker et al. 1972; Nelson et al. 1973; Hsu 1974; Jha et al. 1975; Petrucco et al. 1976). There are many interrelated variables in PHA transformation of lymphocytes. The purity of the lymphocytes used is important, for other cell types like polymorphs and monocytes can affect the response directly or indirectly by consuming the mitogen or liberating suppressive factors. The mode of assessment of lymphocyte transformation, whether by DNA incorporation or by morphological examination, can affect the results. The dose of mitogen used is important for there is an optimal dose for maximal transformation beyond which the mitogen becomes inhibitory. Therefore, dose response curves must be constructed and many of the investigations can be criticised on the grounds that only 1 dose of PHA was used.

Perhaps the most important variable in the context of transformation of maternal lymphocytes is whether the cells are cultured in the presence or absence of autologous serum. It is becoming increasingly evident that suppressive factors in maternal serum are responsible for the apparent depression of maternal lymphocyte response to PHA transformation. Non-pregnant lymphocytes cultured with PHA in the presence of 20% pregnant serum show a depressed response (Leikin 1972; Jha et al. 1975), although 10% pregnant serum in the culture medium appears to be insufficient to cause inhibition (Purtilo et al. 1972). The inhibitory effects of pregnant serum appear to increase as pregnancy progresses and reach a maximum at term (Walker et al. 1972) but are no longer detectable in maternal blood taken seven days after delivery (Yu et al. 1975). Most of the experiments on PHA transformation are performed by culturing maternal lymphocytes in autologous plasma. Even in those experiments without autologous plasma, there is no guarantee that humoral factors are not involved. Maternal lymphocytes may already be coated by serum factors in vivo and these may not have been entirely removed. It has been shown that substantial amounts of serum proteins can be detected on lymphocyte surfaces after three washes which is the usual number employed in most experimental procedures, and traces still remain after six washes (Loke et al. 1976).

Therefore it would appear that in all the in vitro measures of maternal cell-mediated immunity, the observed hyporeactivity of maternal lymphocytes is probably mediated by suppressive factors present in pregnancy serum rather than due to any intrinsic defect of lymphocyte function.

3.3 Lymphocyte populations in pregnant women

At the moment, there is no general agreement as to whether there is any alteration of the lymphocyte populations during pregnancy. The majority opinion seems to be that there is no significant change in the percentage of T- and B-lymphocytes during pregnancy. Using immunofluorescence to detect immunoglobulin-bearing B-lymphocytes, Brain et al. (1972) found no difference in the percentage or total number of B-cells in 34 pregnant women of 6 months gestation age and over, when compared to non-pregnant controls. The percentage of T-lymphocytes as defined by sheep erythrocyte rosettes (E-rosettes) in pregnant women also shows no striking departure from that found in non-pregnant controls, being 45.0% and 47.1% respectively (Campion and Currey 1972). Dodson et al. (1977) found that the percentage of cells bearing receptors for sheep erythrocytes (T-cells) and for C3 (B-cells) remained unchanged throughout pregnancy. Similar results were obtained by Baines et al. (1977) for the first eight months of pregnancy but they did notice a decrease in the percentage of T-cells in the 9th month.

There are two reports of a definite change in the T- and B-cell populations during pregnancy. Strelkauskas et al. (1975) found an inversion of the percentage of T- and B-cells during the early stages of pregnancy, that is, there was a relative drop in T-cells with a relative rise in B-cells while the total lymphocyte count remained as in non-pregnant controls. The authors postulated that this increase in B-cells would assist the acceptance of the foetal allograft by producing blocking antibodies. In this study, T-cells were defined by an indirect rosetting technique, using rabbit anti-human T-cell antiserum and human red cells coated with anti-rabbit light chain antibodies, while B-cells were recognised by a direct rosetting technique, using human erythrocytes coated with rabbit anti-human light chain antibodies. Bulmer and Hancock (1977) observed a decrease in the percentage and absolute number of T-cells throughout pregnancy which became statistically significant at the third trimester. This reduction in T-cells resulted in a relative increase in the percentage of B-cells, as defined by the presence of surface immunoglobulins and their ability to form rosettes with erythrocytes coated with antibody and complement (EAC-rosettes). There was a return to normal proportions six weeks after delivery.

It is clear that further investigations, especially with the help of additional lymphocyte markers, are needed to clarify the situation. Interestingly, a significant decrease in the percentage and absolute number of T-cells has been observed during the menstrual period, which returned to normal a week afterwards (Raptopoulou and Goulis 1977). One wonders whether the intensive hormonal changes during pregnancy can truly affect lymphocyte values.

4

Evasion and suppression of maternal immune response

The preceding section on maternal immunocompetence has shown that there is very little intrinsically defective in the cell types needed to mount an effective immune response. Any hyporeactivity which has been observed seems to be mediated by the suppressive effects of maternal serum. It is not certain what these suppressive factors are, but several possibilities exist.

4.1 Antibody

The evasion of maternal immune response by the conceptus can be compared to the escape from immune destruction by malignant cells. The concept that specific antibody against target cells can paradoxically protect rather than destroy them originated from tumour studies. These non-complement-binding IgG antibodies cover the antigenic sites of the target cells and shield them against attack by host effector lymphocytes (Hellström and Hellström 1969). An analogous situation may occur in pregnancy. It has been demonstrated in mice that lymph node cells from Balb/c mice pregnant by C_3H males reduced colony formation by cultured C_3H embryonic tissue but this inhibitory effect was abrogated by sera from Balb/c mice pregnant by C_3H but not by Balb/c males. This inhibitory factor was present after the first pregnancy but became stronger after several pregnancies (Hellström et al. 1969). The pregnant human mother is frequently sensitised by her conceptus to produce HL-A antibodies of IgG class. These may act as 'blocking' antibodies, especially as trophoblast cells appear to be deficient in antigenic expression. Fixation of IgG antibodies to cell surface antigens which are sparsely distributed, will not readily fix complement because the right 'doublet' configuration is not formed (Linscott 1970).

There is evidence that the inhibition of MLR by maternal serum is also mediated by an IgG antibody (Buckley et al. 1972; Gatti et al. 1973; Robert et al. 1973; Pence et al. 1975). This suppression is specific in that only autologous pregnant serum is inhibitory but not homologous pregnant serum, and this inhibition can be removed by absorption with paternal stimulating cells in MLR between paternal and maternal cells (Pence et al. 1975). It is not clear what specificities are involved, for the inhibition of MLR does not appear to correlate with the presence of HL-A antibodies (Jonker et al. 1977). It may be that these 'blocking' antibodies for MLR are directed against antigens coded by a gene system which is different from that of the HL-A system (Revillard et al. 1972). This MLR system may map with the B-cell antigen system, since certain pregnancy sera containing anti-B-cell antibody are observed to inhibit MLR when stimulated by certain specific stimulator cells (Winchester et al. 1975). The many reports of maternal sera depressing MLR between unrelated pairs (Curzen et al. 1972; Gatti et al. 1973) would seem to indicate there is an additional non-specific element in the inhibition. This is supported by animal experiments which have shown that serum inhibitory factor for MLR is produced in intrastrain pregnant animals carrying syngeneic foetuses, again suggesting that the factor is unlikely to be classical antibody made by the mother against paternal allo-antigens present on foetal cells (Harrison 1976).

Besides masking target cell antigens, protective antibody may completely remove the antigens from the cell surface without killing the cell and thereby prevent host recognition. This process of antibody-mediated antigenic modulation was, again, initially observed in tumour studies where it was found that the surface antigens of mouse leukaemic cells became undetectable after incubation in the presence of specific antiserum (Boyse et al. 1963). This shedding of surface antigens, resulting from interaction with specific antibody, may explain the observation that human lymphocytes sensitised with HL-A antibodies could not be killed by complement if the lymphocytes were incubated for 1—5 hours at 37°C before the addition of complement (Miyajima et al. 1972). Can this process occur in pregnancy? Tiilikainen et al. (1974) examined the HL-A specificities on foetal, maternal and paternal lymphocytes and looked for the presence of HL-A antibodies in maternal sera against a panel of 20 donors. These maternal sera were then tested against foetal and paternal lymphocytes. It was found that maternally derived HL-A antigens were readily demonstrable on foetal lymphocytes but, in contrast, paternally derived antigens were not. However, the expression of paternally derived antigens could be restored if foetal lymphocytes were incubated overnight under tissue culture conditions. Cytotoxic antibodies against paternal HL-A specificities were demonstrable in 19 out of 85 (22%) maternal sera, but these were not cytotoxic to the corresponding foetal lymphocytes in vitro, unless these lymphocytes were first cultured overnight. Thus, this lack of phenotypic expression only of paternally derived antigens may be a manifestation of antigen masking or antigen shedding mediated by specific maternal antibody, and could be an important mechanism for the survival of the conceptus in vivo. However, the role of antibody alone in facilitating tumour escape seems to be gradually losing favour with investigators, because the concept is not generally supported by experimental evidence and especially as it has been shown that bursectomy and the consequent impairment of antibody formation did not affect tumour growth in chickens (Thompson and Linna 1973). It would be of interest to see if women with intact T-cell function but no B-cell function can maintain their pregnancies. At present, there are no definite data on this but it would appear that women with complete absence of immunoglobulins have been observed to give birth to children.

4.2 Antigen

The shedding of antigens in a soluble form by tumour cells has been postulated as another possible mechanism for tumour evasion of host immune attack (Alexander 1974). It is envisaged that these antigens, present in a soluble form in the circulation and therefore relatively non-immunogenic, nevertheless can combine with host antibody or effector cells and thereby abrogate the killing of the tumour cells themselves, a sort of 'smokescreen' process (Currie and Basham 1972). Evidence has also been presented that the rate of shedding of antigens may actually determine the growth pattern of the tumour in vivo so that sarcoma cells, which shed antigens rapidly, are found to metastasise more readily than those with a slow release of antigens (Alexander 1974).

A similar mechanism may operate in the human foetal-maternal interaction. There are three ways by which soluble foetal antigens can accumulate in the maternal circulation. The antibody-mediated shedding of surface antigens has already been discussed in the preceding section. Secondly, antigens can be released by the autolysis of foetal or trophoblast cells. Trophoblast tissue is known to be widely disseminated in maternal blood during pregnancy but to be rapidly lysed, thus providing a ready store of soluble foetal antigens in the maternal circulation. Finally, antigens may be spontaneously released from foetal cells. Water soluble HL-A antigens can be extracted from foetal cells by low frequency sonification (Pellegrino et al. 1970). More of these antigens can be extracted from foetal cells than from a similar number of cells from the corresponding adult organ. Taken in conjunction with the report of Edidin (1966) that embryonic antigens are joined to the cell surface membrane in a less rigid fashion than are adult antigens, it seems that foetal antigens may be more easily solubilised and therefore likely be present in large amounts in the circulation. Soluble histocompatibility antigens have been demonstrated in normal human adult plasma (Charlton and Zmijewski 1970; Van Rood et al. 1970), being associated mainly with the HLD-3 lipoprotein fraction (Aster et al. 1973). These soluble antigens in plasma may have arisen from the continuous shedding of antigen in the form of lipoprotein from membranes of cells exposed to the circulation. In addition to their importance in foetal and tumour evasion of maternal and host immune responses, the possible tolerogenic action of soluble antigens which are continuously shed from a transplanted organ also deserves consideration as a possible explanation of occasional prolonged graft survival (Van Rood et al. 1970).

Naturally-occurring, water soluble antigens like ABH blood group substances may have a similar role to play in protecting the foetus. Water soluble ABH antigens were found to appear in foetal respiratory and digestive tract tissues after the 8th week of gestation (Szulman 1964). Similar antigens were found in the sera of 135 newborn infants and in 11 foetuses of 11—27 weeks gestation age (Hostrup 1963). No soluble blood group substances were detected in 28 group 'O' infants delivered to mothers of either group 'A' or 'B', confirming that these substances were produced by the foetus. Only a very small amount of these A and B substances was sufficient to depress the agglutinating titre of foetal erythrocytes with grouping sera (Constandoulkis and Kay 1962). This suggests that the total amount of A and B substances available within the whole foetus is likely to be sufficient to compete for maternal agglutinins and prevent them from fixing on to similar antigens on foetal tissues.

4.3 Immune complexes

The theory of 'blocking' antibody in tumour immunology was subsequently modified and immune complexes were substituted as the likely protective factors in the sera of tumour-bearing hosts (Sjögren et al. 1971). Similarly, the inhibitory factors detected in their original study on pregnant mice (Hellström et al. 1969) were later also thought to be complexes between embryonic antigens and maternal antibody (Tamerius et al. 1975). In pregnant women, Masson et al. (1977) using a competitive inhibition assay with Clq and rheumatoid factor (Cambiasco et al. 1977), detected the presence of immune complexes in 84 sera collected from 55 women at various stages of pregnancy. These complexes were found to contain IgG, C3, and a substance with molecular weight of about 400,000 which was presumably the antigen. There appeared to be a gradual increase in the amount of these complexes as pregnancy advanced but, surprisingly, the amount fell to non-pregnant levels as early as 3—4 weeks before delivery.

Loke et al. (1975) reported an apparent increase in IgM-bearing lymphocytes in the peripheral blood of pregnant women. Subsequent investigations revealed that this was due to IgM in maternal serum becoming attached to the surface of a certain population of autologous lymphocytes (Loke et al. 1977). On ultracentrifugation, these IgM antibodies were found to occur as relatively large molecules with a sedimentation coefficient of 27S, suggesting they were in the form of aggregates or complexed with antigen. This surface IgM on maternal lymphocytes could only be detected at 4°C or in the presence of sodium azide. It is, therefore, postulated that IgM aggregates or complexes in pregnant serum are constantly fixing on to a population of autologous lymphocytes via surface receptors in vivo. When membrane activity is not artificially suppressed by lowering the temperature or by sodium azide, this IgM together with surface receptors may then be shed, providing a mechanism for the continuous modulation of lymphocyte surface receptors by serum factors during pregnancy.

It may be relevant that, using immune complexes present in the serum of a patient with rheumatoid arthritis and also heat-aggregated

IgG as substrates (Rosenthal 1977), a significant enhancement of the phagocytosis of immune complexes by normal peripheral blood polymorphonuclear leucocytes in the presence of pregnant serum has been observed. These observations suggest that pregnancy serum contains a factor which can aid in the increased clearance of immune complexes. Corticosteroids did not have this effect nor did sera taken from patients on contraceptive drugs, which suggests that this enhancement is probably not hormonally mediated. Whether this mechanism is related to an increased amount of circulating complexes during pregnancy remains to be elucidated. Meanwhile, it may be postulated that this mechanism may be responsible for the improvement in rheumatic diseases so frequently seen during pregnancy.

4.4 Factors liberated by suppressor cells

Maraz and Petri (1974) reported that the supernate from cultures of maternal lymphocytes stimulated by PHA would inhibit DNA synthesis when added to a fresh culture of PHA-stimulated normal lymphocytes. In contrast, supernate generated in a similar way from non-pregnant lymphocytes did not have this inhibitory property. These observations could be interpreted as due to mitogen-stimulated release of soluble factors by a population of suppressor cells which are present in large numbers in maternal blood.

There is evidence to suggest that at least some of these suppressor cells are of foetal origin. Olding and Oldstone (1974, 1976) observed that lymphocytes from human newborns inhibited the division of their mothers' lymphocytes in response to PHA and pokeweed mitogen, and also interfered with maternal B-cells' ability to make IgG in vitro (Oldstone et al. 1977). These inhibitory properties resided in the T-cell enriched population of the infants' cells. Further characterisation has shown that these suppressor T-cells were defined by surface Fc receptors for IgG, whereas those T-cells with Fc receptors for IgM were not inhibitory. Suppressive activity was still present when the two cell populations were cultured across a semi-permeable membrane, but was completely abolished if the foetal cells were irradiated. It may be concluded from these findings that neonatal suppressor T-cell activity is dependent on in vitro cell division and the liberation of a soluble suppressor factor (Olding et al. 1977).

Lawler et al. (1975) have shown that neonatal lymphocytes would also inhibit maternal lymphocyte response when the two cell populations were cultured together in an MLR. This inhibitory effect appeared not to be specific for the neonate's own mother, for cells from unrelated neonates also had similar properties.

Inhibitory activity has also been observed in another foetal cell population. Supernatants obtained from 3-day cultures of cord blood monocytes (surface adherent cells) were found to inhibit unrelated adult lymphocyte response to PHA stimulation and in the MLR. In contrast, this suppressive factor was not produced by adult monocytes (Wolf et al. 1977).

Although all these observations strongly suggest that factors liberated by foetal suppressor cells may be yet another mechanism by which the foetus evades maternal immune response, it is clear that this form of immunoprotection can only come into play after the development of the foetal lymphoid system.

4.5 α-foetoprotein (AFP)

This protein has been the subject of a recent review (Lau and Linkins 1976). AFP is a major plasma protein of the early human foetus, reaching a peak concentration of 2,000—3,000 μg/ml of blood at the 14th week of gestation. Perfusion studies have indicated that the foetal liver is the main site of production, although the abrupt curtailment of synthesis at birth, whether the infant is full term or premature (Gitlin and Boesman 1966), suggests that perhaps the placenta or some other extra-embryonic structures may also contribute to the production of this foetal protein. During pregnancy, this protein can enter the maternal circulation, but in spite of the large concentration gradient from foetus to mother, the amount actuallly transferred to the mother is small, probably less than 450 μg per day. The concentration of AFP in maternal serum progressively rises from the normal adult level of 2—10 ng/ml to about 18—119 ng/ml in the first trimester, to 96—302 ng/ml in the second trimester and to 103—550 ng/ml in the third trimester (Seppälä and Ruoslahti 1972).

Evidence has recently been accumulating that AFP may have similar immunosuppressive properties like other pregnancy-associated serum α-proteins. It was originally suggested by Ayoub and Kasakura (1971) that the observed depression of adult lymphocyte response to PHA by foetal plasma might have been due to the presence of AFP. It may also be relevant that Waldmann and McIntire (1972) reported elevated levels of AFP above 30 ng/ml (range 44—2,800 ng/ml) in patients with ataxia telangiectasia, a disease which is characterised by an immunodeficient state. Elevated levels of AFP were also detected in 54 patients with other immunodeficiency syndromes, and in the parents and siblings of patients with these syndromes. Immunosuppression by AFP was suggested as playing a detrimental role in these diseases.

Availability of preparations of human AFP isolated from foetal liver or from ascitic fluid of hepatoma patients has led to a large number of in vitro investigations. Yachnin (1976) found that human AFP inhibited the in vitro lymphocyte response to a variety of stimuli. Concentrations of 2.5 mg/ml of AFP inhibited the response to PHA, Con A, and rabbit anti-human thymocyte serum but not to pokeweed mitogen (PWM). The inhibition of PHA-induced lymphocyte transformation was confirmed by Gupta and Good (1977). AFP also exerted a profound suppressive effect on lymphocyte response to allogeneic cells in the MLR in concentrations of 150—200μg/ml (Auer and Kress 1977) or 250—550μg/ml (Yachnin 1976), but this was not confirmed by Charpentier et al. (1977) who found that purified human AFP, in high concentration, actually stimulated the MLR. Although it is generally concluded that AFP primarily inhibits T-cell functions, other T-cell properties do not seem to be affected. There is no interference with sheep erythrocyte rosette formation (Baumgarten 1976; Yachnin 1976; Gupta and Good 1977; Littman et al. 1977). If anything, there is an enhancing effect on lymphocyte receptors for sheep red blood cells, for incubation of peripheral blood lymphocytes in AFP resulted in a significant increase in the number of 'active' T-rosettes — that is, rosettes which are formed after centrifugation of lymphocytes and sheep erythrocytes and read immediately without a subsequent period of incubation together (Gupta and Good 1977). The production of MIF by sensitised lymphocytes is not suppressed by human AFP (Littman et al. 1977) nor is there any inhibitory effect on mitogen- or antigen-induced lymphocyte cytotoxicity (Wands et al. 1975). The lack of inhibition of these other parameters of T-cell activity has aroused the suspicion that the suppression of 'blast' transformation in response to stimuli could be an in vitro artefact and is not related to any immunoregulatory function in vivo (Littman et al. 1977).

Before any further conclusions are drawn concerning the immunosuppressive activity of human AFP, what is needed is a standardised preparation of the substance. Even the source from which it is derived is important, for AFP isolated from foetal liver homogenate has a much greater inhibitory capacity than that derived from ascites fluid of hepatoma patients (Yachnin and Lester 1976). It is not clear what is the basis for this biological difference, for the amino-acid and carbohydrate compositions of foetal and hepatoma AFP appear to be indistinguishable (Ruoslahti et al. 1971). The molecule itself does show a degree of heterogeneity. Auer and Kress (1977) purified human AFP from ascites fluid from patients with hepatoma by a method which avoided a low pH or a high salt concentration. Two fractions were obtained of which only one had demonstrable inhibitory activity on in vitro lymphocyte transformation. Lester et al. (1976) also found that human AFP from hepatoma patients contained several electrophoretic variants. The one with the most negative charge had the greatest ability to inhibit in vitro lymphocyte response. This, therefore, indicates that only certain molecular species of human AFP have immunosuppressive properties. This finding of an increased inhibitory activity by the most negatively charged human AFP molecule parallels the finding with mouse AFP, where it is found that immunosuppressive activity is associated with the most sialylated AFP molecules (Zimmerman et al. 1977). It is not clear why there is this requirement for sialic acid residues. Perhaps specific sialic acid receptors on the target cells are involved which trigger off the immunosuppression. It is interesting to note that another powerful immunosuppressive protein present in pregnancy, namely HCG, is also highly sialylated. Furthermore, MIF, produced by sensitised lymphocytes is also dependent on the presence of terminal sialic acid residues for its migration inhibition activity (Remold and David 1971). This aspect of immunosuppression warrants further investigation.

The exact mechanism of immunosuppression by human AFP is not known but investigations with murine AFP may elucidate certain aspects. Binding to lymphocyte cell surface is probably an initial requirement, for mouse AFP has been shown to bind to the surface of murine T-cells (Dattwyler et al. 1975). In man, however, this binding, if it occurs at all, must be of low affinity for in the experiments of Yachnin and Lester (1976), pre-incubation of human AFP with human lymphocytes followed by washing did not impair the ability of these cells subsequently to respond to mitogenic stimulation. Mouse AFP was found to inhibit primary IgM and secondary IgM, IgG and IgA responses by mouse splenic plaque-forming cells to sheep erythrocytes in vitro. A much lower concentration of AFP was needed to suppress secondary IgG and IgA responses than for IgM which was an indication that the suppressive action was directed towards helper T-cells because these cells were more important for cellular events leading to IgG and IgA secretion than for IgM secretion. Addition of AFP after 45 hours of culture did not suppress antibody synthesis, suggesting the action was directed at cellular events earlier than the synthesis of antibody by B-cells, possibly at the level of helper T-cells (Murgita and Tomasi 1975). This may also be applicable to man, for no inhibition of lymphocyte transformation occurred if human AFP was added after DNA synthesis was well advanced at 48—72 hours (Yachnin and Lester 1976). Recent observations that mouse AFP suppresses in vitro antibody response to sheep red blood cells but not to DNP-Ficoll and lipopolysaccharide, further confirm that mouse AFP suppresses T-cell dependent but not T-cell independent immune reactions in vitro (Murgita and Wigzell 1976). Pre-incubation experiments have shown that AFP must interact with the cells involved for at least eight hours for effective suppression. The mechanism, therefore, seems more complex than the mere blocking of receptor sites. This conclusion receives support from work with human AFP where it was found that a large excess of a relatively inactive AFP preparation did not interfere with the capability of a more potent AFP isolate to inhibit lymphocyte transformation (Yachnin and Lester 1977). Perhaps the long incubation time needed with AFP is to generate a population of suppressor T-cells, which then control the level of responsiveness to T-cell dependent antigens (Murgita et al. 1977).

It remains to be seen whether the mechanism of immunosuppressive action of human AFP follows the same pattern as that of murine AFP. Although AFP from different species varies according to structure, electrophoretic mobility and antigenicity, it seems that its immunosuppressive activity can cross species lines. Yachnin (1975) has observed that fetuin, which is a bovine AFP, would inhibit human lymphocyte transformation in response to mitogenic and antigenic stimuli in vitro, so it is hopeful that work with animal AFP can be extrapolated to man.

4.6 Pregnancy-associated proteins

4.6.1 α-macroglobulin

A large number of serum proteins of differing molecular weights and electrophoretic mobilities have been found in the blood of pregnant women. Those that have created most interest in relation to possible immunosuppressive properties are a group of high molecular weight α-glycoproteins. Recent investigations have shown that many of these although variously designated by different investigators as pregnancy zone protein (PZP),α2-pregnoglobulin, pregnancy-associated globulin (PAG), new serum α-macroglobulin, pregnancy-associated α2-globulin, pregnancy-associated α2-glycoprotein, all show immunological identity and therefore probably represent the same protein (Lin and Halbert 1975).

During pregnancy, there is a rapid increase in serum level of this α-macroglobulin at the first trimester, reaching an average concentration of 100 mg/100 ml of blood by the third trimester. After delivery, there is a rapid decrease (Von Schoultz 1974). However, there appears to be a great deal of individual variation, with a few women not reaching more than 4 mg/100 ml of blood throughout pregnancy. Therefore, if this globulin is indeed important in pregnancy, then it would seem that some women need it more than others. Besides pregnancy, a similar α-macroglobulin is also demonstrable in about 18% of normal males and females as well as in patients with disease states like cancer (Horne et al. 1973) and in women on hormonal contraceptives (Davis and Hipkin 1974). The origin of this protein is not known but the placenta is a possible source in pregnancy (Riggio et al. 1971), or peripheral leucocytes and monocytes (Stimson and Blackstock 1975; Stimson 1977).

The pregnancy-associated α-macroglobulin has been found to inhibit T-cell in vitro reactions, like response to stimulation by Con A, PHA, PPD and allogeneic cells, while B-cell reactivity, like response to stimulation by lipopolysaccharide and goat anti-human $F(ab)_2$, is relatively unaffected (Stimson 1976). This substance also blocks antigen-induced inhibition of leucocyte migration and spontaneous sheep red cell rosettes, both of which are T-cell properties. The immunosuppressive potential of this α-macroglobulin can be gauged by the fact that a concentration as low as 6.5 mg/dl would significantly suppress PHA transformation of lymphocytes (Than et al. 1975). It would appear that even the α-macroglobulin found in non-pregnant sera also has demonstrable in vitro immunosuppressive properties. It has been found to inhibit lymphocyte response to non-specific stimuli like Con A and PHA (Chase 1972), as well as to specific antigens like histo-incompatible leucocytes and PPD (Cooperband et al. 1972). Injection of this α-macroglobulin intravenously into animals would prolong skin allograft survival (Mannick and Schmid 1967); and Ford et al. (1973) reported that this substance would block antigen recognition by lymphocytes, as demonstrated by the absence of production of soluble factors by sensitised lymphocytes on macrophage electrophoretic mobility.

The exact mode of action is not known but the diversity indicates that the protein probably acts at the level of the lymphocyte itself, perhaps by coating the cell surface. This hypothesis is consistent with the finding that α-macroglobulin does not interfere with PHA-induced transformation by direct reaction with the mitogen (Yachnin 1972), but acts upon the earliest events of lymphocyte immune responsiveness, at the time of antigen recognition by these cells. A possible mechanism is the competitive blockade of those sites on the lymphocyte surface responsible for antigen recognition (Cooperband et al. 1969). It has also been suggested that an α-glycoprotein from bovine serum acts by inhibition of newly synthesised RNA, thereby interfering with protein synthesis (Milton and Mowbray 1972).

The relationship between pregnancy-associated α-macroglobulin and those found in non-pregnant sera and in sera from patients with a wide spectrum of diseases is not clear. Perhaps they are the same protein and become increased in conditions with longstanding antigenic stimulation. It is, therefore, tempting to speculate that the biological role of this substance is in the regulation of lymphocyte function like some kind of lymphocyte chalone (Miller 1976).

4.6.2 β_1-glycoprotein

Another protein also appears in the sera of pregnant women. This is a β_1-glycoprotein of molecular weight 90,000, which has been designated SP1, an abbreviation from Schwangerschafts-protein (Bohn 1976) or PAPP-C (Lin et al. 1974). The concentration of this protein in pregnant serum increases steadily with advancing pregnancy and may reach a level of 30 mg/100 ml. After delivery, the protein disappears from maternal blood with a half-life of 30—40 hours (Bohn 1976). Unlike the pregnancy-associated α-macroglobulin, the β_1-glycoprotein is claimed to be pregnancy-specific and is synthesised by the syncytial trophoblast cells of both normal and neoplastic trophoblast (Horne et al. 1976b, 1977).

At the moment, interest is mainly focused on this protein for its value as a specific pregnancy marker, but the possibility that it may have immunosuppressive properties is suggested by the report that it inhibited PHA-induced but not Con A-induced lymphocyte transformation (Horne et al. 1976b). It was necessary, however, to pre-incubate lymphocytes with β_1-glycoprotein for 24 hours prior to addition of PHA for inhibition of blastogenesis to take place (Cerni et al. 1977). Furthermore, its localisation to the extracellular surface of the plasma membrane of trophoblast microvilli (Horne et al. 1976b) could imply a local immunoprotective function analogous to that described for HCG.

4.7 Hormones

Pregnancy is associated with profound endocrinological changes due to the production of steroid and protein hormones by the mother or the foeto-placental unit. It is possible that some of these could be responsible for the immunosuppressive properties of pregnant serum.

4.7.1 Steroid hormones

The plasma level of 17-hydroxycorticosteroids rises progressively during pregnancy, sometimes reaching levels which exceed those found in patients with Cushing's syndrome (Bayliss et al. 1955). This high corticosteroid level was thought to be the non-specific factor in maternal serum which blocked MLR between unrelated pairs (Kasakura 1971), but the lack of correlation between plasma cortisol level and inhibitory activity on MLR when individual cases were analysed does not seem to support this hypothesis (Kasakura 1973).

Other hormones like oestrogen and progesterone have also been investigated. It was thought that these hormones could be responsible for the depressed lymphocyte response to PHA stimulation seen in women on oral contraceptives (Hagen and Frøland 1972; Barnes et al. 1974). It was reported that the incorporation of ^{3}H-thymidine by PHA-stimulated human peripheral blood lymphocytes from healthy adult males was significantly suppressed in the presence of diethyl-stilboestrol diphosphate (Ablin et al. 1974). Other investigators, however, found no inhibitory effect on lymphocyte DNA synthesis with these hormones even at concentrations several times greater than physiological plasma levels during pregnancy (Schiff et al. 1975), nor did these hormones prolong skin allograft survival when injected into rabbits (Hulka and Mohr 1969).

Although the evidence concerning the immunosuppressive role of pregnancy steroid hormones is inconclusive, a proper endocrine milieu may still be essential for the maintenance of trophoblast during pregnancy. When trophoblast tissue was transplanted to women suffering from hyperoestrogenism, a considerable degree of trophoblast proliferation was seen in contrast to the rapid destruction of trophoblast similarly transplanted to a group of control women (Lajos et al. 1964). This indicates that oestrogen is important for trophoblast proliferation even when transplanted to an allogeneic host. The action may be an indirect one via the pituitary which is stimulated to produce a placentotrophin (Lajos et al. 1967).

4.7.2 Protein hormones

The placental hormone which has been most investigated is human chorionic gonadotrophin (HCG) and, to a lesser extent, human placental lactogen (HPL). In Chapter 2, we have discussed the local immunoprotective role of HCG on the surface of trophoblast cells. Evidence for the systemic immunosuppressive effects of HCG will now be considered.

Daily injections of HCG into experimental animals have been observed to prolong skin allograft survival (Pearse and Kaiman 1967). This hormone, therefore, may be the suppressive factor responsible for prolongation of skin homograft in pregnant women (Andresen and Monroe 1962). Other observations on the in vivo immunosuppressive action of HCG includes depression of secondary antibody response in mice sensitised to sheep erythrocytes (Younger et al. 1969) and a decrease in the incidence of graft-versus-host disease when Balb/c mice were challenged with C57/B6 spleen cells (Slater et al. 1977). The mechanism of suppression could be by the hormone acting on lymphoid organs, since rats treated by daily injections of HCG had significant reduction of spleen and thymus weights (Nelson et al. 1967). This hypothesis is supported by the observations that lymph nodes of the external iliac chain draining the uterus in pregnant women have very few discernible germinal centres (Nelson and Hall 1964) and that there is an inverse relationship between absolute lymphocyte count and HCG titre in choriocarcinoma patients (Nelson and Hall 1965).

HCG has also been found to depress in vitro transformation of human lymphocytes by PHA (Kaye and Jones 1971; Adcock et al. 1973) and by allogeneic cells in the MLR (Jenkins et al. 1972; Beling and

Weksler 1974). Inhibition can be detected with HCG concentration as low as 10—40 IU/ml which is well within the normal physiological range present in the plasma of pregnant women. This is in the region of 120—160 IU/ml during the first 100 days of pregnancy and 10—80 IU/ml after that (Teoh 1967). Degree of inhibition is related to the concentration of HCG used. A concentration of 200 IU/ml or above resulted in complete inhibition of most types of in vitro lymphocyte transformation. Since HCG is produced by the placenta, this high concentration of the hormone may well be available in the placenta-maternal interface. Dosage of HCG used is obviously an important influencing factor on the results obtained, for Beck et al. (1977) found that while high doses of the hormone suppressed mitogen-induced lymphocyte blastogenesis, low doses actually enhanced the response.

The inhibition of PHA transformation after lymphocytes have been pre-incubated with HCG suggests that the mode of action may be by competition for receptor sites between the hormone and mitogen (Contractor and Davies 1973; Han 1974). This binding to lymphocyte surface, however, appears to be a loose one and can easily be removed by washing (Adcock et al. 1973; Han 1974). An alternative mechanism is suggested by Powell (1974) who argues that since PHA has a known propensity for combining with glycoproteins, the glycoprotein nature of HCG may depress PHA stimulatory capacity by neutralising the effect of the mitogen rather than by competitive inhibition of surface receptor sites.

Early enthusiasm for HCG as an immunosuppressant was somewhat diminished when subsequent studies with purified preparations resulted in many negative findings. Among the earlier investigations, apart from Beling and Weksler (1974), who used HCG with potency of 13,700 IU/mg, all the other experiments employed crude preparations of the hormone with potencies of not more than about 3,000 IU/mg. Analyses of these crude preparations revealed that as much as 75% of the bulk material in these preparations was not HCG (Morse 1976). It is, therefore, important to discover whether the immunosuppressive activity observed in crude preparations of HCG is, in fact, due to the hormone itself or to the presence of contaminating substances. Caldwell et al. (1975) found that crude preparations of HCG depressed lymphocyte response to PHA, but purified HCG had no such suppressive activity even at low PHA doses. There was, in fact, a gradual decrease in suppressive activity of the hormone as its biological potency increased. Similar conclusions were reached by Morse et al.

(1976) who found that crude HCG was several times more inhibitory than purified HCG on lymphocyte response to PHA, pokeweed, PPD, and allogeneic cells. When crude HCG was passed through a Sephadex G-100 column, the fraction that had the most inhibitory activity appeared in the eluate after the major peak of HCG hormonal activity (Morse 1976). Similarly, Maes and Claverie (1977) observed that, while crude HCG depressed T-cell response to PHA, purified HCG did not. Purified HPL also has little inhibitory effect on PHA- and allogeneic cell-induced lymphocyte transformation, except at very high doses of 1,000 IU/ml (Morse 1976).

These data indicate that contaminating factors other than HCG are probably responsible for most of the immunosuppressive activity observed. These substances appear to elute in the region of molecular weight 20,000—40,000 daltons (Morse 1976), so they are unlikely to be pregnancy steroid hormones like oestrogen and progesterone unless they are aggregated or bound to heavier substances. Perhaps they are other pregnancy serum proteins which can exert their effects by neutralising the mitogen (Morse 1968). It has also been shown that crude HCG had marked anti-complementary activity which was found to be due to the presence of immunoglobulin aggregates or complexes in sufficient quantities to convert the third component of complement (Loke and Pepys 1975). In view of the modifying effect of antigen-antibody complexes on lymphocyte transformation and of C3-reactive agents on skin allograft survival, published works on the immunosuppressive action of crude HCG preparations must, therefore, be viewed with caution.

5

Development of immunocompetence in the human foetus

5.1 Ontogeny of cell-mediated immunity

5.1.1 Development of T-lymphocytes

The thymus first appears around the 6th week of foetal development. Its structure, however, remains epithelial until it is populated by lymphocytes at about the 9th week of gestation. There is a constant increase in weight of this organ relative to foetal body weight up till the 3rd trimester, when there is a levelling off. A gradual decline in weight then follows which is already perceptible at birth and continues thereafter (Kay et al. 1962). In animal studies, the period of life in which tolerance to foreign antigens can be most readily induced ceases at a time corresponding to the phase of most rapid growth of the thymus and the attainment of its peak weight ratio relative to foetal body weight. If this is applicable to man, then it would seem that the development of cell-mediated immune responsiveness in the human foetus is well under way long before birth.

At first, the production of lymphocytes is probably by the foetal liver, for this organ contains considerably more lymphoid cells than all the other lymphoid organs combined during the first half of foetal life (Carr et al. 1975). These lymphocytes then migrate to populate the thymus at the 9th week of gestation (Papiernik 1970) and by the 15th week these thymocytes have acquired the T-cell characteristic of rosetting with sheep erythrocytes (Wybran et al. 1972). About 50—96% of thymocytes have been observed to rosette with sheep erythrocytes from 18 weeks gestation onwards (Hayward and Ezer 1974). In an analysis of foetal T-lymphocytes by SRBC-rosettes and by staining with a fluorescent-conjugate of an anti-human T-cell antibody, Asma et al. (1977) found cells which stained with the fluorescent-labelled antibody in foetal liver as early as 5½ weeks gestation age while SRBC-rosetting cells were not detected until after the 9th week when the thymus began to be populated by lymphocytes. There is, thus, a temporal difference in the expression of T-cell surface determinants. It is suggested that those lymphocytes staining by anti-T-cell antibody are cells which are committed to become T-lymphocytes. This commitment can take place outside the thymus, possibly in the liver or bone-marrow (Boyse and Abbott 1975). On the other hand, the expression of receptors for sheep red blood cells is under the influence of the thymus, which explains the appearance of these rosetting cells only after the thymus has been populated.

Small lymphocytes appear in foetal peripheral blood at 7—8 weeks gestation, and by the 10th week these cells make up over 50% of the white cell population (Playfair et al. 1963). Many of these peripheral lymphocytes are demonstrably T-cells but the proportion of these cells (Campbell et al. 1974; Smith et al. 1974; Davis and Galant 1975) and their total number (Diaz-Jouanen et al. 1975) appear to be slightly lower in cord blood than in adults. Halbrecht and Komlos (1976) observed that the proportion of SRBC-rosetting cells in cord blood appeared to be inversely related to that found in maternal blood. When mother's blood had a high percentage of these cells, cord blood had a low count and vice versa. The significance of this finding in relation to the foetal-maternal interaction is not clear.

Dwyer and Mackay (1970) found that the thymus from foetuses of 20—22 weeks gestation age contained cells capable of binding monomeric bacterial flagellar antigens. The mean number of these cells was highest in the foetal thymus, compared to the postnatal and adult organ. An interesting finding was that the surface receptors on these antigen-binding thymocytes could be blocked by anti-μ and anti-light chain sera (Dwyer et al. 1972), suggesting that they may be IgM. The presence of these cells may be indicative of in utero sensitisation of the foetus by maternally-derived antigens.

5.1.2 Response of foetal lymphocytes to PHA stimulation

Proliferation of lymphocytes following culture with PHA is primarily a function of T-lymphocytes. Using a single dose of PHA, Pegrum et al. (1968) observed transformation by thymic cells from foetuses ranging from 16—24 weeks gestation age, but liver and bone-marrow cells did not respond. Kay et al. (1966) established that foetal thymocytes of 14 weeks gestation age could respond to PHA, but this did not occur before 14 weeks (Kay et al. 1970). These studies employed a single dose of PHA which might not have been the optimum and cells were harvested for transformation analyses at one period of time. Stites et al. (1974), measuring time-dose responses, detected foetal thymocyte response to PHA as early as the 10th week of gestation. They also used chromosome markers to confirm that these responsive cells were foetal cells and not transplacentally transmitted maternal lymphocytes. It can be seen, therefore, that there is a remarkably early appearance of at least one functional attribute of foetal thymocytes.

The onset of PHA responsiveness by thymocytes appears at a time when the thymus has differentiated histologically into cortex and medulla (August et al. 1971), but the medulla still occupies a large area of the organ (Kay et al. 1970). On the basis of morphological studies, Papiernik (1970) concluded that the thymic medulla was probably the source of PHA responsive cells. PHA responsive cells appear in the spleen about 2—4 weeks later than in the thymus (Stites et al. 1974), at a time when the small lymphocytes infiltrate the organ in cuffs around the central arterioles to delineate what are called the 'thymus-dependent areas' (August et al. 1971).

At about the same time, PHA responsive lymphocytes are detectable in the peripheral blood of the foetus (Stites et al. 1974). The presence of these cells has been frequently reported in cord blood, although some controversy exists as to whether the extent of this PHA response by cord lymphocytes is different from that of adult lymphocytes. A lower, (Jones 1969), higher (Lindahl-Kiessling and Böök 1964) or similar (Pentycross 1969; Eife et al. 1974; Davis and Galant 1975) PHA response by cord blood lymphocytes compared to adult lymphocytes has been reported. This disparity in the results may be due to the different dosage of PHA employed and the length of culture of the lymphocytes. Carr et al. (1972) and Stites et al. (1972) demonstrated that, at low PHA doses, cord lymphocytes had a significantly higher response than adult lymphocytes but at higher doses, the responses of both were the same. The mean peak response of cord blood lymphocytes also occurred at a lower PHA dose than for adult lymphocytes. The inhibitory effects of serum factors must also be taken into account for it has been observed that foetal sera, like maternal sera, have the capacity to depress PHA stimulation of foetal lymphocytes (Yu et al. 1975).

It is interesting to note that there appears to be a high level of spontaneous transformation without PHA stimulation exhibited by cord blood lymphocytes. These lymphocytes have been found to incorporate 6 to 10 times more isotope on culture without PHA when compared with adult lymphocytes (Carr et al. 1972). Similar findings were reported by Winter et al. (1965), where newborn lymphocytes were more readily labelled with uridine-T and thymidine-T without PHA stimulation compared to adult lymphocytes. Faulk et al. (1973) also found that neonatal lymphocytes have a high autoradiographic labelling index when treated with tritiated thymidine. Morphologically, more medium and large lymphocytes were found in neonatal blood than in adult blood. These observations suggest that foetal lymphocytes at term are already undergoing a low level of stimulation. Maternally-derived antigens crossing the placenta during pregnancy are likely sources for this sensitisation. Siegal (1976) reported that immunoglobulin-bearing B-lymphocytes from children within the first few weeks of life can bind IgG. This is in contrast to the situation in adults where this property is generally found in the so-called 'third population' ($Fc^{+}Ig^{-}$) of mononuclear cells. Perhaps this increased Fc receptor activity on neonatal B-lymphocytes is analogous to the revealing of Fc receptors on activated T-cells concomitant with blast transformation in vitro and is, therefore, indicative that foetal B-lymphocytes are also showing signs of stimulation.

5.1.3 Response of foetal lymphocytes to allogeneic cells

The mixed lymphocyte reaction (MLR) has frequently been used to investigate the response of foetal lymphocytes to allogeneic cells. Cells from foetal thymus of 14—26 weeks gestation can respond to stimulation by adult allogeneic cells in a one-way MLR (Hayward and Soothill 1972). Pegrum (1971) observed that foetal liver, spleen and thymus cells from foetuses of 16—24 weeks gestation could act as both stimulators and responders in a one-way MLR with allogeneic adult lymphocytes. An even earlier response was reported by Ohama and Kajii (1974) who found that foetal thymocytes, splenocytes and blood lymphocytes from 20 foetuses of a length between 76—142 mm, estimated as between 11—15 weeks gestation age, could stimulate and respond to adult allogeneic lymphocytes in a one-way MLR.

It was pointed out by Carr et al. (1973b) that, while foetal liver lymphoid cells can respond strongly to allogeneic cells at a very early age, they do not respond to PHA stimulation. In fact, this MLR response is the earliest cellular immune reaction detected in a human foetus, being present in a foetus of 7½ weeks gestation age (Stites et al. 1974). This raises the possibility that ontogeny of the MLR precedes that of PHA response. It also suggests that PHA and allogeneic cells may stimulate different cell populations. The report that lymphocytes from three children with congenital thymic dysplasia did not respond to PHA while one case responded to stimulation by allogeneic lymphocytes (Meuwissen et al. 1968) is in accord with the postulate of functional heterogeneity within the T-cell system.

The very early maturation of the ability to recognise allogeneic cells by the foetal liver may have an important immunoprotective function. Since the foetal liver is the organ traversed by blood returning from the placenta, this effector function by liver lymphoid tissue could be the mechanism by which the foetus is protected from maternal predator cells (Stites et al. 1974). The identity of these foetal hepatic cells remains obscure. In the concept proposed by Lafferty et al. (1972), allogeneic stimulation and antigen responsiveness are two distinct immune reactions. Allogeneic stimulation depends on the direct stimulation of haemopoietic stem cells by allogeneic lymphocytes; resulting in proliferation. The MLR of foetal hepatic cells may be an example of this.

5.1.4 Cytotoxic activity of foetal lymphocytes

Antibody-mediated cytotoxic activity (K-cell killing) is readily demonstrable in cord blood lymphocytes when allogeneic Chang human liver cells coated with rabbit anti-Chang antibody are used as target cells (Campbell et al. 1974). The mean cytotoxic activity of cord lymphocytes is only slightly lower than for adult lymphocytes, indicating that K-cell activity is well developed at birth. Similarly, surface-adhering cord blood monocytes at term already have a fully developed capacity for antibody-dependent cellular cytotoxicity, as demonstrated by Milgrom and Shore (1977) who used human group 'O', Rh-positive red cells sensitised with optimal concentration of human anti-D and labelled with Cr^{51} as targets. In contrast, Rachelefsky et al. (1973), using HL-A antibody-coated allogeneic lymphocytes as target cells, observed a statistically lower level of killing by newborn lymphocytes. The mean value of Cr^{51} release for newborn lymphocytes was 2.33% ± 1.25 SD compared to adult mean value of 19.5% ± 5.46 SD.

Another form of in vitro cytotoxic killing which has been described, is the non-specific target cell destruction mediated by PHA-transformed but non-sensitised effector cells (Holm and Perlman 1967). These cells appear to be different from K-cells, for it has been found that while antibody-dependent cytotoxicity can be almost completely abolished by passage of the effector cells through an anti-Fc immunoglobulin column, PHA-induced cytotoxicity is little affected (Perlman et al. 1972). Human foetal lymphocytes transformed by PHA have been observed to damage chicken erythrocytes in vitro (Carr et al. 1970). This property is present in the cells of a variety of lymphoid tissues from foetuses of 14—18 weeks gestation age (Stites et al. 1974). It was found that foetal thymocytes failed to produce this kind of xenogeneic target cell destruction, although they could respond strongly to PHA transformation, whereas foetal bone-marrow cells reacted in exactly the opposite pattern. Peripheral blood and splenic lymphocytes responded to both PHA transformation and PHA-induced target cell destruction. Foetal liver lymphoid tissue responded to neither PHA transformation nor PHA-induced cytotoxicity but were responsive to allogeneic cell stimulation. These data further emphasise the marked functional heterogeneity of the lymphocyte population in the human foetus. Different results were obtained by Campbell et al. (1974) who used Chang liver cells as target cells. They found negligible PHA-induced cytotoxicity by cord lymphocytes on these cells.

It is clear that further investigations are necessary before any definite conclusions can be reached regarding the onset of K-cell and PHA-induced cytotoxicity in the human foetus. The relationship of PHA-induced non-specific killing with the rest of cellular immunity is not clear. If this form of lymphocyte activity can be demonstrated to predate the emergence of formal humoral and cellular immune mechanisms, then it may be considered as representing a primitive form of defense in the foetus.

5.2 Ontogeny of humoral immunity

5.2.1 Development of B-lymphocytes

Cells bearing membrane-bound immunoglobulins, which are markers for B-lymphocytes, have been demonstrated in foetal liver at 9 weeks (Asma et al. 1977) and 9½ weeks gestation age (Lawton et al. 1972), so it appears that differentiation of B-lymphocytes begins very early in foetal development, at a time very close to that of thymic lymphopoiesis. Of the two foetal livers studied by Lawton et al. (1972), only IgM-positive cells were seen in one, while IgM- and IgG-positive cells were present in the other. IgA-positive cells were not detected until 11½ weeks. These observations indicate that the order of appearance of cells bearing different immunoglobulin classes is IgM, IgG, and IgA respectively, which is consistent with the sequence IgM → IgG → IgA in immunoglobulin synthesis. Hayward and Ezer (1974), however, detected γ, μ, α and δ heavy chains on foetal lymphocytes and could find no evidence of sequential maturation of lymphocytes bearing different classes of immunoglobulins. It should be pointed out that some of these surface immunoglobulins, especially IgG, may be maternal in origin and could have bound to the Fc receptors of foetal lymphocytes.

Of particular interest is the finding of Rowe et al. (1973a) that there was an unusually large number of IgD-bearing lymphocytes in cord blood (14.5%) compared to that found in adults (3.8%). The authors speculated that IgD might be the foetal immunoglobulin equivalent as haemoglobin F was the foetal haemoglobin. Cells with double IgM and IgD staining could be seen and it was postulated that the sequence of immunoglobulin synthesis might be in the order of $\delta \rightarrow \mu \rightarrow \gamma$ (Rowe et al. 1973b). Vossen and Hijmans (1975), however, disagree. They examined the spleen, liver and bone-marrow of seven foetuses for cells with membrane-bound immunoglobulin and found that μ-positive cells appeared by the 13th week of gestation. This was soon followed by the appearance of δ-positive cells. Furthermore, double staining procedures detected the presence of μ-positive δ-negative cells but never δ-positive μ-negative ones. These findings, therefore, do not support the hypothesis that IgD is the first receptor expressed by lymphocytes but is in agreement with the conclusion of Lawton et al. (1972) that IgM is perhaps the earliest B-lymphocyte receptor. The significance of IgD-bearing foetal lymphocytes, therefore, is unclear at the present moment. The ability of foetal lymphocytes to synthesise surface immunoglobulins of different classes including IgD, may be because repression of these genes is not yet complete. In later life the number of these multiple-immunoglobulin-bearing B-lymphocytes will decrease, possibly as a consequence of some antigen-driven maturation process.

By 14½ weeks gestation age, the percentage of cells in the foetal spleen and blood staining for each class of immunoglobulin has reached a level which is within the range found in the blood from neonates and adults (Lawton et al. 1972). Yet, at this stage of gestation, no cells with cytoplasmic immunoglobulin are detected. Even at later stages of gestation, these cells are rarely seen. Ogra et al. (1971) also did not find any IgG, IgM or IgA secreting cells in various tissues examined from foetuses of 8—22 weeks gestation age. Even during the first few weeks of postnatal life, no plasma cells were detectable in bone-marrow biopsies from 20 normal infants (Bridges et al. 1959). Plasma cells only began to appear in the lamina propria of the ileum and appendix between the 4th and 6th weeks after delivery. These observations indicate that, although the capacity for immunoglobulin synthesis as manifested by the presence of immunoglobulin-bearing B-lymphocytes develops early in gestation, the actual synthesis of immunoglobulins with development into plasma cells only occurs at a very low level.

The attainment of adult proportions of B-lymphocytes bearing surface immunoglobulins so early in foetal life without subsequent maturation into plasma cells implies that the primary development of responsive B-lymphocyte clones occurs as a normal process of differentiation, driven by intrinsic induction factors which are independent of antigenic stimulation. This is in accord with the two-stage model for development of the plasma cell line proposed by Cooper et al. (1971) from the observation that agammaglobulinaemic patients have B-lymphocytes bearing membrane-bound IgM, IgG and IgA which can respond to antigenic challenge by proliferation. Because they cannot complete the second stage of plasma cell differentiation, they cannot make and secrete antibodies. In the foetus, this deficiency in plasma cell maturation may reflect either an absence of antigenic stimulation or an inherent inability to carry out this further stage of B-cell differentiation. The birth of an immunologically normal child to a woman with agammaglobulinaemia provided an opportunity for Bridges et al. (1959) to study this problem. The infant's serum contained very low levels of immunoglobulin at birth because of the lack of maternal transmission. Intensive antigenic stimulation in the form of weekly administration of TAB vaccine did not result in any rise in serum immunoglobulin levels until the 67th day of life. Thereafter, the child's serum immunoglobulin rose to normal levels and was maintained. Serial bone-marrow and lymph node biopsies did not reveal any plasma cell production but these cells appeared concurrently with the capacity to synthesise immunoglobulins. This study, therefore, indicates that the maturation of plasma cells and the production of immunoglobulin is inherently defective in the neonate for the first few months of life. This may explain its vulnerability to infection and its dependence on transmitted maternal antibodies for its defence during this period of extra-uterine life.

5.2.2 Production of immunoglobulins by the foetus

The disparity between cord blood and maternal levels of IgM (Franklin and Kunkel 1958), IgA (Brasher and Hartley 1969; Faulkner and Borella 1970; Virella et al. 1972) and IgD (Leslie and Swate 1972) has usually been considered as suggestive of foetal production of these immunoglobulins rather than of transplacental transmission from the mother. However, it is by no means certain that this is the right interpretation, for the possibility that the levels found in cord sera are due to the differential ability of the various classes of immunoglobulins to traverse the placenta cannot be entirely discounted.

Investigations on immunoglobulin allotypes have provided more definitive evidence. The observation by Martensson and Fudenberg (1965) that some cord sera from infants of Gm(a–) or Gm(b–) mothers contained IgG bearing Gm(a+) or Gm(b+) allotypes respectively is strong evidence that the foetus is capable of synthesising small amounts of IgG. This is confirmed by the reported appearance of an anti-Gm(a) antibody in the serum of a Gm(a–) mother during pregnancy (Fudenberg and Fudenberg 1964). The father was Gm(a+), so the mother was probably sensitised by IgG, bearing the paternal Gm specificity produced by the foetus. Maternal immunisation against Gm specificities have been reported to occur in 28 (1.59%) out of 1,763 normal pregnant women examined (Nathenson et al. 1971). Typing for Am_2 which is a genetic marker for human α_2 heavy chains, Cederqvist and Litwin (1974) found that Am_2 was present in amniotic fluid and in paternal serum but was absent in maternal serum. These findings are, therefore, suggestive of foetal production of IgA2. This receives support from Vyas et al. (1970), who reported that about 15% of recently delivered mothers had anti-IgA antibodies in the sera directed against IgA allotypes.

In vitro studies on cultured foetal tissues are mostly in agreement with the above clinical findings. Van Furth et al. (1965) investigated immunoglobulin synthesis by foetal tissue of 12—31 weeks gestation age. They concluded that the human foetus was capable of synthesising IgG and IgM from about the 20th week of gestation onwards, this production taking place mainly in the spleen. Using a different radioimmunoelectrophoretic assay on cultured foetal tissues, Gitlin and Biasucci

(1969) detected IgG production by embryo cultures of 12 weeks gestation age. Before this, IgG was very low or not detected at all in the cultures, confirming that most of the IgG found in foetal serum at this stage of development is likely to be maternal in origin. Production of IgM was detected even earlier, in cultures from embryos of 10½ weeks gestation age. This is in accord with the concept that the ontogenic sequence of immunoglobulin synthesis begins with IgM.

Two questions need to be clarified in these in vitro studies. Can the immunoglobulins detected be produced by maternal lymphocytes which have crossed the placenta and colonised the foetus? This possibility cannot be entirely excluded with the information available so far, but the large number of IgM-positive cells seen by Van Furth et al. (1965) in foetal tissue would seem to make it unlikely that so many maternal cells have managed to cross the placenta and survived. The other question is whether the immunoglobulins detected in these cultured embryonic tissues represent material secreted by mature plasma cells or whether they are merely shed from the surface membranes of B-lymphocytes bearing these immunoglobulins. Again this cannot be answered with certainty but Van Furth et al. (1965) have observed many medium sized cells with eccentric nuclei and staining for cytoplasmic immunoglobulin in the foetal tissues which they used. These cells had all the characteristics of plasma cells which indicates that at least some of the immunoglobulins detected were secreted. These findings are contrary to those of Ogra et al. (1971) and Lawton et al. (1972) who detected B-lymphocytes with membrane-bound immunoglobulin but no cells with cytoplasmic immunoglobulin. The tissues used by Van Furth et al. (1965) were obtained from foetuses which were born alive but died immediately after birth. They were, therefore, of much later gestation age than in the other studies. Furthermore, some of the mothers had evidence of infection during pregnancy. It may be that antigenic stimulation in utero by maternally transmitted infections was responsible for the presence of some immunoglobulin-secreting plasma cells.

None of the in vitro studies mentioned so far have detected the foetal synthesis of IgA. Perhaps the foetal tissues used were those that did not produce IgA. Petit et al. (1973) analysed gut wall tissue and gut contents from 27 foetuses of 11—32 weeks gestation age. They found secretory IgA in 16 of them. The reactions of complete identity between foetal gut IgA and colostral IgA when tested against anti-secretory IgA and anti-secretory component, confirmed that the foetal IgA detected was secretory IgA. The authors argued that this IgA was synthesised by the foetus and was not of maternal origin. This is certainly supported by the results of clinical studies on IgA allotypes and by the observation by Ogra et al. (1971) that the secretory component was demonstrable in the lungs of the earliest foetuses (8 weeks) studied and became detectable in most secretory tissues by 18—22 weeks of gestation. Nevertheless, the abundant evidence for the presence of maternal immunoglobulins in amniotic fluid (see Chapter 8) cannot be ignored. Swallowing of this fluid by the foetus can, no doubt, make a significant contribution to the immunoglobulin content of foetal gut.

The overall conclusion from the available evidence would seem to be that ontogeny of the B-cell system occurs very early in human foetal development. This is at about the 9th week of gestation around the time when the T-cell system is also developing. Although the proportion of B-lymphocytes bearing membrane-bound immunoglobulin reaches the level found in adults by the 14—15th week of gestation, immunoglobulin synthesis does not begin until about the 20th week of gestation and occurs only at a very low level. This may be a reflection of lack of antigenic stimulation in the relatively sterile uterine environment. However, there is evidence to suggest that, even when stimulated, this phase of immunological development does not reach full maturity until at least after the second month of postnatal life. This inherent immaturity of the humoral immune system may be a factor for the increased susceptibility to infections of neonates within the first few months of extra-uterine life.

5.3 Ontogeny of the complement system

Evidence for foetal synthesis of complement components have been gained by employing several different methods (Adinolfi 1972; Rosen 1974):

(1) Comparison of the mean level of total complement activity in pairs of cord and maternal sera;

(2) Quantitation of individual complement components in foetal sera;

(3) The use of existing complement polymorphism to assess maternal-foetal differences;

(4) Culture of foetal tissues for evidence of complement synthesis in vitro; and

(5) Immunofluorescent localisation of the sites of complement synthesis.

Total complement haemolytic titre in cord blood tends to be lower than corresponding maternal titre, with cord blood containing about 50—80% of maternal values of C4, C3, C5 and Properdin Factor B as found by immunochemical assay. These components reach adult levels by 3 months of age (Fireman et al. 1969). Similar results were reported by Fishel and Pearlman (1961) who found a consistently lower complement activity in cord specimens which was paralleled by a decrease in C1, C2, C3 and C4 components. Ballow et al. (1974) reported a deficiency of all nine complement components in cord serum relative to maternal serum. They confirmed that C1 to C5 components in cord serum were about half that of maternal serum. In addition, C6 and C7 were also present in cord serum at a concentration which was half that in maternal serum. The C8 and C9 components, however, were very low in cord serum, occurring with a titre of only 5—10% relative to maternal titre. Many of these complement components increase dramatically within 4 days of birth. Sawyer et al. (1971) noted that infants with birth weight greater than 2,500 g had normal complement values while 50% of infants with birth weight less than 2,500 g had significant deficiencies of complement components. These observations, therefore, suggest that there is probably a gradual maturation of the complement system which is not complete at birth.

Further evidence for the fœtal synthesis of complement is provided by studies of complement allotypes. Discrepancy noted between cord and maternal blood for C4 and Factor B allotypes indicates that these components are synthesised by the foetus (Bach et al. 1971; Alper et al. 1972). Significant discordance between 25 pairs of maternal and cord blood for C3 allotypes has also been noted by Propp and Alper (1968). In a further analysis of two of these discordant pairs, C3 with mother's phenotype was not found in the newborn's serum and C3 with the newborn's phenotype was not found in the mother's serum. This indicates that C3 does not readily traverse the placenta. This may also be applicable to C2, for Ruddy et al. (1970) described a homozygous C2-deficient foetus whose serum contained a negligible quantity of this component at 18 days of age while maternal C2 levels ranged from 1,980—2,020 units/ml.

In vitro studies of embryo cultures have shown that the human foetus is capable of synthesising β1E (associated with C4) and β1C/β1A (associated with C3) globulins during the second trimester (Adinolfi et al. 1968). Most complement components can be detected from cultures of foetuses as early as at 8 weeks gestation age (Gitlin and Biasucci 1969;

Colten 1972; Kohler 1973). The ability to synthesise complement, therefore, appears to precede that of immunoglobulin production by a significant interval. The ontogeny of the complement system thus reflects phylogeny, for it is thought that this is a more primitive defense system than antibody production.

The site of synthesis for C1 appears to be the columnar epithelium of the intestinal tract, particularly in the colon and to a lesser extent in the ileum (Colten et al. 1968), while C4 and C2 are synthesised in either fixed or wandering macrophages (Colten 1972). Hepatic parenchymal cells are the sites of synthesis for C3, C5, and C1-inhibitor. Thus, the foetal liver, with its content of hepatic cells and fixed macrophages is found to be 20—40 times more active than foetal spleen or thymus in the synthesis of complement components, a finding which agrees with studies that show the adult liver as being the major, if not the only, site of C3 biosynthesis. It has been calculated that 34×10^8 effective haemolytic molecules of C3 were present in the tissue culture fluid after 64 hours incubation of 100 mg of foetal liver of 14-weeks gestation age (Colten 1972).

The maturation of the complement system in man, therefore, follows a very similar course to that of the humoral immune system. While the capacity to synthesise complement components is acquired very early on during foetal development, full adult serum complement levels are not achieved until about the 3rd month of extra-uterine life. The neonate, therefore, will be expected to be somewhat inefficient in complement-dependent immunological reactions.

5.4 Development of phagocytes

Chemotactic response and phagocytosis are important defense mechanisms. This is amply illustrated by the increased susceptibility to infections in conditions which result in the functional derangement of these mechanisms (Baehner 1974; Stiehm 1975). Many stages of these processes are immunologically mediated so it is clear that the development of these activities are intimately related to the ontogeny of immunocompetence in the human foetus.

Neutrophil response to chemotaxis in newborns has been observed to be significantly lower than in adults (Miller 1971; Klein et al. 1976; Pahwa et al. 1977). Chemotactic factors are usually generated from serum by the activation of complement, either via the classical pathway initiated by antigen-antibody interaction, or via the alternate pathway. In the previous sections, we have seen that foetal production of antibody is not well developed until several months after birth and foetal serum is deficient in all the components of complement. It is therefore possible that lack of these serum factors may be responsible for the deficient chemotactic response by neonatal neutrophils. However, neonatal neutrophils have been observed to show a decreased chemotactic migration, even when incubated in the presence of chemotactic factors generated from standard, pooled adult sera (Miller 1971). It would seem, therefore, that the deficient chemotactic response of neonatal neutrophils may be due to both an inherent impaired cellular response to chemotactic stimuli and a diminished ability to generate chemotactic stimuli from serum.

In contrast, cord blood monocytes have been observed to exhibit the same or slightly increased chemotactic response compared to adult monocytes (Pahwa et al. 1977). This was thought to be a compensatory mechanism for the lack of this property in neutrophils. The dissociation in response between the two cell types is difficult to explain on the basis of lack of serum factors, for they both utilise very similar mechanisms, so it must be due to an inherent difference in cellular functional ability to respond. Different results were obtained by Kretschmer et al. (1976) who reported that cord blood monocytes had low chemotactic response. Further investigations are obviously needed to clarify this aspect of cellular activity of the human foetus.

Diminished phagocytosis of bacteria (Tunicliff 1910) and starch granules (Matoth 1952) by cord blood leucocytes in the presence of their own serum is well documented. Again the question arises as to whether this is due to an inherent immaturity of neonatal phagocytes or to a lack of serum opsonising factors. Coen et al. (1969) believed there was an inherent defect and attributed this to inefficient glucose metabolism through the hexose monophosphate shunt in neonatal phagocytes. In contrast, Park et al. (1970) found no abnormality in the functional capacity of the hexose monophosphate shunt in neonatal leucocytes as measured by the nitroblue tetrazolium (NBT) dye reduction test. Even leucocytes from premature infants exhibited only slightly reduced NBT dye reduction. Pross et al. (1977) reported that the percentage of cord blood neutrophils forming EA-rosettes and EAC-rosettes was identical to that for adult neutrophils. This indicates that neonatal neutrophils are as mature as adult neutrophils at least in terms of the expression of surface receptors for antibody and for complement. These receptors for opsonic adherence and immune adherence play an important role in phagocytosis.

Present opinion would seem to favour a lack of serum opsonic factors as the cause of deficient phagocytosis by neonatal neutrophils (Dossett et al. 1969; Forman and Stiehm 1969), for this defect can be corrected by the presence of adult serum (Gluck and Silverman 1957), while sera from newborns incubated with a standard adult neutrophil suspension are deficient in opsonising activity (Miller 1969). Investigations on low birthweight infants with inadequate serum opsonic activity demonstrated a consistent correlation with a deficiency of one or more complement components (Sawyer et al. 1971), especially C3 (McCracken and Eichenwald 1971). It has also been observed that cord sera with low opsonic activity have subnormal concentrations of GBG, a component of the properdin system involved in the alternate pathway of complement activation (Stossel et al. 1973). These observations support the conclusion that hypofunction of complement-dependent opsonisation may be a very important factor responsible for the neonate's inadequate and sluggish phagocytic activity.

5.5 Foetal immunological response to intra-uterine infections

It is well documented that maternal infections during pregnancy can affect the foetus. The foetal morbidity and mortality resulting from maternal rubella infection is an example. What effects do these intra-uterine infective agents have on the foetal immune response?

5.5.1 Evidence of foetal sensitisation

The manifestations of in vitro and in vivo sensitivity to a wide variety of infective agents by the foetus or neonate indicate prior contact with these antigens. It has already been mentioned in a preceding section that the high rate of spontaneous transformation observed in cord blood lymphocytes may be due to antigenic stimulation in utero. Although maternal iso-antigens are likely to be responsible for some of this stimulation, the demonstrable sensitivity of some cord lymphocytes to antigens like staphylococcal filtrate (Leikin et al. 1968) or streptolysin-O (Leikin and Oppenheim 1971) would seem to indicate prior contact with these organisms.

Brody et al. (1968) studied the in vitro lymphocyte response to E. coli extract in two groups of neonates. The first group consisted of those born to mothers with E. coli infections, while the second group included those born to mothers without E. coli infections. Significant mitoses were observed in all 10 cultures of the first group, indicating prior sensitisation. In contrast, nine out of 11 cultures from the second group did not show mitoses while two did show a positive response. Of these two 'false positive' cases, one mother had a previous history of E. coli pyelonephritis during the earlier stages of pregnancy but was now cured. The foetus could have been sensitised then. In vitro neonatal lymphocyte sensitivity to tuberculin (Field and Caspary 1971) and mumps virus (Aase et al. 1972) have also been reported. Astor and Frick (1973) examined six mother/infant pairs by intradermal skin tests and in vitro migration inhibition tests for cellular immunity to three antigens: PPD, Candida, and streptokinase/streptodornase (SK/SD). While there was complete correspondence in the reactions to PPD between mother and infant, only two out of six infants reacted positively to Candida and SK/SD, in spite of their mothers being all positive to these antigens. This suggests that the foetus is more readily sensitised to some antigens in utero than to others. Sensitivity to helminthic antigens has also been observed (Camus et al. 1976). These investigators reported that 13 out of 27 uninfected children of ages 7—34 months born to mothers infected with Schistosoma mansoni developed delayed skin reactions to S. mansoni antigens.

Although these data are generally taken to indicate active sensitisation of the foetus by transplacentally transmitted infective agents or their soluble antigens, alternative explanations must also be considered. It is possible that the observed foetal sensitivity is mediated by the passive transfer of sensitised maternal lymphocytes, either across the placenta or via milk after birth. The adoptive transfer of cellular immunity via milk is receiving much attention and will be discussed in more detail in a later chapter. Instead of intact sensitised maternal cells, transmission of some informational molecules like transfer factor from the mother may also influence the cellular immune response of the foetus. The present evidence is insufficient to permit us to distinguish between these possibilities. Hashem (1972) has demonstrated that lymphocytes from neonates can exhibit in vitro evidence of sensitisation to mixed ragweed and pollen without the corresponding mothers showing similar sensitisation. Animal experiments by Stastny (1965) have shown that infant rats born to mothers sensitised by donor skin cells during pregnancy could display a state of homograft immunity manifested by the accelerated rejection of donor skin graft. This could occur even if the mothers themselves were highly tolerant to donor strain antigens. These observations, therefore, indicate that foetal sensitisation can sometimes occur without evidence of maternal sensitisation. A process of active sensitisation of the foetus by maternally derived antigens is the most likely mechanism in these cases.

5.5.2 Production of specific antibodies by the foetus

It has frequently been observed that congenital infections are accompanied by a raised cord serum level of immunoglobulins, especially of IgM and IgA classes (Stiehm et al. 1966; Alford et al. 1967; Mason et al. 1976). Cederqvist et al. (1977b) reported that infants with congenital toxoplasmosis all had elevated serum IgM and IgA levels but children born to mothers with toxoplasmosis who themselves were not infected did not have raised serum immunoglobulins. This indicates active foetal humoral response to congenital infections. Increased cord levels of IgM and IgA have also been observed following prematurely ruptured membranes, and it is thought that this may be due to foetal response to ascending infection in the mother (Cederqvist et al. 1976).

The specificity of these foetal antibodies has been demonstrated Eichenwald and Shinefield (1963) obtained sera from cord blood in infants with congenital toxoplasmosis contracted as early as the 28th week of gestation, and compared the anti-toxoplasma activity of 7S and 19S fractions with those from mothers (Table 5.1). It can be seen from the Table that the 7S fractions from both cord and maternal sera have high anti-toxoplasma activity but only the 19S fraction from cord sera has this activity. This indicates that IgM anti-toxoplasma antibody was

Table 5.1 Comparison of anti-toxoplasma activity of 7S and 19S globulin fractions from cord and maternal sera.

	Anti-toxoplasma activity	
	7S globulin fraction	19S globulin fraction
Cord sera	++++	+++
Maternal sera	++++	± to ○

With kind permission from Eichenwald, H. F. and Shinefield, H. R. (1963) *J. Pediat.* 63, 870.

probably produced by the congenitally infected foetus while the IgG fraction was entirely or partially transmitted from the mother. This is substantiated by the finding that infants who were not infected with toxoplasmosis but were born to mothers with high titres of anti-toxoplasma antibody showed anti-toxoplasma activity only in the 7S globulin fraction of their sera. Bellanti and Jackson (1967) reported a case of a newborn 8-days-old infant with demonstrable IgM antibody to the somatic 'O' antigen of S. typhosa. The sensitising antigen was thought to be the typhoid-paratyphoid vaccine administered to the mother one day before birth.

However, the human foetus does not invariably mount an active humoral response to congenital infections, for some newborn infants, even with clinically apparent infections, have been observed not to show a rise in cord blood IgM or IgA levels (Miller et al. 1969). Among the Eskimo children with positive cellular immunity against mumps virus reported by Aase et al. (1972), none developed mumps virus neutralising antibodies. Similarly, among the neonates born to E. coli infected mothers and whose lymphocytes showed in vitro sensitisation to E. coli antigens, there was no detectable rise in the levels of IgM or IgA in their cord sera (Brody et al. 1968; Wallach et al. 1969). These findings, therefore, are consistent with the conclusion reached in a preceding section that the humoral immune response of the human foetus does not reach full maturity until several months after birth.

5.5.3 Clinical application of foetal immune response to prenatal infection

A potential clinical application is the prenatal active immunisation of the foetus by administering the antigen to the mother (Gill 1973; Cramer et al. 1974). This will be particularly useful in those areas of the world where infectious diseases early in life are still important causes of infant mortality. Transplacentally transmitted maternal immunoglobulins confer a high degree of protection to the foetus but there comes a time when this passive immunity has to be replaced by the foetus' own active antibody synthesis. This transition period during the first few months of life is when the foetus is most vulnerable. Prenatal immunisation will enable the neonate to mount a more effective secondary immune response to infective agents when it leaves its relatively sheltered intra-uterine milieu for the more hostile environment of the outside world.

In practice, this may be difficult to achieve. The timing is important because, like postnatal immunisation, interference by maternal antibody has to be considered. This obstacle may be circumvented if immunisation can be arranged to be conducted during a time in foetal development before significant amounts of maternal antibody are transmitted across the placenta. On the other hand, the antigen must not be introduced too early before the development of foetal immunocompetence. From what is known about this, a possible compromise may well be sometime during the latter part of the first trimester. Live vaccines are perhaps best avoided but killed vaccines or toxoids may be useful candidates for initial investigations.

A further question that needs to be considered is whether it is at all desirable to augment the foetal immune response at this stage of development. It is now well established that in many diseases the host immune response may contribute towards the inflammatory component of the pathological process. The variation in the lesions seen in congenital syphilis according to the period of gestation when the infection is contracted by the foetus, is such an example. In other cases, the host immunological component may actually cause the disease itself rather than any toxic action of the infective agent. The most frequently quoted example of this is lymphocytic-choriomeningitis virus infection of mice. Here, the relatively incompetent foetus or neonate shows no disease although carrying a heavy load of virus throughout the body but, in contrast, the immunocompetent adult animal suffers from a lethal meningitis probably as a result of immune-complex deposition (Turk 1972). Thus, the possibility that prenatal immunisation may adversely modify certain congenital infections has to be examined further (Silverstein 1972a, b).

Finally, the undesired induction of tolerance rather than sensitisation towards infective agents will be disastrous for the foetus. Fortunately, this phenomenon seems to occur rarely if at all in naturally acquired congenital infections. This is in accord with the observations in a preceding section that exposure of the foetus to maternal isoantigens, even during the early stages of gestation, tends to result in sensitisation and not tolerance. There are, however, some cases of congenital infections with rubella where the neonates continue to shed virus for appreciable periods and yet develop no antibody response nor do they exhibit positive seroconversion after rubella vaccination. Unfortunately, the situation is complicated by the observation that these infants frequently have a low immunological reactivity towards a wide range of unrelated antigens, so it is uncertain whether these cases are examples of specific tolerance to rubella virus or are manifestations of a generalised immune paralysis resulting from the infection.

6

Passage of cells across the human placenta

Although the foetal and maternal circulations are separated throughout human gestation by the placenta, it does not form an impenetrable barrier. Serum proteins and even cells may pass in either direction. This is probably largely due to the structure of the human placenta. It is haemochorial, so classified because only foetal tissues are interposed between maternal blood and foetal capillaries. Maternal layers are absent. This is in contrast to the placentae of other species where, in addition to foetal tissues, maternal layers ranging from 1 to 3 are also present. Within the haemochorial group, the human placenta belongs to the haemomonochorial subdivision. Of the two layers that make up the chorion (an outer syncytial and an inner cytotrophoblast layer), the cytotrophoblast is discontinuous so that only the syncytiotrophoblast effectively intervenes between foetal capillaries and maternal blood (Steven 1975). Thus, the human placenta has the fewest intervening layers between foetal and maternal circulations, a property which is shared by only a few other species like the armadillo, guinea pig, and chipmunk. This may explain the relative ease with which blood constituents are exchanged between the human foetus and its mother.

6.1 Transfer of erythrocytes from foetus to mother

6.1.1 Detection of foetal erythrocytes in maternal blood after birth

The first report of foetal erythrocytes in maternal circulation was that by Chown (1954) who demonstrated by differential agglutination the presence of minute agglutinates of Rh positive cells in a Rh negative mother immediately after delivery of a Rh positive baby. It was therefore assumed that these red cells were from the foetus. Rough quantitation of the agglutinates showed that about 5—10% of the red cells in maternal circulation were foetal in origin so that the amount of foeto-maternal transfusion in this case must have been considerable. The number of Rh positive foetal cells detected in maternal circulation was found to be reduced by half by the 28th day post partum and were not demonstrable at all by the 48th day. Using similar differential agglutination techniques, subsequent investigators have all confirmed the presence of foetal red cells in the maternal circulation. Dunsford (1957) reported a case of a group 'O' Rh negative mother who delivered a group 'A' Rh positive infant. Immediately after birth, some red cells in the mother's blood were agglutinated by anti-A, anti-D, and anti-C. By the 10th day post partum, foetal cells were no longer detectable in the mother's blood. Creger and Steele (1957) examined during labour the blood of 15 group 'A' mothers who subsequently delivered group 'O' babies. A count was made of any unagglutinated red cells in maternal blood after maximal agglutination by anti-A serum. The hypothesis to be tested was that some of these unagglutinated cells were foetal group 'O' erythrocytes, which had gained access into the maternal circulation. A further sample of maternal blood was similarly examined six weeks post partum, when it was assumed that any foetal cells previously present would by now have disappeared. Nine cases of group 'A' mothers who gave birth to group 'A' babies were used as controls. The results are shown in Table 6.1. It can be seen that the average number of unagglutinated erythrocytes in mothers of group 'A' who bore infants

Table 6.1 Average number of erythrocytes unagglutinated by anti-A serum in maternal blood

	Ante partum (per cm)	Post partum (per cm)	Change (per cm)
Group 'A' mothers with group 'O' babies	14,900	7,500	−7,400
Group 'A' mothers with group 'A' babies	6,100	4,400	−1,700

With kind permission from Creger, W. P. and Steele, M. R. (1957) *New Engl. J. Med.* **256**, 158–161.

of group 'O' was higher at delivery and had a greater decline six weeks post partum than group 'A' mothers who bore group 'A' babies. This was therefore considered as confirmatory evidence for the presence of group 'O' foetal erythrocytes in group 'A' maternal blood.

Immunofluorescent techniques with antibodies directed against blood group antigens on foetal erythrocytes which are absent on the mother's have also been used for the differential identification of foetal red cells in the maternal circulation. Using this method, Cohen and Zuelzer (1964) found that in 82 mothers examined, 34 (41.5%) had demonstrable foetal red cells in mother's blood immediately post partum.

Perhaps the most widely used technique is the acid elution method of Kleihauer. This is based on the observation that red cells containing foetal haemoglobin will resist treatment with acid buffers under conditions in which cells with adult haemoglobin will become 'ghosted'. Foetal red cells, therefore, can be picked out from maternal red cells without being dependent on the presence of any antigenic differences. By the artificial in vitro mixing of foetal and maternal red cells in different proportions and then staining by the Kleihauer technique, a rough correlate can be obtained between the number of foetal cells seen in a scan of a maternal blood smear and the amount of foetal blood that this represents. There are, however, many sources of error inherent in the Kleihauer method. The erythrocyte population of the foetus in the later stages of gestation is heterogeneous, and the most recently formed cells can contain more haemoglobin A than haemoglobin F. These cells, therefore, will not stain by the Kleihauer technique, so that in the enumeration of foetal red cells by this method there is a tendency towards underestimation. The premise that all red cells with haemoglobin F found in maternal blood are necessarily of foetal origin may not be correct. It is well established that erythrocytes containing demonstrable quantities of haemoglobin F are found in adult life in a variety of pathological conditions like thalassaemia, sickle-cell anaemia, aplastic anaemia, and leukaemia. It seems that any increased burden on erythropoiesis may result in the persistence of foetal haemoglobin. Even normal adults can occasionally have red cells indistinguishable from foetal red cells (Cohen et al. 1964; Sullivan and Jennings 1966), so that the presence of a few acid-resistant erythrocytes in the maternal blood should be interpreted with this fallibility in mind.

The findings from different groups of investigators are summarised

Table 6.2 Summary of the results from different groups of investigators concerning the post partum detection of foetal erythrocytes in maternal blood by the Kleihauer acid elution method.

Source	No. of cases examined	No. of cases positive for foetal erythrocytes	Estimated equivalent amount of foetal blood present
Zipursky et al. (1959)	42	11 (21%)	0.1–3 ml
Finn et al. (1961a)	200	24 (12%)	1–2 ml
Brown (1963)	165	83 (50%)	Not quoted
Zipursky et al. (1963)	384	106 (27.6%)	0.1–0.2 ml
Cohen et al. (1964)	622	303 (48.7%)	0.004–0.4 ml

in Table 6.2. From this Table it can be seen that, although the frequency and the amount appear to vary, foetal red cells are found in maternal blood with such regularity, at least after delivery, as to suggest that the foeto-maternal passage of erythrocytes is probably a physiological phenomenon.

6.1.2 Detection of foetal erythrocytes in maternal blood during pregnancy

A more relevant finding in relation to the barrier function of the placenta is the demonstration of foetal erythrocytes in the maternal circulation during pregnancy rather than after the separation of the placenta when it might be expected that some blood could spill over during delivery. Employing a differential agglutination method, Weiner et al. (1958) reported the findings in the blood of a group 'A' Rh negative woman examined 2—3 months before her expected date of delivery. When tested with anti-D and anti-C serum, her red cells showed 'small agglutinates in a sea of unagglutinated cells', a picture typical of a mixed field. It was concluded that these agglutinated cells were Rh positive erythrocytes which had gained access to the maternal circulation across the placenta. The mother subsequently gave birth to a baby whose Rh blood group was confirmed as CDe.

Later investigators mainly used the Kleihauer method. The results from different groups are summarised in Table 6.3. From this, it can be

Table 6.3 Summary of the results from different groups of investigators comparing the ante partum and post partum detection of foetal erythrocytes in maternal blood by the Kleihauer acid elution method.

Source	No. of cases examined	Time of study	No. of cases positive for foetal cells	Estimated equivalent amount of foetal blood present
Taylor and Kullman (1961)	40 58	16–42 weeks 2nd day after delivery	7 (18%) 10 (17%)	Not quoted
Fraser and Raper (1962)	240 635	34th week 60 hours after birth	19 (8%) 182 (28.7%)	Not quoted
Woodrow et al. (1965)	200 Same cases	Ante partum Post partum	6 (3%) 40 (20%)	Larger volumes of foetal blood detected after birth
McLarey and Fish (1966)	223	21–42 weeks	121 (54.3%)	Average 0.362 ml
Sullivan and Jennings (1966)	243 562	Ante partum 12–36 hours after birth	27 (11.1%) 188 (33.5%)	Larger volumes of foetal blood detected after birth
Beer (1969)	164 155	3rd trimester 1 hour after delivery	58 (35%) 87 (56.1%)	Volume of foetal blood detected post partum ranged from 0.04 ml to greater than 40.0 ml

seen that nearly all are agreed that the frequency and volume of foetal blood which had gained access to the maternal circulation is greater after delivery than before. It remains to be determined whether the few red cells with haemoglobin F detected during the ante partum period really represent foetal cells or are merely artifacts. 'Foetal' red cells have been detected by the Kleihauer method in the blood of from 2% (Taylor and Kullman 1961) to 12% (Sullivan and Jennings 1966) of normal blood donors. If about 10% of these possible 'false positives' are subtracted from all the data as suggested by Sullivan and Jennings (1966), then the frequency with which foetal red cells are detected in maternal blood during pregnancy will be reduced to insignificant proportions in many cases except for those reported by McLarey and Fish (1966) and Beer (1969). The clinical observations that first pregnancy Rh sensitisation rarely occurs would seem to suggest that, if foetal red cells do succeed in reaching the maternal circulation during early pregnancy, then the volume involved must be too small to induce sensitisation, unless there is some altered immunological state of pregnancy which protects the mother until parturition. The high success rate of protection from Rh sensitisation by giving mothers anti-D after birth further confirms that, for all practical purposes, significant amounts of foetal red cells sufficient to induce sensitisation probably only gain access to the maternal circulation at or perhaps just before delivery.

When foetal red cells are looked for in maternal blood during different stages of pregnancy, it appears that the number of positive observations increases as pregnancy advances (Cohen et al. 1964). This can be seen in Table 6.4. Although there is a marked difference in the incidence of detectable foetal cells between the 3rd trimester and immediately post partum, this does not necessarily indicate that the process of labour, as such, plays a part in forcing foetal blood into the maternal circulation. Duration of labour, method of expulsion of the placenta, and whether the mother delivered naturally or by caesarian section, appear not to influence the frequency of detectable foetal cells in the mother (Brown 1963; Cohen et al. 1964). Perhaps a progressive deterioration of the placental barrier with advancing pregnancy,

Table 6.4 Detection of foetal erythrocytes in maternal blood at different stages of pregnancy

Trimester	No. of cases examined	No. of times foetal red cells detected
1st	15	1 (6.7%)
2nd	113	18 (15.9%)
3rd	491	142 (28.9%)
Immediately post partum	622	303 (48.7%)

With kind permission from Cohen, F. et al. (1964) *Blood* 23, 621–646.

culminating with the complete separation during delivery are the main factors responsible for the increasing leakage of foetal cells into the maternal circulation.

6.1.3 Detection of foetal erythrocytes in maternal blood after abortion

Do abortions, either spontaneous or induced, result in transfer of foetal erythrocytes to the mother? The results concerning spontaneous abortions are conflicting. Matthews and Matthews (1969) believed that the risk of this occurring with spontaneous abortions was small, with only about 6% of the cases having detectable foetal cells in the maternal circulation. The size of the foetal bleeds was estimated to be usually less than 0.02 ml. Katz (1969) found that 23.5—25% of threatened and incomplete abortions had detectable foetal cells in maternal blood. While these figures appear high, they do not differ significantly from the 14.6—24% frequency of detectable foetal cells found in maternal blood during the antenatal period of normal pregnancies recorded by the same authors, so the difference between these figures and those of Matthews and Matthews probably reflects a difference in methodology. In contrast, the data presented by Litwak et al. (1969) showed a definite increase in the incidence of foeto-maternal transfer of erythrocytes after spontaneous abortions compared to normal pregnancy during the same period of gestation. They found 13 (36%) out of 36 women with spontaneous abortions had detectable foetal red cells in their blood. In a subsequent larger study of 98 aborting patients, 31 (32%) had detectable foetal cells in their circulation (Litwak et al. 1970) which therefore confirmed their earlier findings. Of these 31 positive cases, 26 had 0.05 ml or more of foetal blood. At the same time, only three (8%) of 38 normal pregnant controls had detectable foetal cells in their blood.

A further point of controversy is whether surgical intervention, in the form of curettage, after incomplete abortions can increase the frequency and size of foeto-maternal transfer of cells. Litwak et al. (1970) found an increase in foetal cell score after curettage in four out of 11 patients who had incomplete abortions. Of 39 patients with incomplete abortions who had no demonstrable foetal cells in their circulation before curettage, seven had demonstrable foetal cells post-operatively. Katz (1969) reported similar findings. The incidence of detectable foetal cells rose from 25% in incomplete abortions before surgical intervention to 45.5% after curettage, the difference being statistically significant. Four patients had more than 0.2 ml of foetal blood compared to one before curettage. In contrast, Murray, et al. (1970) found 14.2% of women with spontaneous abortions had detectable foetal cells in their circulation compared to 13.6% after curettage. Of 14 cases with 0.1 ml or more of foetal blood, 12 of these had occurred before curettage. The association of foeto-maternal haemorrhage with spontaneous abortions and curettage must therefore await further information before any definite conclusions can be reached.

The incidence of foeto-maternal transmission of erythrocytes following induced abortions has been reported by many investigators. Their data are summarised in Table 6.5. These show that artificial termination of pregnancy frequently results in transplacental haemorrhage. The type of termination is probably of less importance than the stage of pregnancy when termination is performed. Voigt and Britt (1969) found that of 64 vaginal terminations before the 12th week, only 6 (9.4%) had detectable foetal red cells in the mother's blood after

Table 6.5 Summary of the results from different groups of investigators concerning the detection of foetal erythrocytes in maternal blood following induced abortions.

Source	Type of induced abortion	No. of cases examined	% positive for foetal erythrocytes
Matthews and Matthews (1969)	Vaginal termination	118	26
	Abdominal termination	103	25
Normington and Jennison (1969)	Dilatation and evacuation	77	22
	Utus paste	11	45
	Hysterotomy	12	41.5
Voigt and Britt (1969)	Overall for 4 types of termination	212	26.4
Walsh and Lewis (1970)	Vacuum aspiration	98	25.4
	Curettage	28	25
	Hysterotomy	24	25
	Injection of glucose	26	15.1
	Hysterectomy	19	10.5
Queenan et al. (1971)	Suction	404	7.2
	Hypotonic saline	202	20.2

the operation, but of 77 similar terminations after the 12th week, 31 (40.3%) had foetal cells. This is not really surprising for it is to be expected that the larger the area of contact between placenta and uterus, the greater would be the chance of foeto-maternal haemorrhage when the placenta is separated.

Since the main concern in the association between foeto-maternal transfer of cells and various types of abortions is the possibility that Rh sensitisation may result, a more direct and logical approach is to investigate the frequency of this sensitisation following abortions rather than laboriously counting foetal red cells in the maternal circulation. Freda et al. (1970) have approached the problem from this direction. They calculated that while the risk of a Rh negative woman with a Rh positive child in her first pregnancy giving rise to erythroblastosis was less than 1%, this risk increased to 4% if the woman had had a previous abortion. Similarly, Murray and Barron (1971) found that two out of 91 primiparae, following spontaneous or induced abortions, had anti-D in their blood detected by the indirect Coombs' test, with a further seven being positive when tested by an enzyme technique. The overall incidence of 9.4% with detectable anti-D antibodies is therefore high, which indicates that the risk of Rh sensitisation following abortions is significant.

6.2 Transfer of erythrocytes from mother to foetus

6.2.1 Use of radio-active labelled erythrocytes

The passage of red cells from mother to foetus can be studied by injecting labelled cells into pregnant mothers and then monitoring the amount of radio-activity in the foetal circulation. This is the basis of the original study by Naeslund and Nylin (1946) who tagged red blood cells with radio-active P^{32}, injected them into the maternal circulation prior to delivery, and later tested foetal blood for radio-activity. In one case out of six, they were able to demonstrate a significant degree of radio-activity among the infant's erythrocytes and therefore concluded that this indicated the transplacental transmission of maternal red cells to the foetus. However, the data were difficult to interpret because the dissociation rate of phosphorus from the red cells was very rapid and much of the free phosphorus dissolved in maternal plasma could have diffused across the placental barrier to be picked up by foetal erythrocytes. To circumvent this problem, Naeslund (1951) later tried radio-active Fe^{59} which has the merit that, once incorporated into the red cell, the iron tends to remain in the cell for the rest of its life span. There is one serious disadvantage in that red cells do not incorporate Fe^{59} in vitro and will only do so if it is injected in vivo. Unfortunately, this cannot be administered directly into the pregnant woman under investigation, for the iron will find its way into both the red cells and the plasma which may result in free Fe^{59} diffusing across to the foetus. Labelling, therefore, has to be done by injecting the Fe^{59} into donor volunteers of compatible blood group whose washed red cells are subsequently infused into a pregnant woman. Although there is no reason to suppose that these allogeneic erythrocytes would not behave exactly as the pregnant woman's own red cells, it does introduce an additional factor into the experiments. When allogeneic red cells labelled in this way were infused into seven pregnant women, the foetal blood in four cases showed considerable radio-activity (Naeslund 1951).

Similar results were obtained by Mengert et al. (1955). They injected Fe^{59}-labelled donor red cells into blood group compatible pregnant women in the afternoon prior to delivering her the next morning. It was considered that this time interval was insufficient to allow too many of the red cells to reach their natural life span and be haemolysed, and if haemolysis did occur, there was not time for any dissociated Fe^{59} to diffuse across the placenta and be taken up by foetal erythrocytes. Significant radio-activity was observed in the blood of 25 out of 29 foetuses. The amount of radio-activity was calculated to represent an average 4.4 ml of maternal blood having passed to the foetus. The stages of gestation of the subjects ranged from early pregnancy to near term so it would appear that the materno-foetal transmission of red cells can take place throughout pregnancy. Of the 25 women whose foetal blood showed positive radio-activity, 17 were delivered by caesarian section and the foetal blood for examination was obtained from the cord before the utero-placental junction was disturbed. The women in early gestation were aborted therapeutically by abdominal hysterotomy.

Later studies of this kind employed radio-active Cr^{51} which has several advantages (Smith et al. 1961). The pregnant woman's own red cells can be labelled in vitro and then infused back just before delivery. Cr^{51} seems to bind to red cells with great tenacity for after re-injection of tagged cells into the maternal circulation, no free Cr^{51} can be detected in the plasma for at least 24 hours. Any isotope released by destroyed red cells is rapidly cleared by the kidneys and will not re-label other red cells. All these properties therefore ensure that the source of any radio-activity detected in foetal blood is likely to be due to labelled maternal cells crossing the placenta. Using this technique, Smith et al. (1961) detected significant radio-activity in the foetal blood in 13 out of 18 patients after the infusion of labelled erythrocytes 13—18 hours prior to caesarian section. About 0.3—0.9 ml of maternal blood was estimated to have crossed. A lower incidence was reported by Zarou et al. (1964) who observed radio-activity in foetal blood in seven out of 19 cases after similar infusion of Cr^{51}-labelled erythrocytes into the mother. The amount of maternal blood calculated to have crossed the placenta, however, was quite large, ranging from 1—13 ml.

6.2.2 *Use of erythrocytes with hereditary defects*

An alternative approach to radio-active labelling of red cells is to use cells possessing some inherent definitive characteristics which can be recognised in the foetal circulation after infusion into the mother. Hedenstedt and Naeslund (1946) infused elliptocytes into two pregnant women and recovered similar cells in the blood of one of the infants. It could be argued that elliptocytes are not a fair test, for by the very nature of their shape, these cells may not be truly representative regarding their ability to cross the placental barrier. It would be preferable to use cells which have a normal appearance in vivo. The choice, therefore, falls on red cells with the sickling trait for these cells are normal in shape in vivo but can be made to sickle in vitro under conditions of low oxygen tension. Mengert et al. (1955) infused cells from a compatible donor with the sickling trait into two pregnant women at term 21—22 hours before they were delivered by caesarian section. Foetal blood was obtained from the cord while the placenta was still intact, and treated in the appropriate manner to produce sickling. Sickle cells were demonstrable in the blood of both infants.

Further evidence was presented by Macris et al. (1958) who found sickle cells in the umbilical cord blood of the newborn infant in three out of 25 cases where the mother was transfused with whole blood from donors with sickle-cell trait. In one of these cases, the mother herself had sickle-cell trait which obviated the need for artificial transfusion. No sickle cell, however, could be demonstrated in this infant's blood. Although this is only one case, it does raise the nagging suspicion that artificially introduced donor cells might not truly reflect the normal in vivo situation. In a recent study employing examination of 44 placentae from women with the sickle-cell trait, it was found that there was a 100% concurrent incidence of sickling in maternal and foetal blood (Fujikura and Klionsky 1975). The transplacental passage of maternal erythrocytes was inferred because foetal erythrocytes with the sickling trait would not usually sickle because of their high content of haemoglobulin F.

On balance, the evidence would seem to indicate that maternal erythrocytes can frequently cross the placenta into the foetal circulation throughout normal pregnancy, and even relatively large amounts may do so. As with the transmission of red cells in the other direction, the exact mechanism is not known. The surface of the syncytiotrophoblast has absorptive characteristics and it is possible that active pinocytosis could be an initiating transport mechanism. However, in order to survive intact, these red cells have to be protected from the trophoblast's intracellular enzymes but there is no evidence to indicate that transport vacuoles the size of erythrocytes exist in trophoblast cells. A passive mechanism seems more likely with the leakage of blood through breaks occurring in the placental barrier. The amount of blood transmitted will be proportional to the size of the breaks in the barrier and the direction of flow will be dependent on the prevailing pressure differential between the foetal and maternal circulations. It seems that this favours the transmission of cells from the foetus to the mother rather than from the mother to the foetus for Cohen and Zuelzer (1964) found that in 82 pregnant women studied immediately after birth, maternal red cells were demonstrable in foetal blood in only three (3.6%) cases while, at the same time, foetal red cells were found in maternal blood in 34 (41.5%) cases.

6.3 Transfer of leucocytes from foetus to mother

Since there is strong evidence for the transplacental passage of erythrocytes in both directions during pregnancy, it may be supposed that leucocytes are similarly transferred. This, of course, has important immunological implications in view of their surface HL-A antigens and the effector properties of these cells. Desai et al. (1966) studied the foeto-maternal passage of fluorescent-labelled blood following intra-uterine foetal transfusion for erythroblastosis. In 11 instances when this was done, a small number of fluorescent leucocytes and platelets were detected in the maternal blood in all except two cases. The peak number of these presumptive foetal cells were seen in maternal blood 2 hours after the intra-uterine transfusion and cells were no longer demonstrable after 4 hours. This study, therefore, showed that cells administered to the foetal peritoneal cavity could cross the placental barrier into the maternal circulation, but as all the cases were those with erythroblastosis where gross placental pathology was present, it cannot be concluded that similar cell transmission can take place across a normal placenta.

All subsequent studies are based mainly on the identification of male cells in the blood of pregnant women who delivered male infants. The presence of male cells can be evaluated either by stimulating maternal lymphocytes by PHA and analysing the metaphase spreads for those with 46 XY constitutions or by fluorescent staining of the Y chromosomes.

6.3.1 Analysis of metaphase for Y chromosome

Walkanowska et al. (1969) were the first to apply this technique to study the peripheral blood of 30 pregnant women ranging from 14—37 weeks gestation. In 21 cultures, 1—3 XY cells were found. Nineteen of these women subsequently gave birth to boys but two gave birth to girls. Similar studies were reported by Schindler et al. (1972). They examined 16 pregnant women ranging from 12—17 weeks which were therefore relatively early in gestation. Of nine women who subsequently gave birth to boys, four had one male cell after analysis of about 600 metaphases. Of seven women who gave birth to girls, five had 1—3 male cells. The series of Whang-Peng et al. (1973) consisted of 64 pregnant women ranging from 8—39 weeks gestation. Of 34 women who subsequently delivered male infants, 12 had 1—3 male cells in 200 metaphases analysed while two out of 30 women who delivered female infants also had 1 male cell in each of their blood cultures.

Several points emerge from these studies. It is apparent that the frequency with which male cells can be detected in the maternal circulation after birth of a male infant is extremely variable. This may be due to technical reasons or it may be a reflection of the stage of gestation when maternal blood is studied. Walkanowska's patients were mainly at the later stages of pregnancy, while those studied by Schindler were relatively early. However, this explanation seems to be discounted by the data of Whang-Peng who showed a high frequency of detectable male cells during the first trimester. All the metaphase studies were based on PHA cultures for 2—3 days. It is not known how well a few foetal lymphocytes in contact with maternal cells can survive under these conditions. Furthermore, PHA only stimulates a sub-population of lymphocytes which may not be represented by those foetal cells which have crossed into the maternal circulation. All these factors, therefore, may reduce the chance of detecting foetal cells with the present experimental procedures.

Perhaps the most worrying feature of the above studies is the occurrence of varying numbers of male cells in women who subsequently delivered female infants. These 'false positives' raise the question whether the apparent XY cells detected in maternal circulation are really male cells of foetal origin. Especially as only a very small number of these cells are involved, the possibility of chromosome breaks resulting in the formation of a 5th small acrocentric which is not a Y at all should be considered. This has been observed to occur in the blood of non-pregnant women and in women who had never conceived (Jacobs and Smith 1969). An alternative explanation for the occurrence of 'false positive' cases is the persistence of male cells from a previous pregnancy. In one of the cases of Whang-Peng et al. (1973), the mother had a previous male pregnancy three years ago while one of Schindler et al.'s (1972) patients had an abortion seven years previously. Such a long survival of foetal lymphocytes would imply the formation of a foetal lymphocyte clone in the mother. In a previous chapter, we have surveyed the evidence in support of the presence of maternal tolerance towards foetal antigens and it is possible that this tolerance may be sufficient at times to allow foetal cells to establish themselves in the mother. Foetal erythrocytes in those pregnancies in which mother and child have an exceptional degree of blood group compatibility have been observed to persist and colonise the mother for prolonged periods (Cohen et al. 1964). Nevertheless, the persistence of foetal leucocytes with their HL-A antigenic determinants is surprising in view of the frequent appearance of cytotoxic maternal antibodies which would be expected to eliminate most, if not all, of these foetal cells. There may be some special protective mechanism which could influence the survival of foetal leucocytes in the maternal circulation like the observation of Tiilikainen et al. (1974) that foetal lymphocytes have a distinct lack of phenotypic expression of paternally derived HL-A antigens.

6.3.2 Fluorescent staining of Y chromosome

Interest in this technique began around 1968 when it was noticed that certain fluorescent derivatives of acridine would stain the chromosomes of various organisms. Furthermore, one of these dyes, quinacrine mustard made part of the human Y chromosome fluoresce particularly brightly (Nature 1970). Since quinacrine mustard is an alkylating fluorochrome, it was thought that the mode of action could be by alkylation of guanine in the G-C rich areas of DNA. The preferential binding to the human Y chromosome may indicate that this chromosome is particularly rich in these areas (George 1970). In cultured lymphocyte preparations, the largest and brightest fluorescence is over the distal half of the long arms of the Y chromosome (Pearson et al. 1970). Of greater potential practical importance is that male cells can be recognised from a study of interphase nuclei by the presence of a small bright fluorescent spot in about 20—50% of cells from a male subject. The physical dimensions of this male chromatin fluorescent body are similar to those of the fluorescent region of the Y chromosome in metaphase. This technique, therefore, offers a great saving in time for it dispenses with the necessity of culturing cells and the laborious preparation and analysis of metaphase spreads. It is analogous to the identification of XX cells by the Barr body. However, it must be pointed out that some investigators reported finding this Y fluorescent body in lymphocytes from as many as 5% of normal women (Polani and Mutton 1971). Thus, the presence of a small number of these fluorescent cells in the maternal circulation must be interpreted with caution, for they may not be necessarily of foetal origin.

Using this technique, Zimmerman and Schmickel (1971) determined the number of fluorescing Y-bodies in 500—1,000 unstimulated lymphocytes from 32 primiparae. The number of detectable Y-bodies varied from 4.2% to nil with a mean of 1.08% ± 1.2. Unfortunately, the presence of Y-bodies was not related to the sex of the subsequently delivered child, which led the authors to conclude that the presence of male cells could not be determined with sufficient accuracy with this technique.

Schröder and De la Chapelle (1972) performed similar analyses and found Y-bodies in lymphocytes from seven out of nine women who eventually delivered a male infant but similar Y-bodies were also detected in four women who delivered female infants. Of these 'false positive' cases, two women were primigravidae, and one had a previous girl baby so they could not be harbouring male cells from a previous pregnancy. Retrospective studies of the metaphase chromosomes of these four women showed unusually bright fluorescent spots on various autosomes after quinacrine staining. Thus, it would seem that non-specific autosomal fluorescence in some women may result in misinterpretation when interphase nuclei alone are analysed for the Y-body. In a subsequent study, Schröder et al. (1974) discarded all those cases where maternal metaphase smears showed autosomal fluorescence, and only analysed interphase nuclei for Y-bodies in those that did not. They found 34 fluorescent Y-bodies in 240,000 cells analysed from 24 randomly selected primigravidae within 24 hours of delivery. Only one of these Y-bodies was found in the blood of a woman who subsequently delivered a female infant so it appears that the incidence of 'false positives' can be reduced, once the interference from autosomal fluorescence is eliminated. Of those mothers who delivered male infants, 74% had at least one demonstrable Y-body in their blood. These Y-bodies were found in both lymphocytes and granulocytes, indicating that both these foetal cell types can cross into the maternal circulation. This finding has not been established in previous experiments employing PHA stimulation because granulocytes do not enter into mitosis when stimulated by this mitogen. Although the discarding of cases with interfering non-specific autosomal fluorescence had reduced the number of 'false positives' down to insignificant levels, 26% of mothers who delivered male infants still had no demonstrable cells with Y-bodies. Thus, the number of 'false negatives' (i.e. male infants which were not predicted) remained sufficiently high as to preclude the use of this method as a means of antenatal foetal sex determination.

Additional data are available from Grosset et al. (1974) who studied the presence of Y-bodies in PHA-stimulated leucocytes from 86 pregnant women of 14—18 weeks gestation. Their findings are summarised in Table 6.6. It can be seen that the number of correct predictions is notably high but again there is a substantial group of 'false positives'. The transmission of foetal lymphocytes early in gestation is confirmed by Zilliacus et al. (1975) who demonstrated these foetal cells in the maternal blood as early as the 15th week of gestation. The number of foetal cells seems to remain unchanged throughout pregnancy which indicates either a steady turnover of transmission or absence of elimination by the mother. Completely negative findings were reported by Adinolfi (1975) who, in a study of eight women at mid-

Table 6.6 Frequency of correct foetal sex prediction using Y-body analysis of maternal leucocytes.

Sex of infant at birth	No.	Predicted sex: Male (Y-body demonstrated)	Female (Y-body not demonstrated)
Male	45	42	3
Female	41	9	32

With kind permission from Grosset, L. et al. (1974) *Amer. J. Obstet. Gynecol.* 120, 60–63.

gestation and eight at delivery who had male infants, did not find a single cell with fluorescent Y-body among 11,684 cells analysed from maternal blood.

From the preceding review, it is clear that the unequivocal demonstration of foetal leucocytes in maternal blood remains unconvincing with the techniques available at present. This is not really surprising, since only a very small number of foetal leucocytes would be expected to be present. Assuming that a few millilitres of blood are transferred from the foetus to the mother, the dilution factor alone would make the task of detecting foetal leucocytes in maternal blood an extremely difficult one, unless there is a selective process of transfer. Schröder and De la Chapelle (1972) did suggest that foetal lymphocytes might indeed gain access to the maternal circulation by active movements across the placenta, for the number of these lymphocytes detected (0.1—2%) exceeded the number of foetal erythrocytes to such an extent that it was difficult to explain by a passive mechanism of transplacental leakage. The number of foetal leucocytes in the peripheral maternal circulation may be further depleted by the sequestration of some of these cells in maternal organs like the spleen, liver, or lungs. Finally, the population of foetal lymphocytes represented in maternal blood may not be responsive to PHA stimulation and, therefore, will be undetectable by those techniques dependent on stimulation by this mitogen. Schröder (1975) demonstrated that all the cells with fluorescent Y-body detected in maternal blood after delivery, could be removed by passage through a nylon wool column, indicating that these foetal cells behave like B-lymphocytes. These cells, therfore, will not respond to PHA which is mainly a T-cell mitogen. All these factors can combine to interfere with the demonstration of foetal leucocytes in maternal blood and the inconclusive data available at present must not be taken to mean that foetal leucocytes do not cross the placenta.

6.4 Transfer of leucocytes from mother to foetus

In a similar kind of infusion experiment as they used for the study of foeto-maternal transmission of leucocytes, Desai and Creger (1963) reversed the procedure by returning maternal blood treated with a fluorescent label in vitro to the maternal circulation within 15 hours of

Table 6.7 Summary of the results from different groups of investigators concerning the detection of maternal leucocytes in the foetal circulation.

Source	No. of newborns tested	No. of cases where 46 XX cells detected	No. of 46 XX cells present	No. of cells analysed
Turner et al. (1966)	183	2	14	5,490
Angell and Adinolfi (1969) [Cited by Adinolfi (1975)]	18	0	0	6,482
Anderson and Ferguson-Smith (1971)	5	0	0	534
Kay and Margoles (1971)	33	0	0	895
Olding (1972)	14	0	0	1,772
Adinolfi and Gorvette (1973) [Cited by Adinolfi (1975)]	16	1	4	1,600
Schröder (1974)	10	1	4	5,853
Total	279	4	22	22,626

delivery. Out of nine patients, they found fluorescent cells in the cord blood of six cases. Labelled platelets, granulocytes, and lymphocytes were detected, indicating that all these different maternal cell types can cross to the foetus. As a control against free fluorochrome traversing the placenta to stain foetal cells, maternal plasma containing the fluorochrome was injected back into the maternal circulation of three pregnant women before delivery. No labelled cells were detected in cord blood in these cases.

The majority of studies employed the technique of sex determination of the leucocytes in foetal blood. The detection of 46 XX cells in cord blood of male infants is used as evidence for the presence of maternal leucocytes. The results obtained by various groups of investigators are summarised in Table 6.7. It can be seen from this Table that maternal leucocytes are not easily detectable in foetal blood. As in the case of erythrocytes, the pressure gradient between the foetal and maternal circulations probably favours the passage of cells from the foetus to the mother rather than in the reverse direction. The small number of maternal cells that do manage to gain access to the foetal circulation are probably quickly destroyed by the rapidly maturing foetal immunological response.

6.5 Metastases of malignant cells between mother and foetus

6.5.1 Transmission of malignant cells from mother to foetus

Since erythrocytes and leucocytes are exchanged between mother and foetus, it would be logical to suppose that malignant cells would do the same. Yet, surprisingly, metastases of maternal cancer to her foetus occurs very rarely. In a survey of the world literature spanning a period of 100 years from 1866—1966, Potter and Schoeneman (1970) found only 24 reported cases, excluding leukaemias. This is an extremely small number even after taking into account that the conditions of pregnancy and cancer tend to occur in different age groups and, therefore, do not coincide too often. These 24 cases consisted of metastases of maternal cancer to the placenta. In only eight of these cases, was the foetus unequivocally involved as established by autopsy. Eleven of the infants were alive and well from six months to three years later.

Maternal leukaemia also appears to have a similar disinclination to involve the foetus. Bierman et al. (1956) described a case of a mother with subacute lymphocytic leukaemia before, during, and after delivery, but the infant was unaffected. Diamondopoulos and Hertig (1963) followed up 48 children born to 33 mothers with leukaemia and other allied diseases like lymphosarcoma, reticulum-cell sarcoma, and Hodgkin's disease. Although 12 infants subsequently died, autopsy found no evidence of metastatic deposits, so it is possible that these infants could have died from some indirect causes related to the maternal debilitation. All the other 36 children were alive and well at the time of examination, the oldest of whom was over 18 years of age. In a survey of the literature of over 400 cases of pregnancy associated with leukaemia or allied diseases, these authors found only two cases where materno-foetal transmission had definitely occurred, with a further four possible cases. This was also the view of Vitums and Sites (1968) who believed that transmission of maternal leukaemia to the foetus must be either non-existent or extremely infrequent.

Why is the foetus so resistant to invasion by maternal cancer? This lack of foetal involvement may be a manifestation of successful rejection of maternal tumour cells by the foetus. This interpretation is supported by the two cases reported by Aronsson (1963) and by Cavell (1963), where conspicuous tumour deposits of maternal melanoma in the infants spontaneously regressed and both children remained well at 16 months and two years respectively. This rejection of allogeneic maternal tumour cells by the foetus is further confirmatory evidence for the early maturation of immunocompetence in man. When maternal cancer and pregnancy coincide, the fate of the foetus may well be dependent on the stage of gestation when maternal tumour cells begin to metastasise. When this occurs at the later stages of gestation when the foetus would be expected to have reached full immunocompetence, the tumour cells will be successfully rejected. It may be significant that in both the cases of spontaneous regression just described, the mother only developed clinical signs of metastases around the time of delivery.

Another factor which may be protective to the foetus against invasion by maternal tumour cells is the placental barrier. When detailed histological studies are made, many investigators have observed a peculiar distribution of tumour deposits within the placenta (Fig. 6.1). Bender (1950) noticed tumour cells only in the maternal blood spaces with no invasion of the chorionic villi. Horner (1960) similarly did not find any villus invasion, in spite of large masses of tumour cells occupying the intervillous spaces. Freedman and McMahon (1960), after a diligent microscopic examination of 300 sections taken from 20 blocks of

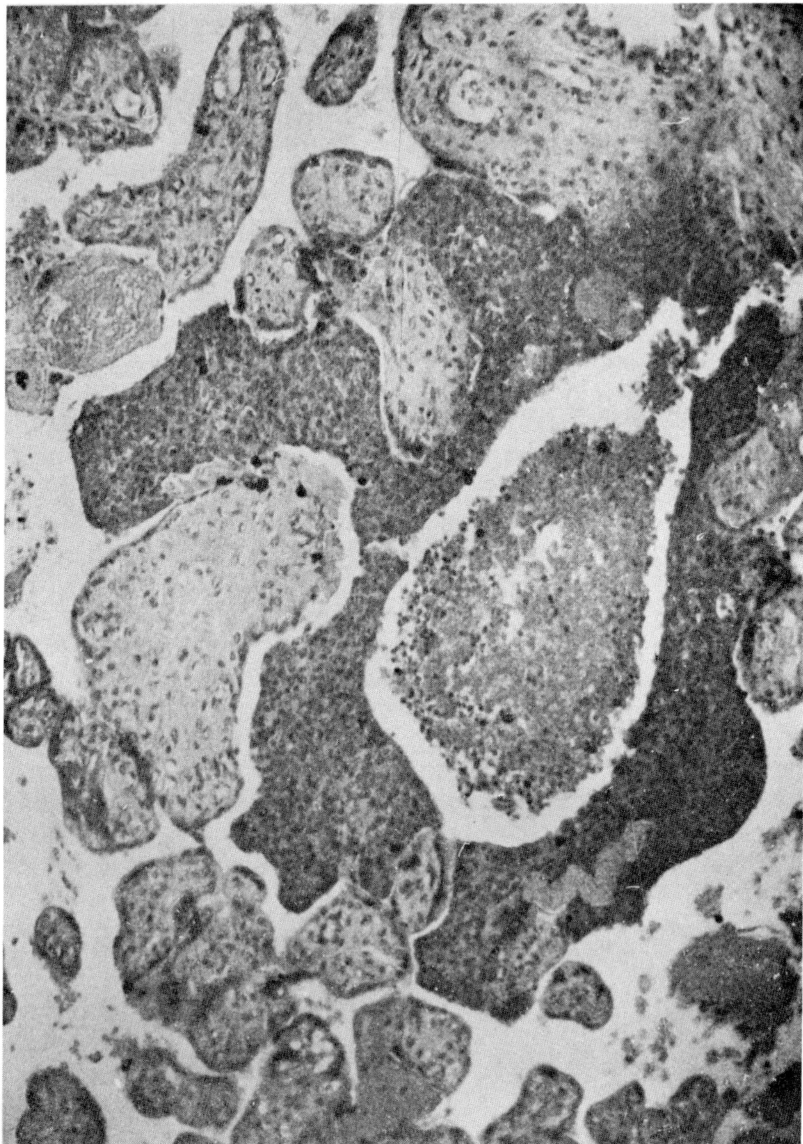

Fig. 6.1 Section of placenta showing tumour masses in intervillous spaces but no invasion of chorionic villi. With kind permission from Potter, J. F. and Schoeneman, M. (1970) *Cancer* 25, 380—388.

placental tissue from a woman who died of metastatic melanoma, also found no evidence of villus invasion.

Leukaemia cells metastasising to the placenta are distributed in a similar manner (Diamondopoulos and Hertig 1963). In the case described by Bierman et al. (1956), leukaemic cells were found in great abundance in the myometrium and also in the maternal portion of the placenta, but none were seen in the foetal portion of the placenta, the cord, or foetal capillaries.

From these histological studies, it would appear that maternal tumour cells, even if they succeed in metastasising to the placenta, are actually prevented from invading further into the foetal side by the trophoblast layer of the chorionic villi. This implies that trophoblast cells may be immunologically competent, a hypothesis which is, to some extent, supported by the experiments of Dancis et al. (1966). They found that injection of suspensions of allogeneic placental cells into irradiated 3 month-old mice resulted in an increased mortality rate. That this did not occur after injection with isogeneic or F_1 placental suspensions indicated that the effect was due to allogeneic differences between injected placental cells and recipient, a situation which is analogous to the graft-versus-host reaction produced by injecting allogeneic immunocompetent lymphocytes into immunologically immature hosts. Guinea pig, rat, and mouse trophoblast cells have been observed to engulf fragments of foetal erythrocytes (Schwartz, J. et al. 1974), and human trophoblast cells in culture have many of the properties required for intracellular digestion of pinocytosed material (Contractor and Krakauer 1976a, b). The intriguing concept that human trophoblast can protect the foetus by actively destroying maternal cells certainly warrants further investigation.

Another interesting feature apparent from the literature survey by Potter and Schoeneman (1970) is the predilection of malignant melanoma to metastasise to the foetus and placenta. Eleven of the 24 reported cases (46%) were melanomas. This is particularly striking in those cases with foetal involvement where seven out of eight cases (88%) were melanomas. According to Potter and Schoeneman (1970), the most frequently encountered malignancies during pregnancy are carcinoma of the breast and carcinoma of the cervix, each comprising 26% of the total. Only 8% of malignancies are melanomas, so there seems to be a definite discrepancy between the distribution of the types of cancer which coexist with pregnancy and those which affect the placenta and foetus. The reason for this selectivity is not clear, for there is no evidence that the malignant potential of malignant melanoma is increased any more than other tumours during pregnancy (George et al. 1960; White et al. 1961). There remains the possibility that the frequent coincidental occurrence of malignant melanoma in both mother and infant is not due to the exchange of tumour cells at all but to the ease in transmission of some inducing agent from mother to foetus. An initial attempt to clarify this issue by studying the sex chromatin of melanoma cells in a male infant was unfortunately unsuccessful (Brodsky et al. 1965).

6.5.2 *Transmission of malignant cells from foetus to mother*

The converse situation, that of metastases of foetal cancer to the mother appears to be equally infrequent. Birner (1961) described a mature stillborn foetus invaded by multiple foci of neuroblastoma but the mother was unaffected. In the two cases of neuroblastoma reported by Strauss and Driscoll (1964), the tumours had metastasised widely, leading to the death of the infants. Tumour cells were found in the foetal vessels of the placenta and yet the mesenchyme of the chorionic villi was not invaded. Both mothers remained well and unaffected by the tumour. Foetal melanoma appears to be similarly confined to the foetal aspect of the placenta (Sweet and Connerty 1941).

It would appear that the placental barrier is equally as effective in preventing the passage of tumour cells from foetus to mother as in the reverse direction. An additional defence is the mother's fully developed immune system which would be expected to deal with any allogeneic foetal tumour cells which may have succeeded in breaching the placental barrier.

There is, however, one notable exception and this is choriocarcinoma. This tumour is derived from trophoblast and is therefore also of foetal origin. Unlike other foetal tumours, choriocarcinoma is highly invasive in the mother. The immunology of these tumours will be discussed more fully in a later chapter. Meanwhile, in relation to the placental barrier, it is clear that, on anatomical grounds, this barrier cannot be as effective with choriocarcinoma as it is for other types of foetal tumours. The two layers of trophoblast cells line the outside of the chorionic villi in direct contact with maternal blood spaces. Any tissue that breaks off will be swept into the maternal circulation with ease, a postulate which is borne out by the frequent demonstration of trophoblast cells in the mother during normal pregnancy.

In contrast, deportation of trophoblast backwards into the foetal circulation has only been reported by one group of investigators (Salvaggio et al. 1960). They demonstrated large multinucleated cells in 32 out of 53 samples of cord blood and also in histological sections of heart and liver from autopsy material of newborn infants who died immediately after delivery. These cells were classified as syncytiotrophoblast on morphological grounds alone, so there is the possibility that other big cells in the blood like megakaryocytes might have been mistakenly identified. Even if these were trophoblast in the foetal circulation, it is by no means certain that they have traversed the placenta during pregnancy rather than after its separation at delivery. In accord with the findings concerning normal trophoblast, invasion by choriocarcinoma backwards into the foetus is also extremely rare in those cases where there is a viable foetus associated with the tumour. There are only about three reported cases in the world's literature (Buckell and Owen 1954; Mercer et al. 1958; Daamen et al. 1968). In a detailed study of two cases of early choriocarcinoma, Brewer and Gerbie (1966) made the observation that, in the infrequent event of the malignant trophoblast tissue succeeding in invading below the basement membrane of the chorionic villi, it consistently failed to penetrate the foetal capillaries in spite of the fact that tumour tissue could lie in direct contact with the endothelium of the foetal capillaries. This is a remarkable finding in view of the ease with which choriocarcinoma can destroy and invade maternal blood vessels. It would appear, therefore, that trophoblast basement membrane as well as foetal capillary endothelium may both contribute towards the barrier effect of the human placenta.

7

Consequence of transplacental passage of cells

7.1 Effects of transfer of leucocytes from foetus to mother

Pregnant women, who have never been transfused, frequently possess detectable leucocyte iso-antibodies (Van Rood et al. 1958). These maternal antibodies will agglutinate leucocytes from the respective newborn infants and also leucocytes from the husbands suggesting that maternal sensitisation is towards paternally derived foetal leucocyte antigens (Payne and Rolfs 1958). The antibodies may be leucoagglutinins or cytotoxic antibodies and mostly belong to the IgG class (Overweg and Engelfriet 1969). Incomplete antibodies, demonstrable by Coombs' consumption test, have also been described (Jensen 1962). From these original observations, pregnancy sera have now become a convenient source of HL-A antibodies (Kissmeyer-Nielsen and Thorsby 1970). A further merit of these pregnancy derived antibodies is that they tend to have a limited specificity, since they are stimulated only by those foetal antigens inherited from the paternal haplotype. Even monospecific HL-A antibodies have been observed in pregnancy sera (Stastny 1972) and it seems that these appear just as frequently in multiparous as in primiparous women (Tongio et al. 1972).

The frequency of these antibodies vary from about 12% in a sample of 1,500 maternal sera tested for cytotoxic antibodies (Tongio et al. 1971) to about 25% in 1,584 samples tested for leucoagglutinins (Zmijewski et al. 1967). It is likely that this difference is a reflection on the sensitivity of the two methods. Carbonara et al. (1974) tested sera from post partum women for leucocyte antibodies by two methods. When tested by complement lysis of paternal lymphocytes at 20°C, they found 15.3% of maternal sera had cytotoxic antibodies. This percentage rose to 41.0% when detection was by antibody-dependent cell-mediated lysis using cells from healthy human donors as effector cells. All the sera found positive by the complement lysis method were also positive by the antibody-dependent cell-mediated lysis, the antibody titre being about two-fold greater in the latter. The greater sensitivity of antibody-dependent cell-mediated lysis is probably due to the fact that this form of cell lysis needs a smaller number of antibody molecules per cell than in complement-mediated lysis. Besides the variation in sensitivity of antibody detection methods, it must also be remembered that results can be further influenced by the leucocyte panel used as target cells. The more antigenic specificities present in the test panel, the more antibodies are likely to be revealed (Ahrons 1971b).

The frequency of multispecific leucocyte antibodies in maternal sera appears to increase with parity. In the study of Zmijewski et al. (1967), leuco-agglutinins were detected in 15.4% of primiparous sera, 24.66% in para II, 26.88% in para III, and 33.15% in para IV and over. Burke and Johansen (1974) found a similar trend for lymphocytotoxic anti-HL-A antibodies in 1,201 maternal sera examined, being present in 10% of primiparous sera, 17% in secundiparous sera, and 22% in the sera of mothers with three or more pregnancies.

In primiparous women, leucocyte antibodies are usually demonstrable by about the 24th week of gestation (Ahrons 1971b) with one report that they may be present as early as 6½ weeks (Van der Werf 1971). These antibodies appear somewhat earlier in multiparous women, around the second month of gestation (Vives et al. 1976). This may be a reflection of previous exposure.

Recently, cytotoxic antibodies directed at an antigenic system apparently distinct from HL-A have been reported in pregnancy sera (Ferrone et al. 1976). These investigators tested 100 sera from pregnant women, chosen for their lack of cytotoxic HL-A antibodies, assayed by the usual methods, and found that 46 sera reacted with a panel of 17 cell lines of cultured B-lymphocytes in the presence of complement. These antibodies were identified to 10 specificities. They were not cytotoxic to human T-cell lines nor to a variety of tumour cell lines tested. The authors, therefore, speculated about the possibility that these antibodies were directed at antigens which were the human B-cell counterparts of murine Ia.

'Cold' auto-antibodies against patients' own lymphocytes have also been observed to occur frequently in pregnancy sera (Naito et al. 1971). Similar auto-lymphocytotoxins have been found in association with many diseases where the patient is subjected to stimulation by diverse antigenic stimuli. It is not known what the biological role of these auto-antibodies are. They may be merely by-products of constant antigen-antibody interactions. On the other hand, they could be regulators of the immune response by acting as 'natural' anti-lymphocyte antibodies.

From the above review, it can be seen that foetal leucocytes can frequently sensitise the mother, about a third of all pregnancy sera being found to contain anti-HL-A antibodies. It is possible that with the use of more sensitive techniques for detection, it will eventually be found that maternal response to foetal leucocyte stimulation is an even more generalised phenomenon. Although the antigenic source for this sensitisation is generally attributed to the transplacental passage of foetal leucocytes, one should bear in mind that other cell types like trophoblast may also contribute. HL-A antigens in soluble form have been detected in plasma, so consideration must be given to the possibility that soluble foetal HL-A antigens could diffuse across the placenta in the same way as blood group substances. Sensitisation by spermatozoal HL-A antigens seems unlikely since nulliparous women with sexual activity usually have no detectable anti-leucocyte antibodies in their blood.

7.2 Effects of transfer of erythrocytes from foetus to mother

7.2.1 Anaemia in the foetus

If large amounts of foetal blood escape into the maternal circulation, this may be an important cause of neonatal anaemia. As high as 5—10% of the red cells in maternal blood has been estimated to be of foetal origin (Chown 1954; Goodall et al. 1958), so in these cases, the foeto-maternal transfusion must be considerable. Woodrow and Donohoe (1968) have also reported a foetal cell score in maternal blood at delivery of over 1,000 which is equivalent to about 170 ml of foetal blood. Such large amounts would probably have to be lost over a long period of time, otherwise the foetus would die in utero.

7.2.2 ABO sensitisation

In the large majority of cases, the amount of erythrocytes transmitted from foetus to mother is small, in the region of about 1 ml or so. The importance of these foetal erythrocytes is in their capacity of acting as antigenic source for maternal iso-immunisation. Maternal sensitisation to foetal ABO antigens has long been recognised. Edgecombe (1930) observed a rise in the titre of maternal iso-agglutinins during the later stages of pregnancy, this rise being most conspicuous in those cases where the baby belonged to a different blood group from the mother. Jonsson (1936), in a systematic study for haemolysins found that 14.5% of sera from 594 group 'O' mothers taken three weeks after delivery haemolysed either group 'A' or 'B' erythrocytes or both. In contrast, similar iso-haemolysins were demonstrable in only 3.5% of 636 group 'O' male controls. This relationship between the presence of iso-haemolysin and heterospecific pregnancy was even more striking when the infant's blood group was taken into account. In those mothers with group 'O' children, the incidence of iso-haemolysins was found to be 7.1%, while the incidence rose to 20.8% for those with group 'B' children and 28.1% for those with group 'A' children. Boorman et al. (1945) also found a considerable increase in anti-A and anti-B iso-agglutinins after the birth of an incompatible ABO infant, the peak antibody titre being reached 10—20 days after delivery. Only eight of 44 cases of heterospecific pregnancy failed to show this rise in iso-agglutinin titre. Similar results were obtained by Smith (1945) who found that in 46 heterospecific pregnancies, 40 had raised titres of anti-A and anti-B iso-agglutinins, while in 154 homospecific pregnancies, only one had raised antibody titre.

It is clear from these observations that a foetus which is ABO incompatible to the mother can stimulate the mother to produce the relevant antibodies. While some investigators have reported a rise in antibody titre occurring during pregnancy (Edgecombe 1930; Smith 1945), others are of the opinion that this only becomes detectable 2—3 weeks after delivery (Boorman et al. 1945; Zuelzer and Kaplan 1954a).

Although the most likely antigenic source for maternal sensitisation is the transplacental passage of foetal erythrocytes, it must be pointed out that, unlike the Rh antigens which are present exclusively on erythrocytes, ABO antigens are found on other tissues. There is still controversy as to whether trophoblast cells express ABO antigens, but if they do, then the widespread deportation of trophoblast tissue during pregnancy should be considered as an important source of these antigens. Furthermore, it is possible that soluble group-specific substances from the foetus have diffused across the placenta to sensitise the mother rather than foetal erythrocytes. Thus, the data of Smith

(1945) showed that, of the 40 mothers who had raised iso-agglutinin titres, all had foetuses who were secretors, while the six mothers who did not have raised titres all had non-secretor foetuses. Similarly Zuelzer and Kaplan (1954ä) found that in each of the mothers who showed a rise in antibody titre, the infant was a secretor. Freda (1958) demonstrated that soluble A, B, and H substances of secretors were readily transported across the placenta and other foetal membranes, in spite of their relatively large molecular size which ranged from 260,000—800,000. Maternal sensitisation to these soluble blood group substances produced by a secretor foetus would provide a logical explanation for the observed excess of secretors in infants affected with ABO haemolytic disease (Wiener et al. 1960).

7.2.3 Rh sensitisation

Although there is a large number of erythrocytic iso-antigens in man, they vary in their immunogenicity and, fortunately, most of them do not evoke a clinically significant level of iso-immunisation. The most important one is the Rhesus (Rh) antigen, so called because of its initial discovery in the Rhesus monkey. This antigen is really a group of antigens C, D, E, of which the strongest one D is responsible for most of the cases of haemolytic disease of the newborn in Rh incompatible pregnancies.

We have seen in the preceding chapter that there is a great variation in the estimations of the quantity of foetal blood present in the maternal circulation. There is a tendency for more foetal blood to be detected after delivery than in the antenatal period. A figure of 0.5 ml of foetal blood in the maternal circulation after delivery with a slightly smaller amount during the antenatal period would probably be a representative average. Is this amount enough to sensitise the mother to the Rh antigen? Surprisingly, few attempts have been made to determine the minimum amount of red cells needed to induce primary Rh immunisation. Zipursky et al. (1963) managed to immunise Rh negative volunteers with repeated injections of 0.1 ml of Rh positive blood. Even smaller amounts have been used by Jakobowicz et al. (1972) who reported the results of injecting 0.01 ml of red cells every two weeks into eight subjects. Anti-Rh antibodies were detected in two subjects after only three injections (i.e. a total of 0.03 ml of red cells). However, both these subjects were women who had pregnancies several years previously, so they could already have been primed to Rh antigens. The only male subject in the series who developed anti-Rh antibodies did so after his 6th injection which was about three months after the start of the series of injections. Since it usually takes a month or two for the appearance of demonstrable antibodies, it is possible that the dose needed to initiate primary sensitisation could be less than the total of 0.06 ml injected.

Taking into account that some individuals respond more readily than others to the Rh antigen, it seems that about 1 ml of Rh positive blood should be enough to sensitise all those who are capable of responding (Mollison 1973). Transplacental haemorrhage of this order is certainly achieved in many pregnancies. It must also be remembered that the estimation of foetal cells in maternal blood is measured at one point in time which does not take into account any previous or subsequent haemorrhagic episodes. There is, therefore, no reason to doubt that the amount of foeto-maternal transfer of red cells in many normal pregnancies is sufficient to act as Rh sensitising stimulus to the

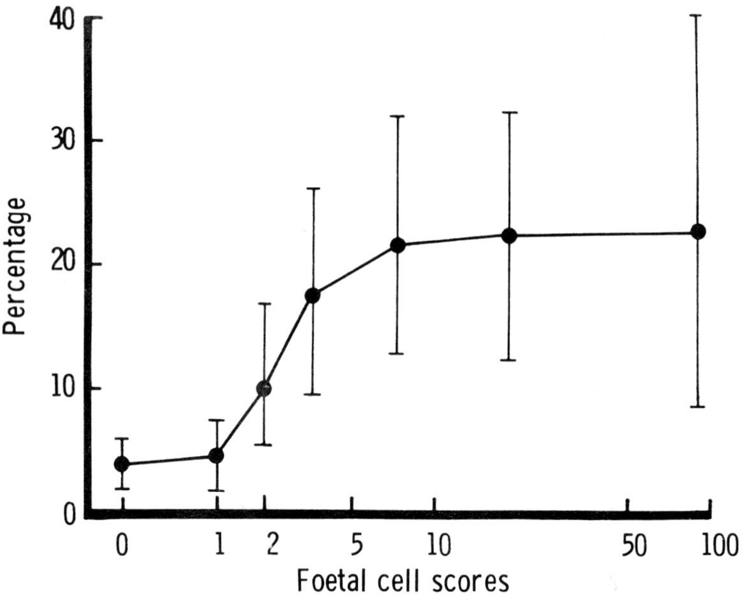

Fig. 7.1 Relation between the foetal cell score in maternal blood after delivery of an ABO-compatible Rh-positive baby and the percentage of mothers who developed anti-D during the subsequent six months. The 90% confidence limits on the percentages are given. With kind permission from Woodrow, J. C. and Donohoe, W. T. A. (1968) *Brit. med. J.* 4, 139—144.

mother. Since transplacental haemorrhage can occur as early as the first trimester of pregnancy (Zipursky et al. 1963), it may be that in a small proportion of women primary sensitisation is already well established by the time of their first delivery.

There is a relationship between the number of foetal cells found in the maternal circulation at the time of delivery and the incidence of serologically detectable anti-Rh antibody in her plasma six months later (Woodrow and Donohoe 1968). This can be seen in Fig. 7.1, where there is a close relationship up to a foetal cell score of around 10 which is estimated to be equivalent to about 0.4 ml of foetal blood. It is remarkable how low the foetal cell score is in women who subsequently developed anti-Rh antibody. An equivalent of 0.1 ml of foetal blood appears to be sufficient. This is in support of the conclusion from experimental findings that an amount of less than 1 ml of Rh-positive foetal blood should be sufficient antigenic stimulus for maternal sensitisation.

7.2.4 Interaction between ABO and Rh antigens

Since nearly all individuals possess 'natural' anti-A and anti-B isohaemagglutinins, it would be expected that foetal erythrocytes which are ABO incompatible to the mother will have a shorter survival time and be, therefore, less frequently detectable in maternal blood than compatible red cells. This is confirmed by several investigations as shown in Table 7.1. It can be seen that all the data reveal a definite decrease in the frequency with which ABO incompatible foetal cells are detected in the maternal circulation when compared to ABO compatible cells. There is no reason to suppose that the actual incidence of transplacental transmission is different in the two groups, so the most likely explanation is that ABO incompatible red cells are rapidly removed from the maternal circulation.

It is logical to assume that the longer foetal red cells survive in the mother, the more chance they will have to induce sensitisation. An extension of this concept will be that the incidence of Rh sensitisation should be lower with Rh positive foetuses who are also ABO incompatible to the mother than with those who are ABO compatible. That this, in fact, does occur has been observed over 30 years ago by Levine (1943) who pointed out that there was a statistically higher frequency of Rh negative women with Rh antibodies in a series of homospecific pregnancies as compared with heterospecific pregnancies. In

Table 7.1 Summary of the results from different groups of investigators comparing the frequency with which ABO-compatible and ABO-incompatible foetal erythrocytes are detected in maternal blood.

Source	No. of cases examined	ABO compatibility between foetus and mother	No. of cases positive for foetal erythrocytes in maternal blood
Fraser and Raper (1962)	535 100	Compatible Incompatible	161 (31%) 16 (16%)
Sullivan and Jennings (1966)	277 49	Compatible Incompatible	106 (38.2%) 5 (10.2%)
Woodrow and Donohoe (1968)	2000 417	Compatible Incompatible	1120 (56%) 103 (24.7%)
Joint European Study [Cited by Tovey and Maroni (1976)]	5678 1048	Compatible Incompatible	(28.6%) (15.4%)

other words, in matings which were ABO incompatible, there was a considerably reduced risk for those couples, if also Rh incompatible, to have infants affected with erythroblastosis. It was estimated by Woodrow and Donohoe (1968) that anti-D was 8.5 times more likely to appear in the antenatal period after first ABO compatible pregnancies than after ABO incompatible ones. The protection from Rh sensitisation by ABO incompatibility has also been confirmed experimentally by Stern et al. (1956). They found that injection of Rh negative male volunteers with Rh positive blood was approximately six times more likely to result in production of Rh antibodies when the blood was ABO compatible for the recipient than when it was ABO incompatible. Furthermore, ABO incompatible Rh positive cells were also less able to stimulate the secondary response in Rh sensitised individuals (Stern et al. 1961). Thus, this is one example in the human foetal-maternal interaction where genetic incompatibility at one locus can protect against the harmful effects due to incompatibility of genes from a different locus.

The simplest mechanism for this protection would be the rapid elimination of incompatible red cells by maternal natural' iso-haemagglutinins. However, the problem remains as to how these foetal red cells are eliminated without first sensitising the mother. Complement-binding antibodies like the 'natural' anti-A and anti-B iso-agglutinins appear to bring about the destruction of red cells in the liver, and it is thought that sequestration of the cells in this organ rather than the spleen is less likely to be immunogenic (Mollison 1973) because the liver contains less immunocompetent tissue.

An alternative mechanism could be that anti-A or anti-B attached to foetal red cells may interfere with the expression of Rh antigens. This hypothesis, however, is not supported by the results of experiments performed by Stern et al. (1961) in which 'A' Rh positive red cells were first coated with anti-A in vitro and then injected into 'A' Rh negative volunteers. These coated red cells remained efficient stimuli for anti-Rh production.

It is also possible that a mechanism involving some kind of antigenic competition could be involved, in that the simultaneous exposure to ABO and Rh antigens may result in a situation that is not favourable for the development of Rh antibodies. If this were a significant factor, one might expect that Rh negative male volunteers injected with ABO incompatible Rh positive blood would develop high titres of immune anti-A or anti-B at the expense of anti-D, but this was not observed (Stern et al. 1961). These investigators postulated a variation of this hypothesis designated as 'clonal competition for antigen', which was based on the clonal selection theory of antibody formation. The basic concept of this hypothesis presupposes that the presence of large numbers of a clone of antibody-forming cells for one red cell factor may interfere with the antibody response to another factor on the same cell. Thus, in the situation where ABO incompatible Rh positive blood is introduced into Rh negative individuals, the more numerous cells belonging to the clone which produces anti-A or anti-B will take up most of the introduced red cells, leaving little opportunity for them to come into contact with and stimulate the few cells bearing appropriate Rh receptors.

The investigations by Woodrow et al. (1975) using another red cell antigenic system, 'Kell', may be relevant to the present discussion. They gave 62 Rh negative Kell negative male volunteers two successive stimuli of 1 ml of Rh positive Kell positive blood each. To half of this group, they also gave 13—14 μg of IgG anti-Kell immediately after each stimulus. The other half acted as controls. They found that 11 of 31 controls eventually developed anti-D but only one of 31 of those who had anti-K did so. The protection was probably due to rapid elimination of the Rh positive Kell positive red cells by the anti-Kell antibody for it was found by Cr^{51} labelling studies that virtually all the injected cells were cleared from the peripheral circulation within 24 hours. Surface pulsing over various viscera recorded considerable excess activity over the spleen which suggested that sequestration of the cleared red cells was predominantly in this organ; this is in contrast to the clearance of ABO incompatible red cells by 'natural' iso-agglutinins which is in the liver (Mollison 1973). Maybe this is a reflection of a basic difference in immunoglobulin class, with IgM coated cells being filtered off by the scavenging cells of the liver, while IgG coated cells are bound by the Fc-receptors on the surface of splenic macrophages and thereby may be diverted from cells bearing the appropriate Rh antigen receptors.

Woodrow et al. (1975) also found that when D-positive K-positive cells were treated with an excess of anti-K in vitro, they could still be agglutinated by anti-D in the normal way. This lends further support to the conclusion of Stern et al. (1961) that antibody directed at other red cell antigens do not protect against Rh sensitisation by steric hindrance or any kind of interference with the expression of the Rh antigens.

From the available evidence, therefore, it would seem that, although it may not be the sole mechanism, the rapid elimination of ABO incompatible Rh positive foetal red cells by maternal iso-antibodies is certainly an important process leading to the suppression of Rh sensitisation of the mother.

7.2.5 Artificial suppression of Rh sensitisation

If survival of foetal red cells is an important factor in maternal sensitisation, then it should be possible to prevent sensitisation by artificially destroying any Rh positive cells which may have gained access to the maternal circulation. Based on this line of reasoning, a group of investigators from Liverpool devised a method for Rh prophylaxis by administering anti-D to a mother immediately after delivery of a Rh positive child in order to destroy any foetal red cells present in maternal blood before they could induce sensitisation. Initial experiments with male volunteers were promising (Finn et al. 1961b). They injected Rh positive, ABO compatible blood tagged with Cr^{51} into six Rh negative male and gave three of these 10 ml of anti-D intravenously 30 minutes later. In the men not given anti-D, the transfused Rh positive cells survived normally, but in the three men given anti-D, over 50% of the transfused cells had disappeared within

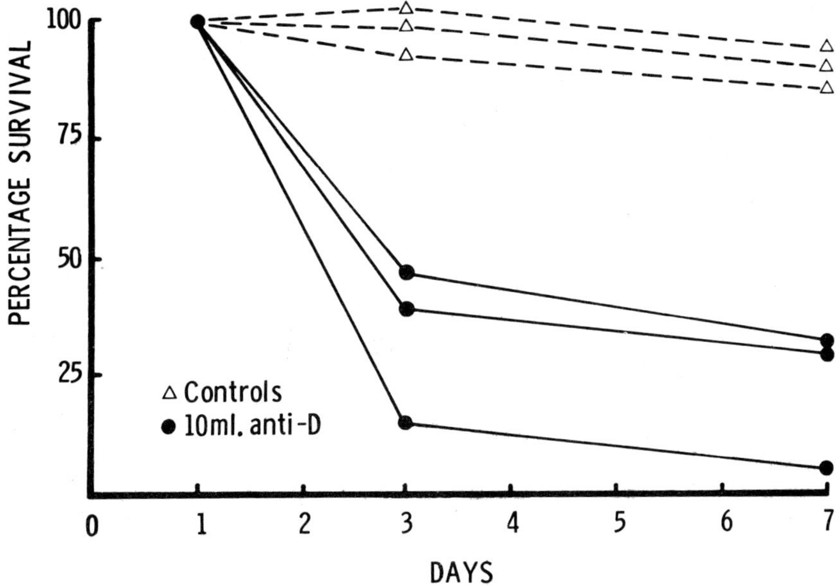

Fig. 7.2 Remaining percentage radio-activity at various times after injection of Rh-positive blood tagged with Cr^{51} into 6 Rh-negative male volunteers. With kind permission from Finn, R. et al. (1961b) *Brit. med. J.* 1, 1486—1490.

two days (Fig. 7.2). A similar procedure was also effective in rapid clearance of transfused Rh positive foetal cells into postmenopausal Rh negative female volunteers (Woodrow et al. 1965).

A clinical trial based on this procedure was launched from various centres in Britain and the United States (Combined Study 1966). In the trial were 156 Rh negative primiparae shown to have foetal erythrocytes in their blood after delivery of a Rh positive child. Half of this group were each given an intramuscular injection of 5 ml of γ-globulin containing high titres of incomplete anti-D, while the other half served as controls. All the women were tested for anti-D production 6 months later. It was found that of the 78 women given anti-D at delivery, none developed Rh-antibodies while 19 in the control group did so. Furthermore, of 18 treated women who subsequently had a second Rh positive ABO compatible baby, none developed anti-D. This lack of a secondary response is of greater significance because it provides a more stringent test for the absence of initial sensitisation than the mere absence of antibody production.

Since these early studies, clinical experience in many countries has confirmed the efficacy of this method of Rh prophylaxis. Freda et al. (1977) have recently reported that after 10 years of use in their clinic, the incidence of sensitisation among Rh negative mothers has fallen from 14% to 1%.

Although extremely successful, the protection is not complete. There is a failure rate of about 1.7% (Medical Research Council Working Party Report 1974). Two major reasons may account for this. One is the difficulty in estimating the dose of anti-D required in individual cases. The most commonly used dose of 200—300 μg of IgG anti-D is probably sufficient to prevent immunisation in the vast majority of women, but there may be a few with very large foeto-maternal haemorrhages when this dose is inadequate. The second reason is that foetal red cells may already have crossed into the maternal circulation early on in gestation so that the administration of anti-D after delivery may very well be too late to prevent sensitisation. In order to protect these cases, consideration has to be given to the possibility of giving anti-D treatment during pregnancy rather than waiting until after delivery. Initial apprehension regarding giving anti-D to pregnant women appears to be unfounded, for doses of the order of 100 μg given to the mother from about the 28th week of gestation onwards will be unlikely to have any effects on the foetus but will be sufficient for the suppression of Rh immunisation (Mollison 1973). Such antenatal therapy of 145 μg of anti-D given to 260 Rh negative women about the 34th week of gestation was observed to have no ill-effects on either the mother or baby (Buchanan et al. 1969).

The mechanism of protection by anti-D (Clarke, C.A. 1971) may be the same as that mediated by 'natural' iso-haemagglutinins in ABO incompatibility. Nevertheless, there is reason to believe that the two mechanisms may not be exactly comparable. Reaction of 'natural' IgM anti-A or anti-B with incompatible red cells leads to immune lysis. The remains of the cells are then sequestered by macrophages in the liver, an organ which is deficient in antibody-producing cells. In contrast, 'incomplete' IgG anti-D merely coats the Rh positive erythrocytes and this appears to lead to sequestration of the coated cells in the spleen, an organ which is known to be a highly favourable site for antibody production. Furthermore, since anti-D is directed at the D antigen itself, it is conceivable that some additional antigen-specific mechanism may come into play. In recent years, there has been a great deal of interest in the physiological role of antibody in the induction and control of the immune response, with extensive studies directed at antibody-mediated immunosuppression. Two major mechanisms are available by which anti-D may interfere with the induction of sensitisation. One is afferent inhibition, where anti-D blocks or masks D antigenic sites and thereby interferes with their expression. The other is a central inhibition, where antibody directly suppresses the proliferation of antibody-synthesising cells in a form of negative feed-back mechanism. Although the immunological principles for the above two mechanisms have been established in animal studies by use of different antigen/antibody systems, there is, as yet, no direct evidence that these mechanisms are relevant to Rh suppression by anti-D. Masking of antigenic sites is not supported by the work of Mollison and Hughes-Jones (1967) who calculated that the removal of 99% of red cells within 24 hours required an amount of anti-D which was sufficient to occupy only about 10% of the antigenic sites. The low level of anti-D needed for suppression is also against the postulate of a negative feed-back mechanism because this form of central inhibition usually demands the presence of excess antibody.

Thus, it seems that the mechanism of action of anti-D may be more complex than it would at first appear. Tovey and Robinson (1975), when analysing those women who failed to be protected by anti-D prophylaxis, observed there was a tendency for their subsequent infants to be clinically less severely affected than would be expected. This suggests that anti-D may have protective effects on subsequent pregnancies, even when it fails to protect against primary sensitisation. It is not clear how this is mediated. The failure of anti-D from a monozygotic twin to suppress Rh immunisation in a co-twin, as observed by Hummel (1972), indicates that a genetic difference between the anti-D of donor and recipient is necessary for suppression to take place. The author postulated that the possible mode of action of homologous but not isologous anti-D was by coating Rh positive cells and giving them a new antigenic 'face' of Gm-Inv or other immunoglobulin allotype specificities. As a result, these coated red cells would come into contact with those clones producing antibody against allogeneic anti-globulin specificities rather than those producing anti-D. This diversion of antigen away from the relevant Rh antigen-sensitive cells is, therefore, analogous to the 'clonal competition' theory proposed by Stern et al. (1961) for the suppression of Rh sensitisation by ABO incompatibility. Thus, perhaps the mechanism of suppression of Rh sensitisation by anti-D and ABO incompatibility may be very similar after all.

7.3 Effects of maternal leucocytes on the foetus

7.3.1 Leucocyte chimerism

There is evidence that, occasionally, maternal leucocytes that have crossed to the foetus may survive for a considerable time. The reports of XX/XY chimerism in newborn male infants who had not been transfused could be examples of this phenomenon (Kadowaki et al. 1965; Taylor and Polani 1965; El-alfi and Hathout 1969; Githens et al. 1969). The conclusion that the XX cells in these infants were of maternal origin was supported by the finding in one case where XX/XY chimerism was found only in cells cultured from peripheral blood leucocytes and not from any other foetal tissues, indicating that the foetus itself was not a mosaic (Kadowaki et al. 1965). In the case described by El-alfi and Hathout (1969), the two populations of XX and XY cells detected in a male infant at 39 weeks of age had reverted to a pure XY karyotype by five months, suggesting that the XX cells detected earlier were probably migrants from the mother. Lymphocyte chimerism has also been detected in a female child by HL-A typing (O'Reilly et al. 1973). The child's father carried HL-A2 and W15 on one chromosome and W14 on the other. Her mother carried HL-A1 and 8 on one chromosome and HL-A3 and W10 on her second chromosome. Lymphocytotoxicity typing of the child showed her to possess HL-A1, 2, 3, 8, W10, and W15. Thus, the child's lymphocyte population carried all four antigens from the mother as well as the antigens from one chromosome of the father. Platelet complement-fixation typing confirmed the same antigens in the parents but the child demonstrated only antigens HL-A2, 3, W10 and W15. The results, therefore, show that, while platelet typing is consistent with the inheritance from one chromosome of each parent, the child's lymphocytes are probably made up of two populations. Those possessing HL-A1, 3, 8 and W10 are of maternal origin, while her own set presumably carry HL-A3 and W10 from her mother and HL-A2 and W15 from her father.

7.3.2 Maternal leucocytes as tolerogens

It has been well established that acquired immunological tolerance to foreign antigens can be evoked experimentally in certain species by the injection of leucocytes into foetal or neonatal animals during a period when the animals have not passed beyond the critical period in their immunological maturation. That the natural exchange of cells between two individuals early on in gestation can also lead to the subsequent development of tolerance has been documented in transplantation studies of twin calves where it has been found that skin grafts exchanged between dizygotic cattle twins which are blood chimeras can survive for long periods and sometimes even indefinitely.

These observations raise the question whether a similar tolerance induction can result from maternal leucocytes reaching the foetus at an appropriate stage during human gestation. Peer (1958) found that maternal skin grafted to her child survived for as long as 15 months while father's skin grafts were rejected within 20 days. This tolerance to maternal skin allografts could last for many years as demonstrated in two cases where mother's skin grafted to her 7- and 12-year-old male children survived for 78 and 253 days respectively. These findings are consistent with the development of acquired tolerance in the foetus to maternal antigens, possibly as a result of materno-foetal transmission of cells in utero. Woodruff and Lennox (1959) described reciprocal skin graft studies in a pair of unlike-sex twins with demonstrable leucocyte and erythrocyte blood chimerism. Grafts survived in both twins for the whole of the 6-months observation period. It would be of interest to note the behaviour of a second-set graft but this was not done because the authors felt it was unjustifiable to impose a futher burden on their subjects.

The advent of the practice of intra-uterine transfusion and postnatal exchange transfusion for erythroblastosis has provided an opportunity to study the development of artificially induced tolerance in the human neonate. Fowler et al. (1960) test-grafted 12 newborn infants following exchange transfusion with adult skin. Rapid graft rejection was observed in six infants who were exchanged with blood which had been stored for 48 hours or more. The number of viable leucocytes in these blood specimens were probably too low. In contrast, marked prolongation of graft survival was found in six infants who received transfusions of fresh blood and were grafted with skin from the corresponding blood donor. This tolerance, however, was incomplete as illustrated by the varying degrees of rejection seen when three of the infants were subjected to second-set grafts.

The available evidence, therefore, would seem to indicate that the transfer of viable leucocytes to the human foetus in utero, or even to the newborn, can interfere to some extent with its immunological mechanism for allograft rejection. Whether this partial tolerance extends to other kinds of immunological response is not possible to say. Although none of the six children in Fowler's series who manifested tolerance to homologous skin grafts showed any immediate pathological reactions, two of them later developed major infective episodes from which one died. One is left with the uncomfortable feeling that these infections might not be mere coincidental findings but could have resulted from the development of a generalised non-specific immune paralysis.

7.3.3. Graft-versus-host reaction (GVHR)

Maternal lymphocytes are immunocompetent cells. Besides acting as potential antigenic or tolerogenic stimuli, these cells can mount a reaction against the foetus, giving rise to a graft-versus-host reaction (GVHR). This reaction has long been recognised in animal studies (Streilein and Grebe 1976) where the most common form, 'runt disease' is induced in an immunologically immature animal by the transfer of immunocompetent cells from an histoincompatible donor. The clinical importance of this syndrome in man was first brought to light when GVHR was reported in certain patients with congenital immunodeficiency or whole body irradiation who were treated with allogeneic bone-marrow transplants. The other situations where GVHR has been observed to occur are following intra-uterine transfusions or exchange transfusions of foetusus or neonates for erythroblastosis (Cohen et al. 1965; Naiman et al. 1966, 1969; Parkman et al. 1974). There is still some doubt as to how often this occurs. Jones (1968b) reported two cases of intra-uterine transfusions performed between 29—32 weeks of gestation where there was not clinical evidence of GVHR in spite of the fact that, in one case, donor lymphocytes were found to make up 50% of the peripheral lymphocyte population. Similarly, the 14 cases of intra-uterine tranfusions with maternal blood reported by Hutchinson et al. (1971), did not show any evidence of GVHR, although maternal lymphocytes were found to persist for longer than two years in the peripheral blood of four of the infants. From the experience of Parkman et al. (1974) in Boston, no case of GVHR has been observed in infants treated with exchange transfusions since 1947 and only two cases of GVHR were reported in 81 cases treated with intra-uterine transfusions. It would appear then, that the incidence of GVHR following transfusion procedures in infants is infrequent.

There is very little information available concerning maternally induced GVHR in human gestation. Data from animal studies show that this can indeed occur. Fisher female rats grafted with incompatible DA strain skin 27—34 days before delivery can incite a GVHR in their (Fisher x DA)F_1 offsprings which results in 94% of the infants dying four weeks after birth. This GVHR can be similarly achieved in (Fisher x DA)F_1 offsprings by the adoptive transfer of 100 million lymphoid cells obtained from Fisher donors specifically sensitised to DA allo-antigens. Although it has not been unequivocally demonstrated that these runted offsprings are lymphoid chimeras, the results strongly indicate that transplacentally transferred maternal lymphocytes sensitised to the paternally derived component of foetal antigens are the probable mediators of the observed GVHR. Even weak immunogenic disparity that does not involve the major histocompatibility complex is sufficient to induce GVHR if the recipients are particularly vulnerable, like adults after X-irradiation or the foetus in utero (Beer and Billingham 1973).

Since experiments similar in design to that described above have resulted in runt disease in mice, guinea pigs, hamsters, and rabbits, it seems likely that the human foetus may be similarly affected during pregnancy. So far, there is no conclusive evidence that this, in fact, occurs. Perhaps all affected foetuses are aborted early in gestation and are, therefore, not recognised as having runt disease. The two cases of XX/XY lymphoid chimerism described by Kadowaki et al. (1965) and Githens et al. (1969), where the foetuses suffered from thymic alymphoplasia and immunological deficiency, may be examples of maternally-induced GVHR, and so may the case reported by Grogan et al. (1975) of a female infant who had never been transfused, with signs of combined immune deficiency syndrome and evidence of GVHR. It could be argued, however, that the lymphoid chimerism in these cases was the result of foetal immunodeficiency rather than the cause of the GVHR syndrome.

There may be less overt manifestations of GVHR which are not initially recognised as such. Observations on animals have shown that GVHR across weak histocompatibility barriers may lead to a 2- to 4-fold increase in the incidence of lymphomas in mice injected at birth with adult incompatible spleen cells (Walford 1966). Therefore, the possibility should be considered that certain lymphomas in children and even in adults like Hodgkin's disease (Green et al. 1960) may be manifestations of a subclinical runt disease due to persistence of a maternal lymphocyte clone established at a stage in utero when the foetus' immunological system is relatively immature. It is postulated that these lymphocytes can remain dormant for prolonged periods within the foetus, ultimately becoming the progenitors of malignant lymphocytes. Turner et al. (1975), in a follow-up of children who had been given intra-uterine transfusions, found that one child developed acute lymphoblastic leukaemia at 4½ years of age.

In this context, cytogenetic studies of Burkitt's lymphoma by Manolov et al. (1970) are of interest. They found that the chromosomes of a tumour from a phenotypic male had a female karyotype. This was corroborated by autoradiographic studies which demonstrated a late replicating X chromosome. The chromosomal abnormalities observed in other samples of Burkitt's lymphoma may be further examples of sex discrepancy between the tumour and the host. In one tumour from a male patient described by Jacobs et al. (1963), all cells had 46 chromosomes but one chromosome from group G was missing, while there was an extra medium-sized chromosome. Although it was felt that the missing chromosome was an autosome, there is the alternative possibility that it could have been a Y and the additional chromosome an X. In other words, it could have been a female karyotype. The case described by Tomkins (1968), where the cell line from a Burkitt's tumour derived from a male patient, showed the presence of an extra C-group and a missing G-group chromosome could be similarly interpreted as a female karyotype. Further indirect evidence that Burkitt's lymphoma could have developed from cells transmitted from another host, is seen in the relatively strong immunological response mounted by the host against the tumour, and in the dramatic response to chemotherapy, a property which is also seen in that allogeneic tumour par excellence, choriocarcinoma. Where do these allogeneic cells come from? They could be transmitted directly by mosquitoes, a hypothesis which has the merit of conforming with the geographical distribution of the disease. If this were the case, one would expect also to find male tumours in female patients but, so far, this appears not to have been recorded. Alternatively, these cells could be maternal cells which have traversed the placenta during pregnancy. However, direct evidence in support of this hypothesis is lacking, for histocompatibility typing of the tumour cells in the case described by Manolov et al. (1970) and peripheral lymphocytes from the patient's mother showed marked discordance in antigens.

The mechanism responsible for tumour induction in GVHR has not been satisfactorily explained. That neoplastic change is probably a sequel to GVHR is suggested by the histological study of Armstrong et al. (1967). These investigators produced GVHR in mice by injecting them at the age of six weeks with allogeneic spleen cells. The animals were killed at regular intervals from one week to 15 months afterwards. On histological examination, their lymphoid tissues showed a continuous spectrum of changes, progressing to a condition of exuberant hyperplasia difficult to distinguish from neoplasia. There are many theories to explain why tumours should arise. The immuno-depression caused by GVHR may render the host more susceptible to oncogenic agents. However, this appears not to be the primary factor, since those donor-host combinations of GVHR with the highest incidence of lymphomas have the least degree of immunosuppression as tested by various antigens and by their capacity to reject allografts (Solnick et al. 1973). In some of these lymphomas, the cells comprising the tumour appear to be of donor and not host genotype. This observation suggests that over-stimulation of donor lymphocytes by host antigens in GVHR may be the initial mechanism for the induction of lymphomas (Cornelius 1972a). The theory which commands a wide following is that GVHR causes the release or activation of an oncogenic virus (Cornelius 1972b; Armstrong et al. 1973; Nemirovsky and Trainin 1973). Viruses have been observed to appear in suspensions consisting of a mixture of lymphocytes from parental and F_1 mice but not when either lymphocyte population was incubated by itself. When lymphocyte transformation was blocked by treating parental lymphocytes with mitomycin, viruses did not appear (Hirsch et al. 1972). Since this mixed lymphocyte reaction can in certain aspects be regarded as an in vitro analogue of GVHR, it seems a fair supposition that viruses may similarly be released or activated by GVHR in vivo. It is not clear why oncogenic viruses should be activated but it is possible that these viruses replicate better in mitotically active lymphoblasts than in inactive lymphocytes (Hirsch et al. 1970). Thus, the formation of lymphomas following GVHR is probably governed by a complex interplay of factors which include histocompatibility differences between donor and recipient, immune responsiveness of donor lymphocytes towards recipient antigenic challenge, and the inherent susceptibility to oncogenic viruses once these are activated (Gleichmann et al. 1972).

It has been postulated that maternally-induced GVHR could also be a basic mechanism for the induction of auto-allergic diseases (Schwartz 1974) where antibodies directed at 'self' antigens are produced by maternal cell clones.

Although the evidence presented is not conclusive, it does emphasise that consideration should be given to the possibility that maternal lymphocytes colonising the foetus during a stage in utero may subsequently become responsible for some of the diseases in children and even adults. This has prompted Schwartz (1974) to call these maternal cells 'Trojan Horse lymphocytes'. That these diseases occur relatively infrequently is perhaps testimony for the integrity of the human placental barrier and the early maturation of immunocompetence in the human foetus.

7.4 Effects of maternal erythrocytes on the foetus

Unlike lymphocytes, maternal erythrocytes are not immunocompetent cells. The expected consequence of materno-foetal transfer of these cells will be dependent on whether maternal erythrocytes act as tolerogenic or immunogenic stimuli to the foetus.

7.4.1 Maternal erythrocytes as tolerogens

As discussed in the preceding section concerning the effects of maternal leucocytes on the foetus, experiments have shown that animals can be rendered tolerant if antigens are introduced sufficiently early during development. Maternal erythrocytes, therefore, may have similar effects on the foetus if transplacental transfer of cells occurs early in gestation. This tolerance may be long-lasting. On this basis, a Rh negative foetus exposed to maternal Rh positive red cells in utero can be rendered tolerant to the Rh antigen and will remain tolerant even in adult life. Is this the explanation for why certain Rh negative women are not immunised even after successive births of Rh positive infants?

If this hypothesis is correct, two features of Rh disease will be apparent (Bowley and Dunsford 1957):
(1) there will be an excess of Rh positive maternal grandmothers among normal Rh positive children born to multiparous Rh negative women who fail to produce anti-D antibodies; and
(2) there will be an excess of Rh negative maternal grandmothers among children with erythroblastosis due to anti-D.

Several studies have been done to test if these two criteria are met. Booth et al. (1953) pooled the results from four centres in Britain with reference to the Rh blood group of the maternal grandmothers of children with erythroblastosis. Out of 113 maternal grandmothers, 67 were Rh positive and 46 were Rh negative. These figures were precisely equal to the expected number as calculated from gene frequencies. A study of 173 Rh negative women with anti-D in their sera who gave birth to afflicted infants of varying severity (Ward et al. 1957) also revealed no significant deviation from the expected figure regarding the Rh group of maternal grandmothers. There was also no correlation between the Rh group of maternal grandmother and severity of erythroblastosis, nor with the anti-D titre in the mother.

The observations on the development of haemolytic disease, therefore, do not favour the concept of in utero induction of tolerance by the transplacental passage of maternal Rh positve erythrocytes. However, using the onset of erythroblastosis as a yardstick to measure the presence or absence of tolerance may be too extreme for, after all, it is maternal response which is in question and not the result on the foetus of that response. Owen et al. (1954) provided evidence indicating that Rh negative women who developed Rh antibody in a first, second, or third pregnancy but whose babies did not develop clinically recognised haemolytic disease were, in a disproportionate number of cases, the daughters of Rh negative mothers. In contrast, Rh negative women who did not develop anti-Rh antibody in their first three Rh positive pregnancies were, more often than chance would suggest, the daughters of Rh positive women. These results, therefore, indicate that relative tolerance as manifested by the production of antibodies in successive pregnancies, does seem to be related to the Rh blood group of the maternal grandmothers. Unfortunately, Owen's data may be faulted in that no correction was made for foetal-maternal ABO incompatibility. This can greatly affect the survival of foetal red cells in the maternal circulation and, ultimately, the frequency of maternal sensitisation.

7.4.2 Maternal erythrocytes as immunogens

With present knowledge about the early maturation of immunocompetence in the human foetus, it seems highly unlikely that the 'null' period in foetal immunological development would be sufficiently extensive for the induction of tolerance by maternal antigens. What is more likely to happen is foetal sensitisation. In the context of Rh antigen, an observation which has always puzzled investigators is the occasional production of anti-D antibodies during pregnancy by Rh negative primigravidae who have not been previously sensitised by abortions or blood transfusions. Most cases of sensitisation occur at the second or subsequent pregnancies. Foetal red cells may have leaked into the maternal circulation very early in gestation so that maternal sensitisation has developed by the time of the first delivery. An alternative explanation which has been offered is that the mother was sensitised in a previous generation, i.e. the primary sensitisation was due to exposure of the woman, while still a foetus in utero, to the Rh positive red cells of her own mother. Thus, the data for the Rh blood group of maternal grandmothers in support of this hypothesis would be exactly the reverse of those needed for induction of Rh tolerance (Beasley 1953).

Available evidence would seem to confirm this in utero sensitisation hypothesis. Scott and Beer (1973) studied eight women who developed anti-D before delivery of their first child and found five of the women had Rh positive mothers while two had Rh negative mothers with one unknown. Taylor (1967) reported that after three Rh positive ABO compatible pregnancies, women with Rh positive mothers were more likely to have children affected with erythroblastosis than women with Rh negative mothers. Observed in another way, 78.65% of children with Rh positive maternal grandmothers had erythroblastosis while only 60.29% of children with Rh negative maternal grandmothers were affected. If Rh negative foetuses are sensitised in utero by maternal Rh positive cells, then it is to be expected that some of them may produce anti-D antibodies. This has, indeed, been found by Hindemann (1973) who reported that about 5% of Rh negative neonates born to Rh positive mothers already had demonstrable anti-D in their sera six months after birth.

Foetal immune response to maternal ABO antigens has also been reported. Anti-A and anti-B iso-agglutinins of IgM class which do not readily cross the placenta have been demonstrated in neonatal sera (Chattoraj et al. 1968). In seven out of 33 cases, the blood groups of the newborns and mothers were such that the iso-agglutinins must be produced by the foetus and not transmitted from the mother (Table 7.2). Thomaidis et al. (1969) detected anti-A and anti-B iso-agglutinins in the sera of 79 out of 137 (57%) full-term newborns. In 31 of these, the antibody was IgM. In five infants, the iso-agglutinin reacted against maternal red cells which was further support for the foetal origin of these antibodies. A 'cold' agglutinin with anti-I specificity has also been found in a high percentage of cord sera (Adinolfi 1965). Evidence that

Table 7.2 Blood groups of neonates and their mothers which suggest iso-agglutinin in neonatal serum is not transmitted from mother.

Newborn		Mother	
Blood group	Iso-agglutinin	Blood group	Iso-agglutinin
O	anti-A	A	anti-B
O	anti-B	B	anti-B
B	anti-A	A	anti-B
O	anti-A	A	anti-B
O	anti-A	A	anti-B
O	anti-B	B	anti-A
O	anti-A	A	anti-B

With kind permission from Chattoraj, A. et al. (1968) *Vox Sang.* **14**, 289–291.

this antibody was foetal in origin was provided by several observations. The antibody was characterised as IgM. In infants tested repeatedly, there was no variation in antibody titre. This is, therefore, in contrast to that seen for maternally-derived IgG which is usually quickly catabolised. The titre of antibody in cord serum was not related to the titre in maternal serum. In one case, the antibody was present in cord blood but absent from the respective maternal sample. Although all these agglutinins found in neonatal sera may be 'natural' antibodies, the possibility that they are iso-antibodies resulting from maternal erythrocyte stimulation in utero cannot be entirely discounted.

The available evidence, therefore, favours the view that erythrocytes transmitted across the placenta from the mother result in foetal sensitisation rather than tolerance. The foetus will be able, therefore, to deal effectively with any maternal cells that may have breached the first line defence of the placental barrier. Perhaps the early onset of immunocompetence in the human foetus has been developed for just such contingencies.

8

Transmission of immunoglobulins from mother to foetus before birth

8.1 Detection of antibodies in maternal and cord sera

A vast amount has been written about the detection of various kinds of antibodies in pairs of maternal and cord sera ever since the beginning of the century. These findings have often been used as supporting evidence for the transmission of antibodies from mother to foetus before birth. Since much of the work is old and rather repetitive, it would be more profitable to discuss them in a general way, rather than to try and include them all individually merely for the sake of completeness. Readers who would like to pursue the bibliography in greater detail are advised to read the review by Freda (1962), where individual reports are classified in tabulated form, and also the relevant chapter in Brambell's (1970) monograph.

The overall conclusion from the available data is that, although a large number of maternal antibodies will readily pass into the foetal circulation, not all of them do so. Antibodies to bacteria or their products like antistreptolysin (Gordon and Janney 1941; Vahlquist et al. 1950; Murray and Calman 1953), diphtheria antitoxin (Neill et al. 1932; Barr et al. 1949; Osborn et al. 1952) and tetanus antitoxin (Ten Broeck and Bauer 1923; Chandra 1976) are all readily transmitted. So are antibodies to many viruses like influenza (Mantyjarvi et al. 1970), polio (Aycock and Kramer 1930; Gelfand et al. 1960a) and smallpox (Kempe and Benenson 1953). It seems that there may be a difference in the transmissibility of antibodies to the three different strains of polio virus. Lipton and Steigman (1957) performed neutralising antibody titrations for the three polio virus serotypes in maternal and cord blood at 48 deliveries. They found disparities of 4- to 64-fold in 14 individuals, the maternal titre being always higher. The disparity most frequently detected was with antibody to Type 3 polio virus. Gelfand et al. (1960b) also observed a tendency for the transfer of antibody to Type 3 polio virus to be less efficient compared with antibody to Type 1 and 2.

In Chapter 5, evidence has been presented to show that the foetus can respond to a certain extent to congenital infections. The question therefore arises as to how many of the antibodies found in cord serum are, in fact, of maternal origin. Good and Zak (1956) observed that the baby of an agammaglobulinaemic mother was also agammaglobulinaemic at birth and during the neonatal period. The serum electrophoretic patterns of both maternal and cord sera lacked a γ-globulin peak, with concentrations of this protein estimated to be only about 11 mg/100 ml (Bridges et al. 1959). By about the second month of life, the infant began to synthesise γ-globulins normally, indicating it had not inherited its mother's genetic defect. The corollary to this finding is that elevated levels of immunoglobulins have been observed in infants born to mothers with high levels of γ-globulins in countries where there is a high endemic rate of infectious diseases. This dependence on maternal serum levels offers clear evidence that most of the immunoglobulins detected in foetal and neonatal sera are likely to be of maternal origin.

It has also been observed that the IgG Gm phenotype of the newborn is always similar to that of the corresponding mother, even when the infant's genotype is different (Grubb and Laurell 1956; Linnet-Jepson et al. 1958; Lawler 1960; Morell et al. 1971). McKay and Thom (1971) compared 92 mother infant pairs for Gm 1, 2, 4, 5, and for Inv 1. They found no discrepancies, suggesting that antibodies present in foetal sera were probably derived from the mother.

8.2 Evidence that transmission of antibodies is selective

8.2.1 Selection according to molecular weight of the antibody

Blood group iso-antibodies show a great variation in their ability to be transmitted. The initial demonstration of Rh antibody was by the classic agglutination method in a saline medium. The failure to demonstrate Rh antibody by this method in many cases of erythroblastosis foetalis had puzzled investigators until it was discovered that another 'incomplete' Rh antibody was present (Race 1944; Wiener 1944) which was not demonstrable by the usual saline agglutination. The critical observation was made that these 'incomplete' antibodies were readily transmitted while the saline antibodies were not, and it was thought that the reason might be that these 'incomplete' antibodies had a lower molecular weight. This was subsequently confirmed. Campbell et al. (1955) demonstrated that the Rh saline agglutinins were indeed associated with those serum fractions which sedimented near 18 Svedberg units while the 'incomplete' albumin agglutinable Rh antibodies sedimented near 6.5 Svedberg units. Franklin and Kunkel (1958) examined the macroglobulin content of maternal and cord sera by ultracentrifugation and by immunological estimation using an antiserum specific for normal serum 19S γ-globulin fraction. Maternal sera were found to contain 50—100 mg/100 ml of 19S γ-globulins by ultracentrifugation but none were detected in 13 out of 14 cord sera examined, while one had a small amount. Immunological estimation confirmed maternal levels of 35—70 mg/100 ml while in most cases cord sera only had levels of 2.5 mg/100 ml. Therefore, it appears that the transmission of 19S γ-globulins from mother to foetus occurs only slightly, if at all, and the small amounts detected in foetal blood may well be autologous.

It has been shown that all the ABO iso-agglutinins were γ-globulins with sedimentation values of either 7S or 19S (Fahey and Morrison 1960), so the variability of transmission of these antibodies may similarly reflect their heterogeneity. This is supported by the results of Kochwa et al. (1961) who found that the ABO iso-agglutinin activity of 33 specimens of cord sera was restricted to the serum fraction containing 7S γ_2-globulin. In contrast, maternal serum ABO iso-agglutinins were encountered chiefly in the macroglobulin serum fractions. Examination of paired specimens of maternal and cord sera obtained at delivery revealed that the 7S-associated iso-agglutinin existed in equilibrium in both. Thus, in the same way as for Rh, it is the maternal ABO agglutinins of 7S molecular size which are readily transmitted to the foetus, while those associated with the macroglobulin fractions are not. This may explain the disparity in titres of 'natural' anti-A and anti-B observed between maternal and cord sera (Tovey 1945), for these antibodies are macroglobulins.

The association between molecular weight and transmissibility is also applicable to the 'H' and 'O' agglutinins to Salmonella typhi. In a study of 59 paired maternal and infant sera, Timmerman (1931) found that 44 mothers had 'H' agglutinins which were also present in 28 of their offsprings but whereas 43 mothers also had 'O' agglutinins, this antibody was present in only one infant. The 'H' agglutinins, therefore, were more readily transmitted than the 'O' agglutinins. It was subsequently shown that 'H' agglutinins were to be found in the serum fraction which corresponded to 6.6S γ_2-globulins while the 'O' agglutinins were present only in the fraction containing 18S γ-macroglobulins (Fahey 1960).

8.2.2 *Selection according to immunoglobulin class*

Further investigations have shown that transmissibility is related more to the class of immunoglobulin than to its molecular weight. Many maternal serum proteins of the same size or even smaller than 7S γ_2-globulins do not appear in significant amounts in the foetal circulation. Ceruloplasmin is an example. This protein is an α-globulin with a molecular weight of approximately 150,000. It is, therefore, no larger than 7S γ_2-globulin and yet the concentration of ceruloplasmin in maternal serum is about 7—8 times that of cord serum (Scheinberg et al. 1954; Usategui-Gomez et al. 1966). The levels of α- and β-globulins have also been found to be lower in cord sera compared to maternal sera (Longsworth et al. 1945; Moore et al. 1949).

These observations are supported by experimental findings. In experiments using injection of labelled serum proteins into pregnant Rhesus monkeys, it was found that the materno-foetal transmission of γ-globulin exceeded that for albumin by about 15—20 times, in spite of the fact that the molecular weight of γ-globulin is about twice that of albumin (Bangham et al. 1958). Globulins of α- and β-mobility were not transferred at all. Similar results were obtained on human subjects by Dancis et al. (1961). They injected I^{131}-labelled albumin, β-globulin and γ-globulin into maternal circulation during the first trimester of women scheduled for termination of pregnancy. In estimating foetal blood for these proteins, they found more γ-globulin than albumin or β-globulin transferred from the mother. The lack of transfer of β_2M-globulin may be explained on the basis of molecular size for this protein has a molecular weight of nearly 1,000,000 but β_2A-globulin has a sedimentation constant in the range of 7S so the selectivity against this protein is clearly not because of size.

The 7S γ_2-globulin molecule can be hydrolysed by papain into three major polypeptide fragments of approximately equal sizes. When these fragments are labelled and injected into pregnant animals, it is found that, despite the reduction in molecular size, only the Fc fragment reaches the foetal circulation at the same rate as the whole molecule, whereas the other two fragments pass at only about a tenth of this rate (Brambell et al. 1960). Using human subjects, Gitlin et al. (1964a) injected I^{131}-labelled 7S γ-globulin, Fc fragments and Fab fragments into women at the last trimester and estimated the amounts of these proteins in foetal blood at delivery. They confirmed that the concentration of labelled Fc fragments in foetal blood was 4—10 times greater than labelled Fab fragments, but that both these fragments were less readily transmitted than the whole 7S γ-globulin molecule. Also, very little albumin, transferrin or fibrinogen was detected in foetal blood, when similarly labelled and injected into the maternal circulation.

From these observations, it is clear that the transmission of antibody from mother to foetus during pregnancy is dependent, not so much on the molecular size of the antibody, but mainly on the class of immunoglobulin involved, with a particular selection for the γ_2-globulins. Thus, in man, IgG is found to occur in dynamic equilibrium between the foetus and its mother (Cochron and Good 1974) and it frequently is present in a higher concentration in foetal serum than in maternal serum (Virella et al. 1972), with a mean cord serum level of 1,512.5 mg% compared to 1,260.1 mg% in maternal serum (Kohler and Farr 1966). At present, the data concerning the materno-foetal transmission of IgG subclasses are conflicting. Hay et al. (1971) measured the concentrations of IgG subclasses in matched pairs of maternal and cord sera. They found that while IgGl, IgG3, and IgG4 were present in similar amounts in both mother and infant, IgG2 was about three times less in cord sera than in maternal sera. Similar results were presented by Wang et al. (1970) who observed that IgG2 was present only in trace amounts in foetal sera. Using more sensitive radio-labelled antigen-antibody methods, Morell et al. (1971) observed that the level of all four IgG subclasses were low during the early part of gestation but rose steadily, so that by the 33rd week the foetal-maternal ratio for all four IgG subclasses approached unity. Chandra (1976) found that the bulk of IgG in foetal serum at 16 weeks gestation consisted of IgG1 but by the 22nd week, there was a significant rise in all the other subclasses. However, when the concentration of IgG subclasses in foetal serum were expressed as a percentage of total serum IgG, the distribution gradually approached the adult pattern except for IgG2 which remained low (Table 8.1).

Table 8.1 Geometric mean levels of IgG subclasses in foetal sera expressed as percentage of total serum IgG.

Gestational age (weeks)	IgG1	IgG2	IgG3	IgG4
16	97	2	0.5	0.5
20	79	20	0.8	0.2
24	76	17	5.3	1.7
28	79	11	8.4	1.6
32	70	19	8.9	2.1
36	67	23	7.7	2.3
40	66	24	7.6	2.4
40+	68	21	8.0	3.0
Adults	60	30	7.2	2.8

With kind permission from Chandra, R. K. (1976) In: *Maternofoetal Transmission of Immunoglobulins*, Ed.: Hemmings. Cambridge University Press, pp. 77–87.

It may be concluded that all four subclasses of maternal IgG are probably transmitted to her foetus with perhaps a slight deficiency in the transfer of IgG2. This does not appear to be due to a differential catabolic rate for it has been found that it is IgG3 which has the shortest half-life of 7.1 days compared to 21 days for IgG1, IgG2, and IgG4 (Morell et al. 1970).

The concentration of IgM in foetal blood is low (Virella et al. 1972), being about 10 times less than in maternal serum (Cochron and Good 1974). About 2.5 mg/100 ml of IgM is found in most cord sera compared to maternal levels of 35—70 mg/100 ml (Franklin and Kunkel 1958). The transmission of this immunoglobulin in man, therefore, is inefficient and is in contrast to the situation in rabbits where maternal IgM can readily be transferred to the foetus (Hemmings 1973; Shek and Dubiski 1975).

The concentration of IgA in foetal blood is also low (Virella et al. 1972), or even completely absent (Cochron and Good 1974). Stiehm and Fudenberg (1966) reported that IgA was absent in two-thirds of cord specimens tested, while the rest had only trace quantities. This was confirmed by Brasher and Hartley (1969) who detected a mean concentration of 2.6 mg/100 ml of IgA in 29.9% of 97 unselected cord sera by immuno-electrophoresis. More sensitive methods can increase the frequency of detection of IgA in cord sera but, even then, the concentrations still lie within the range of 0.15—2.15 mg% (Faulkner and Borella 1970). These observations indicate that transmission of maternal IgA to the foetus, if any, is relatively inefficient, and the small quantities found in some foetal sera may be produced by the foetus itself in response to intra-uterine infection. However, the report of a foetus developing anti-IgA antibodies (Vyas and Fudenberg 1970) would seem to suggest that, in certain circumstances, perhaps in the event of minor damage to the placenta, sufficient amounts of maternal IgA may reach the foetus to result in sensitisation.

IgD was not detected in normal cord serum by Rowe et al. (1968), but a later investigation by Leslie and Swate (1972) found detectable IgD in 4.5% of 90 unselected cord specimens. Again, the disparate results are probably due to the sensitivity of the techniques employed. Using a haemagglutination inhibition method, Cederqvist et al. (1977a) detected IgD in 84% of cord sera tested with a mean value of 0.5 ± 0.4 mg/100 ml. There is no correlation between cord and maternal IgD levels, the level of IgD being very much higher in maternal blood (Leslie and Swate 1972; Cederqvist et al. 1977a). This discrepancy, therefore, indicates poor transmissibility of this immunoglobulin. In Chapter 5, we have discussed the possible role of IgD surface receptors on foetal lymphocytes. The function of circulating IgD has also not been established. Cederqvist et al. (1977a) observed that there was no correlation between cord IgD level and levels of IgM or IgA. Since the latter two immunoglobulins are usually produced by the foetus in response to congenital infections, this suggests that the presence of IgD in cord serum does not reflect foetal synthesis of specific antibody in response to antigenic challenge. It has been observed that 41% of women at delivery have IgD levels at the higher ranges (Klapper and Mendenhall 1971). No explanation is available for this observation but the possibility that this immunoglobulin may play a role in foetal-maternal interaction warrants further investigation.

Although the original studies of Ratner et al. (1927a) and Ratner and Gruehl (1929) showed that immediate hypersensitivity of guinea pigs could be passively transferred from mother to young in utero, the weight of evidence is against any significant transmission of IgE in humans. This was established almost 50 years ago by Bell and Erickkson (1931) who studied five women with asthma or hay-fever. The ability of their sera to give rise to local transfer skin reactions by the

Prausnitz—Küstner (P-K) test on normal individuals was present in a dilution of 1 in 40 to 1 in 320, but in no case could similar properties be shown in the cord sera of their children. This was confirmed by the observations of Sherman et al. (1940) that skin-sensitising antibodies of human allergy, even when present at high concentrations in the mother, were not transmitted to the foetus, while blocking antibodies (presumably IgG) in hay-fever patients immunised with pollen were freely transmitted. Similar conclusions were reached by Kuhns (1965), who studied the immediate hypersensitivity reactions of eight Schick negative pregnant women given repeated injections of fluid diphtheria toxoid, by monitoring the appearance of reaginic antibodies in their sera and in their ability to form immediate wheal reactions when challenged with intradermal toxoid. It was found that although seven out of eight mothers were positive for both tests, this was not mirrored by their infants. That this was not due to an inherent hyporeactivity of neonatal skin was controlled by the demonstration that the immediate wheal reaction could be elicited in both infant's and mother's skin when they served as recipients for passive transfer P-K tests with reaginic antibodies derived from an alternative source. In a study of serum IgE levels, Johansson (1968) found a marked disparity in levels between cord and maternal blood, the former containing a mean IgE level of 36 ng/ml which is about 15% of adult mean level.

From these observations, it can be concluded that maternal IgE is not readily transmissible to the human foetus. The small amounts present in cord sera are probably produced by the foetus itself as a result of maternally transferred allergens. The production of Type 1 immediate hypersensitivity by active sensitisation in utero has been demonstrated in guinea pigs (Ratner et al. 1927b). That this may also occur in man is illustrated by the findings of Kaufman (1971) in a 3-hour-old infant who exhibited an immediate skin reaction to mixed grasses. A P-K test on a normal recipient with the infant's serum was also positive to grass pollen antigens. The infant's serum level of IgE at birth was 71 ng/ml which is twice the normal mean cord level. The mother was unreactive to similar antigens which indicates that the skin-sensitising antibodies in the foetus are unlikely to be passively transferred from the mother. The sensitising antigen must have been inhaled by the mother and then transmitted to the foetus without affecting the mother. This development of Type 1 hypersensitivity by the foetus in response to maternally transmitted allergens is further evidence for the early onset of immunocompetence in man.

8.2.3 Selection according to antibody specificity

Analyses of HL-A specificities of IgG eluted from the placenta have revealed several interesting findings (Doughty and Gelsthorpe 1974; Tongio et al. 1975; Doughty and Gelsthorpe 1976):
(1) placental eluates contained cytotoxic antibodies with the same HL-A specificities as the antibodies found in the corresponding maternal serum;
(2) when maternal serum was cytotoxic to her infant's lymphocytes, IgG with the same HL-A specificities as maternal serum could be eluted from the placenta; in this situation, no HL-A antibodies were demonstrable in foetal serum;
(3) when maternal serum did not contain cytotoxic antibodies to her infant's lymphocytes (i.e. not relevant to the present pregnancy), placental IgG eluate did not have any demonstrable anti-HL-A activity; in this situation, anti-HL-A antibodies were found in foetal serum which had the same specificities as those in maternal serum.

Therefore, it would appear that when the foetus possesses the corresponding HL-A antigen to which maternal antibody is directed, this antibody is found in placental eluate but not in foetal serum. Conversely, when the foetus lacks the corresponding antigen, then antibody with anti-HL-A activity is demonstrable in foetal serum but not in placental eluate.

These findings have led to the postulate that placental antigens may act by absorbing out all maternal antibodies which are potentially harmful to the foetus and prevent them from reaching the foetal circulation. Only those antibodies which are not directed at any foetal antigenic specificities are allowed to cross. This capacity of the human placenta to act like a sponge (Swinburne 1970) may therefore be an important selective mechanism in the transmission of antibodies from mother to foetus.

In this context, it may be reiterated that human placental cells have been shown also to express ABO antigens, so it is possible that a similar mechanism may be operative regarding maternal 'immune' anti-A or anti-B iso-antibodies. In a study of anti-A and anti-B iso-agglutinins in cord blood, Zuelzer and Kaplan (1954b) found that in group 'A' or group 'B' infants born to group 'O' mothers, the maternal antibody which was potentially antagonistic to the foetus was usually absent from cord sera. Although it is generally thought that this is due to neutralisation by ABO antigens on foetal tissues or by soluble blood group substances, it may be that the relevant maternal antibody has completely failed to cross the placenta.

8.3 Route of transmission of immunoglobulins

The transfer of immunoglobulins from mother to foetus varies in different species. While this has been observed to occur in primates, rabbits and guinea pigs, the main transfer in mice, rats, cats, and dogs, appears to take place after birth via the milk. In ungulates, this process of transfer is more restricted, being confined to suckling during a period immediately after birth (Brambell 1970).

On the basis of experimental studies in rabbits, Brambell (1966, 1970) established that the route of transmission is via the foetal yolk-sac and not the placenta in this species. However, a consideration of the development and final arrangement of the placenta and foetal membranes in man indicates that, on purely anatomical grounds, transmission is unlikely to be by this route. The human allantoic cavity is vestigial and the yolk-sac is rudimentary. At the final stage of development of the embryo, foetal tissue is separated from maternal tissue at all points by the chorion. Thus, all traffic between mother and foetus must take place via the chorionic trophoblast. The most direct route from maternal to foetal circulation is, of course, via the chorio-allantoic placenta where substances in maternal blood can pass across the trophoblast layer covering the chorionic villi, and be absorbed by the rich foetal capillaries beneath. However, an alternate route of transfer via the amniotic cavity is also possible. Maternal immunoglobulins transfered to the amniotic fluid can be swallowed by the foetus and then absorbed via the foetal intestine into the circulation. This route has the attraction of involving absorption by the gut which is an endodermal structure, a feature which occurs, as far as is known, in all other animals. The placenta, on the other hand, is derived from mesoderm which makes its involvement unique to man and other primates.

8.3.1 Transmission via amniotic fluid

The presence of immunoglobulins and other serum proteins in amniotic fluid is well documented. Steigman and Lipton (1958) reported that human amniotic fluid at birth could neutralise the cytopathic effects of three polio virus serotypes. Since γ-globulins were also detected, the authors inferred that this neutralising property was due to specific antibodies. Anti-D has also been detected in amniotic fluid (Wild 1960; Usategui-Gomez and Stearns 1969).

Most investigators favour the view that these antibodies in amniotic fluid are probably derived from the mother. In a comparative study of the protein pattern of maternal serum, foetal serum and amniotic fluid by paper electrophoresis, Abbas and Tovey (1960) observed a low concentration of proteins moving in the α_2 region in amniotic fluid relative to maternal serum concentration. They suggested that the proteins in amniotic fluid represented a dialysate from maternal serum, with the high molecular weight α_2 proteins being filtered off. Further evidence in support of this hypothesis was provided by dialysing maternal serum across corresponding foetal membranes in vitro. The resultant dialysate protein pattern was found to be identical to that of amniotic fluid. Similar conclusions were reached by Usategui-Gomez et al. (1966) who used disc electrophoresis combined with quantitative immunodiffusion to distinguish individual proteins. They found that amniotic fluid contained mainly IgG, transferrin and albumin. Since the larger molecules like β-lipoprotein, α_2-macroglobulin, and IgM, all of which have molecular weights exceeding 300,000, were not detected, this supports the filtration theory postulated by Abbas and Tovey (1960). Derrington and Soothill (1961), in a quantitative immunochemical study of amniotic fluid proteins, were also of the view that these proteins arose by ultrafiltration from maternal serum.

Perhaps the most conclusive evidence for maternal origin of amniotic fluid proteins is provided by studies on proteins which exhibit genetic polymorphisms. Usategui-Gomez et al. (1966) observed that the genetic variant of haptoglobulin 1-1 was present in all amniotic fluids derived from mothers of this type but this protein was absent from the corresponding cord serum. This prompted them to extend this type of study to include another protein, the Gc protein, which also has three genetic variants 1-1, 1-2, 2-2 (Usategui-Gomez and Morgan 1966). They compared 12 amniotic fluids with the corresponding maternal sera and foetal sera and found that in six cases where maternal and foetal Gc patterns differed, the amniotic fluid pattern invariably reflected the maternal pattern. This was confirmed in further studies by Ruoslahti et al. (1966) who reported that where mother and child belonged to different Gc variants, the Gc type of protein in amniotic fluid was always that of the mother.

Thus, the weight of evidence is in accord with the hypothesis that amniotic fluid proteins, including immunoglobulins, are derived from the mother. However, the demonstration of bilirubin in amniotic fluid in cases of erythroblastosis foetalis (Wild 1961) and of α-foetoprotein in amniotic fluid but not in maternal serum (Gitlin and Boesman 1966), indicates that perhaps the foetus, occasionally, may make some contribution towards the protein content of amniotic fluid.

Are maternal immunoglobulins in human amniotic fluid transferred to the foetal circulation by swallowing and absorption via the intestine like in many animal species (Brambell et al. 1954)? Relevant clinical observations were made by Wasz-Höckert et al. (1956) who described six infants born with oesophageal atresia. These infants could not have swallowed amniotic fluid in utero. Diphtheria antitoxin levels in maternal and infant sera were compared and it was found that, while two mothers and their respective infants had no demonstrable antitoxin, the other four infants had antitoxin levels equivalent to that found in their mothers' sera. Steigman and Lipton (1958) observed that antipolio antibody could be found in foetal serum without these antibodies being present in the corresponding amniotic fluid. Taken together, these observations indicate that the principal route of materno-foetal transmission of immunoglobulins in man is unlikely to be by swallowing of amniotic fluid.

A small amount of amniotic fluid immunoglobulins may be transferred to the foetal circulation. In two infants with oesophageal atresia described by Abbas and Tovey (1960), although γ-globulin was detectable in the sera of these infants, the level was much lower than in normal infants. In experimental studies of pregnant monkeys, Bangham et al. (1958) injected homologous I^{131}-labelled proteins directly into the amniotic cavities and studied the presence of these proteins in foetal sera after caesarian section 8 and 24 hours later. Only very small quantities of labelled proteins were found in foetal sera. Similar studies were conducted in human subjects by Dancis et al. (1961) who injected labelled γ-globulin into the amniotic cavities of two pregnant women in the first trimester scheduled for termination 24 hours later. Radio-activity was detected in foetal blood but in a much lower concentration than in amniotic fluid. They also investigated four women at term by injecting 5 ml of human serum containing high titres of tetanus antitoxin into amniotic fluid. At caesarian section 18—24 hours later, no antitoxin was detectable in cord sera.

From both clinical and experimental data, it may be concluded that, while some maternal proteins can reach the foetal circulation via the amniotic fluid and intestinal absorption, this mode of transmission appears to account for only a small fraction of the total transfer. In man, therefore, the bulk of the maternal immunoglobulins must gain access to the foetus by another route. The chorioallantoic placenta is well suited for this task.

8.3.2 Transmission across the placenta

Both light-microscope (Wislocki and Bennett 1943) and electron-microscope studies (Tighe et al. 1967; Boyde et al. 1968) of the human placenta have revealed features which indicate that this organ does indeed have the capacity to act in the functional role of transporting material from the maternal circulation to the foetus. The syncytial trophoblast is covered with microvilli (Fig. 8.1). At the bases of the microvilli, the surface of the syncytial trophoblast invaginates to form pinocytotic vesicles. The peripheral cytoplasm is filled with vesicles or cisternae, mitochondria and various organelles like large multivesicular bodies, phagosomes and autophagous vacuoles. The syncytial trophoblast may, in parts, come to lie directly on the basement membrane without the intervention of a layer of cytotrophoblast. Here, the basal layer of the syncytium is provided with many finger-like processes like the surface microvilli but less regularly arranged. In these

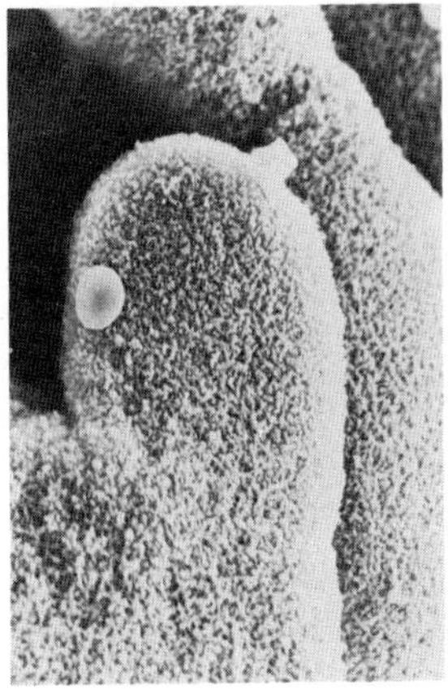

Fig. 8.1 Scanning electron micrograph of human chorionic villus showing microvilli. Kindly supplied by Dr. C. D. Ockleford.

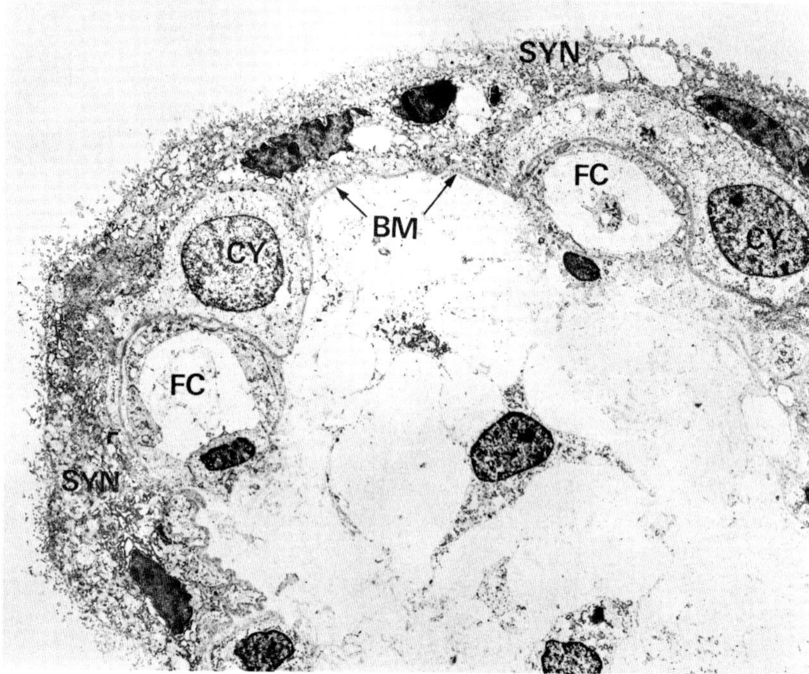

Fig. 8.2 Transmission electron micrograph of human placenta showing relationship between trophoblast and foetal tissue. SYN — Syncytiotrophoblast; FC — foetal capillary; CY — cytotrophoblast; BM — basement membrane. With kind permission from Ockleford, C. D. and Whyte, A. (1977) *J. cell. Sci.* 25, 293—312.

areas, the endothelium of the foetal capillaries is in close proximity to the syncytial trophoblast, separated from each other only by a layer of basement membrane (Fig. 8.2). From these descriptions, it is apparent that the syncytial trophoblast of human placental villi can present a large absorptive surface where pinocytotic activity may occur. In this respect, it bears a remarkable resemblance to the cellular epithelium of rabbit yolk-sac or mouse intestine, two organs which are involved in materno-foetal transport in these species.

On the basis of animal experimental work, Brambell (1966) formulated the hypothesis that the first stage of immunoglobulin transmission by yolk-sac endoderm is by the active absorption of these proteins by pinocytosis. In order to explain the selective nature of this transmission, it is further postulated that the protein to be transmitted

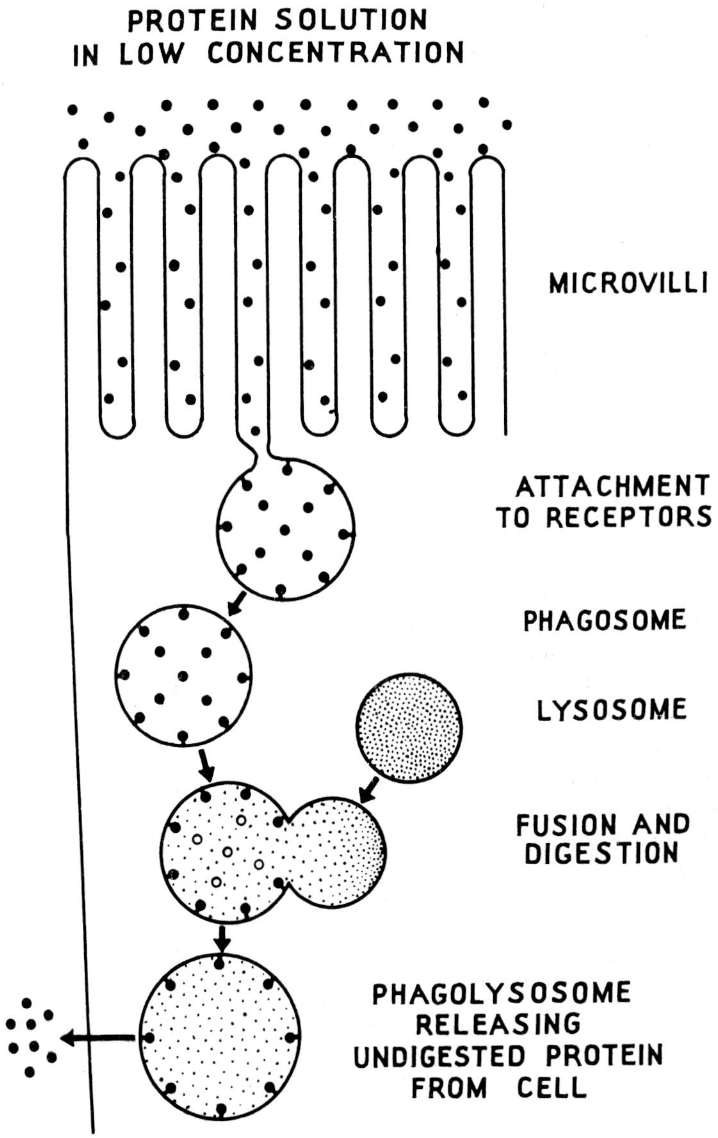

PROTEIN SOLUTION
IN LOW CONCENTRATION

MICROVILLI

ATTACHMENT
TO RECEPTORS

PHAGOSOME

LYSOSOME

FUSION AND
DIGESTION

PHAGOLYSOSOME
RELEASING
UNDIGESTED PROTEIN
FROM CELL

Fig. 8.3 Proposed mechanism for γ-globulin transmission by the cell. With kind permission from Brambell, F. W. R. (1966) *Lancet* 2, 1087—1093.

becomes attached to specific receptors on the walls of the pinocytotic vesicles and this attachment protects it from degradation. Proteins which are not so attached are degraded by lysosomal enzymes. The transported proteins are ultimately released intact from the cells into the foetal tissue spaces to be absorbed into the foetal circulation (Fig. 8.3).

A modification of this hypothesis has recently been presented by Wild (1976) who proposes that instead of selection being an intra-cellular event taking place within pinocytotic vesicles, this selection occurs at the yolk-sac cell surface by protein binding to receptors over certain areas which are subsequently carried in by invagination to form coated micro-pinocytotic vesicles. These vesicles then move to the basal region of the cell, fuse with the basal membrane and discharge their protein contents. It is suggested that the 'bristle-coat' of the coated vesicles prevent fusion with lysosomes during migration inside the cell so no degradation takes place. The remaining proteins which are not bound to receptor sites are pinocytosed into macro-pinocytotic vesicles. These fuse with lysosomes with the resultant degradation of the protein content (Fig. 8.4). A reason which has prompted this alternative hypothesis is the observation that the common proteolytic cellular enzyme, cathepsin D, which is associated with macropinocytotic vesicles, is not detectable in or below the basement membrane. This is interpreted as being due to the fact that phagolysosomes do not discharge their contents into these extracellular sites as envisaged by Brambell's original hypothesis.

Hemmings and Williams (1976) have also questioned Brambell's hypothesis on the basis of two discrepancies between prediction of the hypothesis and experimental observations. Using ferritin markers and electron-microscopic examination, these authors did not detect any pinocytosed protein attached to the periphery of pinocytotic vesicles as would be expected according to the hypothesis. Instead, proteins appeared to lie free in the cytoplasm. It would also be expected that when more protein enters the cell more of it will be left free in the lumen of the vesicle once receptors are saturated and, therefore, more protein will be degraded. However, it was observed that the proportion of protein broken down was largely independent of concentration fed. These authors, therefore, postulate that proteins entering the cell by pinocytosis are unselected. Some of these proteins are released into the cytoplasm from the pinocytotic vesicles indiscriminately and it is this fraction which undergoes onward transport by diffusion to the basement membrane. It is at this stage that selection takes place,

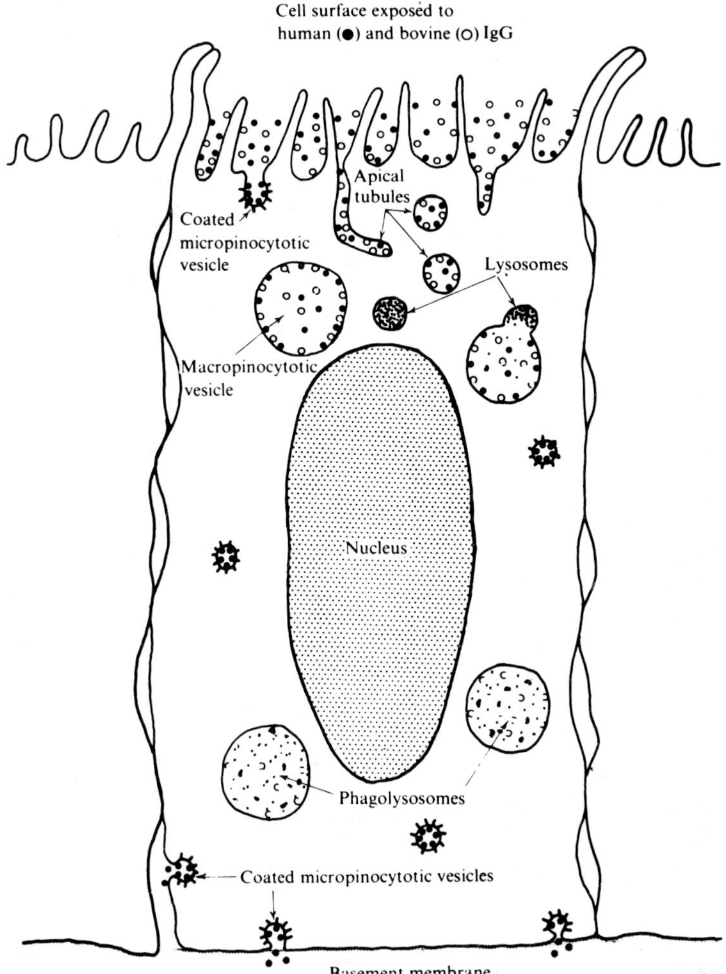

Fig. 8.4 Diagrammatic representation of a hypothetical mechanism of selective transport of immunoglobulins across the rabbit yolk-sac endoderm. With kind permission from Wild, A. E. (1976) In: *Maternofoetal Transmission of Immunoglobulins*. Ed.: Hemmings. Cambridge University Press, pp. 155—167.

although the mechanism for this is not clear. Thus, this hypothesis is different in that it proposes a transport mechanism whereby the protein diffuses freely across the cell cytoplasm instead of packaged in intracellular vesicles, and also that selection takes place at exit rather than on entry.

It is not known to what extent these proposed models for materno-foetal transmission of proteins across transporting membranes in animal systems are applicable to the transfer of immunoglobulins across the human placenta. With the availability of techniques for the separation and preparation of purified plasma membranes from the human placenta, many investigations have recently been carried out to study the binding capacity of these membranes to various proteins. Gitlin and Gitlin (1976) observed that the average amounts of radio-iodinated proteins bound to human placental membranes varied (Table 8.2). It is apparent that there is marked selectivity in the binding of different proteins and it is possible that the rate of transport of these proteins across the placenta may be dependent upon the degree of this binding. It is generally thought that human insulin does not pass readily from mother to foetus, at least during the early stages of gestation (Gitlin et al. 1965). The observation of significant binding of insulin to placental membranes, therefore, suggests that, while binding of proteins is a necessary initial step for transplacental transport, an additional mechanism may be necessary to complete the transfer. Perhaps some release mechanism is required when the bound protein reaches the foetal side. Jones and Waldmann (1972) observed that rat intestinal cells bound IgG selectively at pH 6.5 but lost their ability when pH was raised to 7.4 or more. It is suggested that this could be a

Table 8.2 Binding of different proteins by human placenta membrane fractions

Protein	Amount bound (%)
Bence–Jones protein	10.6
Human insulin	9.3
Human IgG	6.3
Guinea pig IgG	5.4
Bovine IgG	2
Human IgE	1.7
Human albumin	0.4

With kind permission from Gitlin, J. D. and Gitlin, D. (1976) In: *Maternofoetal Transmission of Immunoglobulins*, Ed.: Hemmings. Cambridge University Press, pp. 113–119.

mechanism for the release of bound IgG when it comes into contact with foetal serous fluid which has a pH of around 7.4. Thus, the reversible nature of binding determined by pH changes can influence not only the selectivity but also the efficiency of transport. Those proteins that can bind but do not release at the right pH will, therefore, not be transported efficiently (Rodewald 1976). In the studies of Balfour and Jones (1976), they found that human placental membranes bound labelled IgG to a greater extent at pH 6.6 than at pH 7.8, but it is not known if this higher pH is, in fact, present on the foetal side of the trophoblast basement membrane.

It appears that the binding of IgG by human placental membranes may be via the Fc region of the immunoglobulin molecule. Balfour and Jones (1976), in a study where membrane-rich fractions of full-term human placentae were incubated with radio-iodinated IgG, found that the Fc piece bound to a much greater extent than the Fab fragments. This is in agreement with in vivo findings in both animals and man. Brambell et al. (1960) noticed that the non-antibody reactive fragments of rabbit IgG were transported from mother to foetus with greater efficiency than the antibody reactive fragments. Similar results were obtained by Gitlin et al. (1964a) by injecting I^{131}-labelled fragments of human IgG into pregnant women and then measuring the quantity of these proteins in foetal blood after delivery. They found the concentration of Fc fragments was 4—10 times greater than Fab fragments. It must be pointed out that in this type of study, the observed disparity in concentration in foetal serum of different protein fractions after injection into the mother is not necessarily a measure of the differential rate of transfer. It could be accounted for by a differential rate of degradation. In an attempt to correct for this, Gitlin et al. (1964b) repeated their original experiments but this time measured the concentration of labelled protein fragments in foetal serum relative to that found in maternal serum (i.e. concentration in the foetal serum over concentration in maternal serum) expressed as a function of time. Calculated in this way, they found that both Fc and Fab fragments were, in fact, transported equally readily. The data from Gitlin and Gitlin (1976) that Bence Jones proteins — which consist entirely of immunoglobulin light chains and thus have no Fc region — bind readily to human placental membranes, would seem to indicate that receptor sites for more than one area of the immunoglobulin molecule may be available.

Nevertheless, the concept that binding via the Fc region is an initial step in the transport of immunoglobulins in man is attractive in that it offers a logical explanation for selectivity according to the different classes of immunoglobulins. There are many reports on the presence of Fc receptors on human trophoblast cells. Matre et al. (1975) using frozen sections of term placentae, demonstrated rosettes with indicator red cells sensitised with IgG (EAIgG) of rabbit, guinea pig and human origin. No rosettes were formed with EAIgM or EAIgA indicating a specificity towards IgG of both homologous and heterologous origin. The reaction was dependent on complete IgG molecules, as shown by the lack of reactivity with indicator red cells sensitised by the $F(ab')_2$ fragments even in agglutinating doses. Neither rabbit nor human $F(ab')_2$ fragments inhibited the rosette reactions but, in contrast, there was marked inhibition with IgG Fc fragments. No inhibition was detected with C3. These results, therefore, indicate that the human placenta, like human spleen and liver tissues (Tønder et al. 1974) possesses receptors for the Fc portion of IgG. A study of porcine placentae by the same investigators revealed no Fc receptors which agrees with the concept that no transmission of immunoglobulin takes place in the pig before birth. Thomas et al. (1976) confirmed that Fc receptor activity for human placental tissue was greater at all degrees of EA sensitisation compared with other tissues tested like breast, skin, muscle or kidney.

In a study of rosette formation directly on tissue sections where relatively large areas may be covered by indicator cells, it is difficult to be certain that it is the trophoblast layer which is reacting. Johnson et al. (1975) have reported that it are the endothelial cells of foetal stem vessels rather than trophoblast in cryostat sections of normal full-term human placentae which could bind fluorescein-labelled aggregated human IgG. Aggregated IgM or IgA were not bound. This binding was blocked by heat-aggregated Fc fragments from IgG1, IgG2, IgG3, and IgG4 but not by aggregated light chains, Fab, or $F(ab')_2$, indicating that the receptors are probably Fc receptors (Johnson et al. 1976). It was suggested that these endothelial cell receptors might function to prevent immune complexes, formed by the reaction of maternal antibodies against incompatible foetal allo-antigens, from entering the foetal circulation. These Fc receptors, therefore, have no bearing on the transplacental transport of immunoglobulins. The expression of Fc receptors by placental endothelial cells was recently confirmed by Matre (1977) but it was emphasised that these receptors were also detected on trophoblast cells.

McNabb et al. (1976) studied the binding of IgG to placental membrane preparations and found that the affinity of this binding for the different IgG subclasses was IgGl = IgG3 > IgG4 > IgG2. This differential binding is in accord with IgG transport studies where IgG2 appears to be transmitted with least efficiency. IgA and IgM were found not to bind. The purity of the membrane preparations was checked only by histological examination of the resultant centrifuged pellet to ensure that no intact cells like macrophages were present which could contribute to the IgG binding. Nevertheless, it would be difficult to conclude, without the use of additional membrane markers, that it was trophoblast plasma membranes which were involved in the binding assay.

Recently Jenkinson et al. (1976) have devised a method for the demonstration of EA rosettes on separated human placental cells obtained by trypsinisation of placental material. Differential centrifugation over Ficoll provided confirmatory evidence that EA rosettes were contributed mainly by cells with the appearance of syncytial trophoblast (1—4 nuclei), together with a few cytotrophoblast and Hofbauer cells. Receptors for IgG on placental Hofbauer cells as well as cells resembling monocytes have been observed by Moskalewski et al. (1975).

The expression of Fc receptors by human trophoblast, therefore, may be related to its capacity to function as a transport membrane for the selective transmission of immunoglobulins from mother to foetus. These receptors may have an additional role to play in protecting the placenta against maternal immunological attack. Ockleford (1977) has suggested that Fc binding of maternal IgG will leave insufficient IgG for specific $F(ab')_2$ binding directed at foetal antigenic determinants and thereby abrogates maternal humoral response against the placenta. In this context, it is of interest to note that tumour cells have also been shown to express Fc receptors (Tønder et al. 1974).

9

Effects of maternal antibodies on the foetus

9.1 Transfer of passive immunity

Although the human foetus is capable of mounting an immunological response to a variety of antigens at birth, it is clear that its main protection at this stage of development is conferred by the passive transfer of maternal antibody. This homologous antibody is gradually catabolised over the first few months of life to be replaced by the infant's own actively acquired antibody which is developed as a result of coming into contact with antigens in the environment. The importance of this passive immunity is illustrated by the increased susceptibility to infections for the first few months of life which occurs in normal infants born to mothers with hypogammaglobulinaemia (Zak and Good 1959). In tropical areas of the world with a high prevalence of endemic diseases (e.g. malaria), detectable parasitaemia in newborn infants of mothers from endemic areas is very rare, but these infants become increasingly susceptible to malaria after the first week of life. In contrast, infants of non-indigenous infected mothers frequently have congenital malaria (WHO Techn. Report 1968). These observations indicate that the initial immunity seen in infants born to indigenous mothers is likely to be due to passively transferred maternal antibody.

Unfortunately, not all maternal antibodies are beneficial to the foetus. Those directed at foetal antigenic specificities can lead to diseases of varying severity, the most important of which is erythroblastosis foetalis, but there may be other less overt manifestations.

9.2 Erythrocyte antibodies

By far the most important 'immune' blood group antibodies found in pregnant women are anti-Rh, followed by anti-A or anti-B. The incidence of 'immune' antibodies directed at other red cell antigens is less than 1% of the total (Mollison 1967). Our discussion on the effects of maternal erythrocyte antibodies on the foetus may, therefore, be restricted to the three antibodies mentioned.

9.2.1 Haemolytic disease caused by anti-Rh

Almost all examples of anti-Rh, the most important being anti-D, are IgG so they are readily transmitted from mother to foetus. Since the D antigens are present exclusively on erythrocytes, these cells will bear the brunt of the action of these specific antibodies, resulting in haemolytic disease of the newborn. Anti-D do not bind complement, possibly because the D antigens are too far apart on the red cell surface to allow co-operation between two attached antibody molecules. Anti-D has no obvious damaging effects on Rh-positive red cells in vitro, so its mode of action is unlikely to be via the classical complement pathway of immune lysis. It is thought that Rh antibodies probably bring about the destruction of red cells in vivo by causing the red cells to adhere to macrophages and subsequently to be engulfed (Mollison 1973). This is supported by the finding that, although anti-D can belong to any of the IgG subclasses, the predominant subclasses are IgG1 and IgG3 (Mollison 1973), both being very efficient antibodies to bring about opsonic adherence. The engulfed red cells are then sequestered in the spleen (Jandl et al. 1957).

9.2.2. Haemolytic disease caused by anti-A or anti-B

Maternal 'natural' anti-A or anti-B iso-agglutinins do not usually affect the foetus as they are IgM antibodies and are not readily transmitted to the foetus. On the other hand, maternal 'immune' blood group isoantibodies stimulated by incompatible foetal red cells during pregnancy are IgG and these may cause haemolytic disease of the newborn as with anti-D. The production of 'immune' anti-A or anti-B occurs especially frequently in group 'O' mothers (Kochwa et al. 1961) which may explain the excess of haemolytic disease in group 'A' or group 'B' infants born to group 'O' mothers compared to all types of

ABO foetal-maternal incompatibility. Thus, Rosenfield (1955) found that among 39 infants with a positive direct antiglobulin test, 38 had group 'O' mothers. This was confirmed by Munk-Anderson (1958) who found that in 43 out of a series of 45 cases of ABO haemolytic disease, the mother was group 'O'. Freda and Carter (1962) have found that antibodies from group 'O' mothers seemed to be transmitted to the foetus more readily than when she was either group 'A' or 'B'. In addition, haemolysins occurred with greater frequency in group 'O' mothers with a prevalence of 67% compared to 34% in group 'A' and 32% in group 'B' mothers. When haemolysins were present in the mother, the chance that the foetus would also have them was 5—10 times greater when the mother was group 'O' than when she was group 'A' or 'B'. From these observations, it is therefore not surprising that in practice, the incidence of ABO haemolytic disease is virtually confined to babies of group 'O' mothers and is hardly ever found in other foetal-maternal ABO incompatible situations.

Compared to Rh haemolytic disease, the clinical effects of haemolytic disease due to ABO incompatibility tends to be mild and only in rare cases are they severe enough to require treatment. It is generally believed that this is because ABO antigens are present also in many other foetal tissues (Högman 1959; Szulman 1964) and occurring in soluble forms in body fluids and serum (Hostrup 1963). These antigens will combine with much of the available maternal antibodies (Tovey 1945) and therefore divert the attack away from foetal red cells. Kochwa et al. (1961) have produced evidence that resistance to neutralisation by soluble blood group substances by some 'immune' anti-A or anti-B is associated with severe haemolytic disease. Another factor which may afford some protection to the foetus is the apparent relative deficiency of ABO antigens on foetal erythrocytes compared to adult erythrocytes. Constandoulkis and Kay (1962) found that erythrocytes from foetuses of 3—7 months gestation age absorbed less anti-A or anti-B than the corresponding adult cells, in spite of the relatively large size of the foetal cells. Grundbacher (1964) estimated the degree of haemolysis by rabbit anti-A of A1 human red cells and found that, while 57% of adult cells were lysed, only 27% of cord red cells were affected.

When severe and mild forms are all included, then the frequency of ABO haemolytic disease is similar to or even exceeds that due to Rh incompatibility. Halbrecht (1944) was the first to point out that jaundice developing early in the neonatal period was frequently associated with ABO incompatibility. The incidence of this jaundice was 1 in 180 births

(Halbrecht 1951). A similar frequency of 1 in 140 births was reported by Hsia and Gellis (1954), while Valentine (1958) found 1 in 70 newborn infants to be affected. When laboratory evidence for haemolysis was used instead of clinical signs of jaundice, an even higher proportion of 1 in 30 newborn infants were found to be affected by mild ABO haemolytic disease (Rosenfield and Ohno 1955). These figures may be compared to the incidence of haemolytic disease due to Rh incompatibility which is quoted to be in the region of 1 in 150 to 1 in 200 births (Mollison 1967).

ABO haemolytic disease can affect first-born babies in contrast to the natural history of Rh haemolytic disease, where usually the second or subsequent babies are affected. It has, therefore, been suggested that there may be two clinical types of ABO haemolytic disease. One is caused by the presence in a few mothers of 'natural' blood group antibodies belonging to IgG class which can affect first-borns. With the development of 'immune' antibodies, subsequent infants are affected, perhaps more severely, and it is these infants which occasionally develop typical signs of erythroblastosis.

Crawford et al. (1953) observed that maternal serum was able to haemolyse her infant's red cells in vitro in every one of 11 cases of haemolytic disease due to anti-A. This suggests that the pathogenic mechanism for producing foetal red cell destruction in ABO haemolytic disease in vivo may be by complement-dependent intravascular haemolysis. However, it is by no means certain that this is the right conclusion for, as we have discussed in Chapter 5, the deficiency in complement components in foetal blood may not permit this form of cell lysis to occur. Alternatively, it has been suggested that the mechanism of red cell destruction by anti-A or anti-B may be the same as that produced by anti-D, via opsonic adherence and engulfment by macrophages. Surprisingly, in the case of ABO haemolytic disease, it is extremely difficult to demonstrate the fixation of the relevant antibody on the surface of incompatible foetal erythrocytes by the direct antiglobulin test, and only a modification of the test involving centrifugation can give rise to positive results (Rosenfield 1955). This seems to be due to the extremely small amount of antibody attached to the red cells, for it was estimated by Mollison (1973) that the amount of anti-A or anti-B on the infant's red cells was usually not greater than 0.5μg antibody/ml of red cells, this amount being scarcely sufficient to give a direct antiglobulin test. The association of a haemolytic syndrome with such small amounts of antibody on the red cell would seem to indicate that IgG 'immune' anti-A or anti-B are relatively more effective than IgG anti-D in bringing about red cell destruction (Romano et al. 1973).

9.3 Leucocyte antibodies

We have seen in a previous chapter that mothers are frequently sensitised to their foetal leucocyte iso-antigens during pregnancy. The resultant antibodies, which are mainly IgG, will be expected to have some effect on foetal well-being in the same way as erythrocyte antibodies. Surprisingly, clear-cut associations between maternal anti-leucocyte antibodies and foetal pathology have been difficult to establish and only meagre, often conflicting evidence is available.

Stefanini et al. (1958) described two cases of transitory neonatal neutropenia with the bone marrow showing hyperplasia and maturation arrest of the granulocyte series. In one case, the mother's serum contained a demonstrable leucoagglutinin. Both mothers also suffered from similar neutropenic syndromes so it seems that these cases are mediated by maternal auto-allergic leucocyte antibodies rather than iso-antibodies. The same authors described two other cases of mothers with neutropenia and demonstrable serum leucoagglutinins and yet their infants were not affected.

The case described by Hitzig and Gitzelmann (1959) may be an example of iso-immunisation. They reported an infant who developed infection and severe neutropenia shortly after birth. Haematological investigations revealed no neutrophils at all in a differential white cell count. The mother's serum contained strong leucocyte agglutinins which agglutinated the child's and father's leucocytes but not her own. At six weeks, the infant's serum also had these leucoagglutinins which decreased at a rate very similar to the catabolic curve of normal transplacentally transmitted IgG, and by 10 weeks had completely disappeared. The infant recovered fully. These observations suggest that the neonatal neutropenia may be caused by transfer of maternal leucocyte agglutinins directed against paternally derived antigens of the foetal cells. Jensen (1960) described a case where leucocyte antibodies with identical specificities were detected in both maternal and cord serum and both sera agglutinated the infant's leucocytes. After birth, the infant developed pronounced leucopenia and died of overwhelming infection. A whole family with multiple cases of neonatal neutropenia has also been reported (Lalezari et al. 1960) where the first child died of severe infection, the second was symptomless, while the third and fourth child suffered from mild agranulocytosis which lasted about 10 weeks. A potent leucoagglutinin was detected in the mother's serum which agglutinated leucocytes from the father and all three available children but did not react with her own cells. An identical leucoagglutinin was found in the serum of the last baby which disappeared within a few weeks.

Other investigators were unable to confirm the association between maternal leucocyte antibodies and foetal leucopenia. Abilgaard and Jensen (1964) followed up a group of 44 infants born to mothers with leucocyte antibodies but found no reduction in mean leucocyte or granulocyte counts two weeks after birth. Of the 44 cord sera, leucoagglutinins were demonstrable in 10 (23%). The antibody in cord sera all had similar specificities as the antibody in maternal sera, as demonstrated with a panel from six different donors. Furthermore, maternal sera in 22 out of 28 (80%) cases agglutinated corresponding foetal leucocytes. Thus it would appear that the presence of leucocyte antibodies in maternal serum and in cord serum, even when they are directed at foetal antigenic specificities, does not seem to lead to any damaging effects on the foetus. It may be argued that in this series, haematological investigations were not done until two months after delivery by which time any transient depression in leucocyte count could have returned to normal. This criticism does not apply to the series of Payne (1964) who did haematological examinations on newborn infants within the first four days of life. He compared 39 newborn infants born to mothers with leucoagglutinins with 79 infants born to mothers without leucoagglutinins and found no significant difference in total leucocyte or differential counts. Overweg and Engelfriet (1969) looked for cytotoxic leucocyte antibodies in pregnant sera and found them to be present in 15 out of 116 women. No case of granulopenia or lymphopenia was seen among the infants although maternal serum was cytotoxic to her foetal white cells in vitro.

The contradictory results may be due to the fact that the outcome to the foetus could be determined by additional factors like antibody titre and class of antibody rather than the mere presence of leucocyte agglutinins. Jensen (1962) observed that leucoagglutinins were detectable in cord serum only when the titre in the corresponding maternal serum was 1 in 8 or higher. In 34 cases where maternal serum had 'complete' antibody, no case of neutropenia was seen among the infants but in four cases where the mothers had 'incomplete' antibody, an appreciably lower leucocyte count was detected in all the children. Braun et al. (1960) reported a mother who was given a transfusion of fresh blood from her husband and subsequently delivered three infants with neutropenia out of seven pregnancies, the other four infants being symptomless. It was suggested that this could be due to the presence of a high titre of leucocyte antibody in the mother resulting from initial sensitisation by husband's blood and with each successive pregnancy acting as a further booster. The fact that of the seven children some were affected while others were not, point to the leucocyte antibody being directed at allo-antigens on the infant's neutrophils.

It can be seen from the above review that the evidence relating to the association between maternal leucocyte antibodies and neonatal neutropenia is unconvincing. Leucocyte counts usually vary widely in neonates, so it can be difficult to distinguish a pathological leucocyte count from one which may be at the lower limit of physiological variation. The picture may be further confused by the fact that the leucocyte pool in bone marrow is very large in contrast to the erythrocyte pool, so that any mild destruction is easily compensated. Nevertheless, the conclusion would seem to be that, unlike erythrocyte antibodies, maternal leucocyte antibodies appear to have very little effect on foetal white cells, and any abnormalities that may result are usually mild and transient.

9.4 Platelet antibodies

The platelet is another blood cell which expresses allo-antigens including some HL-A specificities, so it is a potential target for iso-immune reactions.

Harrington et al. (1953) reported two cases where babies born to normal mothers developed thrombocytopenia shortly after birth. Anti-platelet agglutinins were present in both children's sera. In one case, maternal serum had demonstrable agglutinins which reacted against the child's platelets plus six other unrelated platelet suspensions, but not with the mother's own platelets, indicating that the antibody was directed at foetal allo-specificity which was not possessed by the mother. There was no history of a previous transfusion so she could have been sensitised by her pregnancy. Schulman et al. (1954) reported another three infants born to a normal mother, all of whom developed purpura with thrombocytopenia within two hours of delivery, but returned to normal after two weeks. After the third pregnancy, the mother's serum was found to contain a strong platelet agglutinin which reacted with platelets from her husband, the infant and a group of normal controls. The infant's serum also contained agglutinins which reacted with its own platelets. The case, however, was complicated by the finding of an auto-agglutinin in maternal serum which reacted with her own platelets, in spite of her being clinically normal. It is, therefore, not possible to decide whether this case involved the transfer of an auto-antibody or an iso-antibody or both.

A serious difficulty in the investigation of platelet agglutinins is the tendency for these cells to agglutinate spontaneously. A method has been devised to circumvent these difficulties by Sell et al. (1969), where the fixation of antibody on the test cells is monitored by the formation of mixed cell clumps formed by the test cells and antibody-coated indicator red cells in the presence of an antiglobulin bridge. Using this method, Garrett et al. (1960) investigated the serum of a normal mother who gave birth to an infant with generalised petechial rash developing after delivery. An anti-platelet antibody was detected in the mother's serum which reacted with the platelets from the father and from 10 normal controls to a dilution of 1 in 320. There was no reaction with the mother's own platelets, even at dilutions as low as 1 in 2 and 1 in 20.

Complement-fixation has been used to detect anti-platelet antibodies in the sera of four normal mothers who had given birth to six children between them, all of whom developed neonatal purpura (Shulman et al. 1962). In two families, they found foetal-maternal incompatibility for a platelet antigenic system which they had previously defined as PL^{A1}, while in the other two families there was foetal-maternal incompatibility for a PL^{B1} system.

From these results, it can be seen that maternal anti-platelet antibodies, produced as a result of iso-immunisation during pregnancy and directed at foetal antigenic specificities, can occasionally damage foetal platelets. There is another group of neonatal thrombocytopenic purpura where both the infant and the mother are affected. Epstein et al. (1950) described five mothers with thrombocytopenic purpura who delivered children all of whom had evidence of depressed platelet counts and three had clinical manifestations of petechial haemorrhages. A review of the literature revealed reports of 39 other such pregnancies with about half the children born being affected. All the affected children usually returned to normal within a few months which supported the suggestion that the neonatal thrombocytopenia was due to some factor which had come from the mother. Many other similar cases have since been described (Vandenbroucke and Verstraete 1955; Jones et al. 1961). In most of these cases, anti-platelet antibodies were detected in the infant's serum as well as the mother's serum and these antibodies reacted with both infant and maternal platelets. These antibodies, therefore, are probably maternal auto-antibodies which have developed during some auto-allergic process and not iso-antibodies. The fact that in all the cases described, the neonatal thrombocytopenia was invariably transient with rapid spontaneous recovery of the infant, suggests that transmission of maternal anti-platelet auto-antibody is likely to be the causative factor rather than some shared hereditary predisposition to this disease by mother and offspring.

9.5 Auto-antibodies

The observation in the preceding section that maternal auto-antibodies can damage foetal platelets raises the question whether other types of auto-antibodies may lead to similar consequences. Many diseases are accompanied by the appearance of antibodies in the patient's serum which are directed at his own cellular components. Although most of these antibodies are generally considered as merely side-effects of an underlying immunological derangement and have not been directly incriminated as actually causing the disease, it is possible that they may play a part in maintaining some of the secondary inflammatory manifestations. The materno-foetal transmission of these antibodies and their effects on the foetus will therefore provide a natural in vivo opportunity to study the role of these antibodies in the pathogenesis of auto-allergic conditions.

9.5.1 Auto-antibodies associated with connective tissue disorders

A variety of auto-antibodies appear in the sera of patients suffering from connective tissue disorders like systemic lupus erythematosus (SLE) or rheumatoid arthritis. Since the original observation of the LE phenomenon, it has been subsequently shown that this is mediated by an antibody to the patient's nuclear material. This activity of lupus serum lies in its IgG fraction and is thus able to be transmitted from mother to foetus. There have been numerous reports on the presence of the LE factor in the sera of infants born to mothers with SLE (Bridge and Foley 1954; Berlyne et al. 1957; Burman and Oliver 1958; Mijer and Olsen 1958; Nathan and Snapper 1958; Beck and Rowell 1963). At birth, the titre of this antibody in the newborn's serum is as high as that in the mother. The concentration gradually falls with a half-life roughly equivalent to that of γ-globulin catabolism, and is usually no longer demonstrable in the infant's serum by about the 7th week. These findings, therefore, support the maternal origin of the LE factor in newborn sera. None of the infants showed any clinical signs of SLE, when examined, up to six months of age. Although it could be argued that this follow-up period is too short to conclude that these infants will not develop SLE in later life, it does indicate that the presence of the LE factor does not lead to any immediate effects in the foetus. This is in accord with current thoughts about the role of the LE factor in the pathogenesis of SLE. Since the nuclear antigen against which the LE factor is directed is intracellular in location and is, therefore, inaccessible to the antibody in vivo, it seems unlikely that this antibody can play an aetiological role in the immunological disorder. It is more reasonable to suppose that the LE factor is produced as a response to the liberation of nuclear material which is not rapidly degraded due to the widespread cellular destruction accompanying the SLE disease process.

The LE factor may also be present in rheumatoid arthritis, but the rheumatoid factor is detected with a greater regularity in the sera of these patients. The rheumatoid factor is a high molecular weight substance, probably an IgM antibody, so it is not expected to be readily transmitted to the foetus. This was confirmed by Den Oudsten et al. (1958) who reported a mother with rheumatoid arthritis whose blood contained the LE factor as well as the rheumatoid factor but only the LE factor was detected in the sera of her newly delivered twins. In another series of six women with rheumatoid arthritis, the rheumatoid factor was consistently absent in the cord blood of their newborns.

In addition to the LE factor and rheumatoid factor, there are other auto-antibodies associated with connective tissue disorders which have been shown to be unequivocally destructive. These antibodies are directed at the patient's own haemopoietic tissue resulting in auto-haemolytic anaemia, leucopenia, or thrombocytopenia which are frequently associated lesions in SLE or rheumatoid arthritis. Transmission of these maternal auto-antibodies will, therefore, be expected to affect the foetus. In the case described by Nathan and Snapper (1958), a mother had SLE with thrombocytopenia. At delivery, the child also had thrombocytopenia but not SLE. Serological investigations demonstrated the presence of LE factor and platelet agglutinins in cord and maternal sera. Another case, of a mother with SLE who developed haemolytic anaemia with a positive Coombs' test, together with leucopenia and mild thrombocytopenia, was reported by Seip (1960). The newborn infant was affected by similar but transient haematological symptoms with complete recovery by three and a half months of age. Although not directly related to SLE, the case reported by Chaplin et al. (1973) further confirms that transmission of maternal auto-antibody can result in auto-haemolytic disease in her infant. They described a woman with a history of auto-immune haemolytic anaemia who delivered an infant with mild hyperbilirubinaemia and a fall in haemoglobin value to 50% of the normal cord blood level by the 8th week. On serological investigation, both maternal and cord blood erythrocytes were found to be coated with IgG, with free auto-antibody demonstrable in cord serum. This antibody was not directed at any blood group specificity. Comparison of maternal and infant red cell phenotypes revealed none of the incompatibilities commonly responsible for iso-immune haemolytic disease of the newborn. These observations therefore indicate that the infant was probably affected by a red cell auto-antibody. Review of the literature for the past 50 years revealed another 19 cases of pregnancy occurring in women with auto-immune haemolytic anaemia. Of 11 infants who survived, three had definite evidence of severe postnatal haemolysis.

9.5.2 Auto-antibodies associated with thyroïd disorders

Auto-antibodies to several normal thyroid constituents can be detected in the serum of patients with a variety of thyroid diseases. These may be conveniently discussed under separate headings:

(1) those antibodies associated with destructive thyroid lesions; and
(2) those antibodies associated with stimulatory thyroid lesions.

The destructive thyroid lesions in Hashimoto's disease are frequently accompanied by the appearance of auto-antibodies directed at various thyroid components like thyroglobulin or microsomal antigens of the epithelial cell cytoplasm. Although it has been suggested that the glandular destruction may be mediated by these auto-antibodies, the exact mechanism involved is not clear. A similar lesion to Hashimoto's thyroiditis can be produced in experimental animals by immunisation with homologous thyroid antigens, but injections of anti-thyroid antibodies into normal animals have failed to evoke any glandular damage. The transmission of these auto-antibodies from mother to foetus has provided a natural experimental situation for the study of the effects of passive transfer of these antibodies in man. Beierwaltes et al. (1959) tested the sera of a family with cretins for the presence of thyroid antibodies by haemagglutination, complement-fixation and precipitation techniques in comparison with a control group. Their study failed to support the hypothesis that transmission of thyroid auto-antibodies from mother to foetus can result in congenital hypothyroidism. The findings of Parker and Beierwaltes (1961) are in agreement with this conclusion. They found that thyroid auto-antibodies detected in the sera of nine mothers at the time of delivery were also detected in eight of their infants' cord blood. These antibodies gradually disappeared from the infants' circulation during the first three months after birth suggesting they were of maternal origin. None of the infants, however, had any clinical signs of hypothyroidism and the levels of serum protein-bound iodine at birth were within normal limits.

One variety of auto-antibody present in Hashimoto's disease has been shown to have cytopathic effects on human thyroid cells grown in culture, and it is possible that only this antibody has a pathogenic significance and not the others. Blizzard et al. (1960) tested the sera of mother/infant pairs for thyroid auto-antibodies by haemagglutination, precipitation, complement-fixation and Coon's immunofluorescence. Antibodies were detected in the sera of five mother/infant pairs. Of these infants, three were normal but two were cretins. The sera of the mothers of the two cretins contained a cytotoxic antibody against cultured human thyroid tissue in addition to the other varieties of auto-antibodies. Sutherland et al. (1960) similarly described a hypothyroid mother who gave birth to two hypothyroid infants. The mother's serum also contained an auto-antibody which was cytotoxic to thyroid tissue in vitro.

Thus, it would appear that, of the many thyroid auto-antibodies demonstrable by different methods in the sera of patients with destructive thyroid lesions, only the cytotoxic antibody may have an aetiological significance. It has been suggested that the in vivo damage to thyroid cell surface may be initiated by sensitised lymphocytes (Doniach and Roitt 1968), while the cytotoxic auto-antibody then leads to further destruction.

It has long been suspected that many instances of hyperthyroidism may also have an auto-allergic basis, with the auto-antibody acting in a stimulatory capacity on the thyroid cell surface rather than causing cell destruction. The sera of patients with thyrotoxicosis frequently contain a substance given the name of 'long-acting thyroid stimulator (LATS)' which can mimic the biological effects of pituitary thyroid-stimulating hormone (TSH) when assayed in an animal system, the main difference being the longer time course of the action of LATS. That LATS and TSH are two different substances is supported by the findings that LATS cannot be extracted from the pituitary and is not inactivated by anti-TSH serum. On gel filtration, LATS activity is recovered in the 7S peak while TSH is in the 4S peak. Further characterisation of LATS revealed it to possess many of the characteristics of a thyroid-specific antibody. Its activity resides in the IgG fraction and only Fab or $F(ab')_2$ fragments are stimulatory and not the Fc. This activity can be absorbed preferentially with thyroid microsomes and can be subsequently eluted under acid conditions like other antigen-antibody reactions.

Since the discovery of LATS, the presence of another substance, given the name of 'LATS-protector (LATS-P)' has been described in the serum of LATS-negative patients with thyrotoxicosis (Adams and Kennedy 1967, 1971). This substance also appears to be an IgG and has the ability to interfere with the inhibition of LATS by an extract of human thyroid gland, hence the origin of its name. LATS-P itself has also been shown to stimulate colloid droplet formation in human thyroid gland but not in mouse or rhesus monkey thyroid. Thus, the presence of either LATS or LATS-P type of auto-antibody in almost all cases of thyrotoxicosis provides strong support for the auto-allergic basis of this disease (Hoffenberg 1974). The antibody may operate via the adenyl cyclase system after stimulating receptors on the surface of the thyroid cells. This concept of antibodies stimulating cells rather than damaging them is not unique to thyroid diseases but can be seen in other situations like the blast-transformation of lymphocytes by anti-lymphocyte or anti-IgG allotype sera.

If LATS or LATS-P type of IgG auto-antibody are indeed the cause of adult hyperthyroidism, then the potential effects on the foetus of trans-placental transmission of these substances must be considered as a real threat to foetal well-being. Early investigators reporting on the occurrence of neonatal thyrotoxicosis in infants born to thyrotoxic mothers, were uncertain of the pathogenic mechanisms involved (Koerner 1954; Javett et al. 1959), but the possibility that some of the cases might have been due to the transplacental passage of some maternal thyroid-stimulating substances was discussed (Sclare 1960). The original suggestion that maternal TSH might be responsible is discounted by McKenzie (1964) for several reasons. Excess TSH is not usually associated with hyperthyroidism. When the clinical features of the cases described in the literature are analysed, it is found that the average duration of the neonatal hyperthyroid state is 1—3 months. This is too long for what is known about the half-life of thyrotropin in the circulation. Finally, experimental work on animals has indicated that TSH appears not to cross the placenta, so it is perhaps improbable that it can do so in man.

With the discovery of LATS in association with adult hyperthyroidism, investigators began to look for the presence of this substance in neonatal thyrotoxicosis. Rosenberg et al. (1963) were the first to report a case of neonatal thyrotoxicosis with demonstrable LATS in the infant's serum which rapidly disappeared. This was followed by the demonstration of LATS in the sera of a further five children with neonatal Grave's disease and in the sera of their mothers by McKenzie (1964). The half-life of LATS in the sera of these children was about 1—2 weeks. Up till 1971, there were a total of 13 reported cases of neonatal hyperthyroidism, associated with demonstrable LATS in the foetal circulation ranging from 89—264 units (Samuel et al. 1971). The relatively short half-life of LATS in the neonate's serum of 4—8 days (Maisey and Stimmler 1972) is suggestive of maternal origin. In those cases of neonatal thyrotoxicosis where LATS is not demonstrable, it seems that LATS-P is present instead. Thus, in the case originally reported by Thomson and Riley (1966), where no LATS was found in the serum of the mother or the affected infant, subsequent assay of the mother's serum found LATS-P to be readily detectable (Thomson et al. 1975). Two further cases of neonatal thyrotoxicosis associated with LATS-P but not LATS were reported by Dirmikis et al. (1974) and Nutt et al. (1974).

It can be seen, therefore, that transmission of maternal LATS or LATS-P can affect the foetus, resulting in hyperthyroidism which is usually transient. It must not be concluded that all cases of neonatal thyrotoxicosis are necessarily due to this pathogenic mechanism. Hollingsworth et al. (1972) described seven newborns and young infants with Grave's disease with many features which were not readily explainable by the transfer of maternal factors. The infants' hyperthyroidism was not transient but could last as long as five years which was the maximum period of observation. The mother of one of the children did not have Grave's disease while two other mothers developed the disease subsequent to the birth of their children. All the cases occurred in families with a high incidence of Grave's disease among the relatives. These observations prompted the authors to suggest that an inherited predisposition to the disease might be responsible.

9.5.3 Auto-antibodies associated with pernicious anaemia

Two distinct antibodies directed against gastric antigens may be found in the sera of patients with pernicious anaemia. One is the parietal cell antibody and the other is the intrinsic factor antibody. Fisher and Taylor (1967) reported three mothers with circulating parietal cell antibody who were suffering from gastric mucosal disease. These antibodies were also detected in the cord sera of their infants but were not found in the infants' gastric juice. One infant also had a high titre of intrinsic factor antibody in his serum but not in his gastric juice. All three infants were healthy, indicating that the presence of these maternal antibodies in the foetal circulation has no detrimental effects on foetal B12 absorption. This is in accord with the findings in adult pernicious anaemia where it has been shown that circulating intrinsic factor antibody has no effect on the absorption of B12 but that it is the locally produced antibody in the stomach, possibly of IgA class, which can bind intrinsic factor and thereby inhibits absorption of the vitamin. It is, therefore, interesting to note that megaloblastic anaemia has been reported in infants who were breast-fed by mothers with pernicious anaemia (Zuelzer and Rutzky 1953; Lampkin et al. 1966). Although this was attributed to a deficiency of vitamin B12 in breast milk of these mothers, the alternative explanation that this could be due to transmission of maternal IgA intrinsic factor antibody locally to foetal stomach should also be considered.

9.5.4 Auto-antibodies associated with myasthenia gravis

Myasthenia gravis in newborn infants occurs in two forms. One is a persistent illness which occurs in children of normal mothers. The other is a transient illness which occurs in children born to mothers affected with myasthenia gravis. It is this latter group, known as neonatal myasthenia gravis, which is relevant to our present discussion. In a survey of the literature. Namba et al. (1970) found 80 neonates reported to be affected by this form of myasthenia gravis and added two more cases of their own. It was estimated that about 12% of babies born to mothers with myasthenia gravis were affected, with the disease lasting a maximum of 47 days. A complete recovery was usual.

The transient nature of the neonatal disease and the invariable presence of the disease in the mother suggest the transfer of some maternal factors to the foetus, but as yet, there is no indication what these factors are. The sera of some myasthenia gravis patients, particularly the IgG fraction, have been found to bind to striations of skeletal muscle. Since IgG can readily traverse the placenta, it has been suggested that this maternal auto-antibody may be responsible for the neuromuscular block in both the mother and her infant (Brit. med. J. 1966). Unfortunately, there is no complete correlation between the presence of this antibody and the disease and in one of the mother/infant pairs described by Namba et al. (1970), muscle striation-binding globulin was positive in the serum of the mother but was absent in the infant.

Thus, although there is reason for suspecting myasthenia gravis to be caused by some immunological derangement, it would be premature to incriminate the anti-muscle antibody as the aetiological agent. It may well be that the auto-antibodies in myasthenia gravis, like those found in many other auto-allergic conditions, are merely immunological markers of an underlying disease process.

9.6 Allotype suppression

Immunoglobulins possess a number of genetic markers which are inherited in allelic forms from both parents. It has been shown in animals that anti-allotype antibodies directed against a paternally derived allele which is absent in the mother can lead to suppression in the production of immunoglobulins with paternal specificities by the foetus (Dray 1972). This deficiency may be compensated by an increased production of immunoglobulins bearing maternal allotypes so that the total immunoglobulin level in the foetus remains unchanged. During allotype suppression, the cells secreting the relevant allotype antibody cannot be detected in the circulation, which indicates that the mechanism of suppression is probably by preventing the development of lymphocytes which secrete immunoglobulins of the target allotype, rather than by interference with the secretion of immunoglobulin of the relevant allotype (Catty and Lowe 1976). A state of chronic suppression can be maintained for an extensive period, even in the absence of further sources of anti-allotype antibody. It is generally believed that this persistence of suppression may be due to the presence of specific regulatory T-cells inhibiting the development of those B-cells responsible for secreting immunoglobulins belonging to the suppressed allotype (Jacobson et al. 1972).

At present, there is no conclusive evidence that allotype suppression occurs in man, for although anti-allotype antibodies have been detected in maternal sera, their effects on foetal immunoglobulin synthesis have not been documented. Human immunoglobulins carry genetic markers on their light and heavy chains. The markers for IgG heavy chains are designated as Gm, for IgA heavy chains as Am, and for light chains as Inv. Fudenberg and Fudenberg (1964) reported the appearance of an anti-Gm(a) antibody in the serum of a Gm(a—) mother during the third trimester of her fourth pregnancy. The father was Gm(a+) and since the newborn was found to produce small amounts of Gm(a+) immunoglobulin in his serum, it must be this foetal immunoglobulin which had immunised the mother to produce anti-allotype antibody directed towards paternal Gm specificity. Vyas et al. (1970) observed that about 15% of mothers of recently delivered babies had anti-IgA in their sera which might be directed against Am allotypes. Since these women had not received any form of parenteral IgA, it was thought that the antigenic source for maternal sensitisation was IgA bearing paternal allotypes produced by the foetus. A case of immunisation by foetal immunoglobulin light chain Inv allotype in a primiparous Inv (I—a—) woman who had never received a blood transfusion has been reported by Faulk et al. (1974b). Both the child and the father were found to be Inv (I+a+). The maternal anti-Inv antibody was an IgM suggesting it was probably a primary response. Examination of the placenta revealed it to be grossly abnormal, being large, pale and oedematous. A subsequent child which was also Inv (I+a+), did not result in further sensitisation of the mother. The placenta of this second child was normal. These observations suggest that perhaps only when the placenta is abnormal resulting in impaired control of placental traffic, can a sufficient amount of foetal immunoglobulin reach the maternal circulation to induce sensitisation.

It is interesting to note that, as well as maternal sensitisation to foetal immunoglobulin allotype, it seems that the reverse can also occur. Foetal sensitisation by maternal Gm allotype has been reported (Faulk et al. 1974b) where a Gm(a—) newborn of a Gm(a+) mother was found to develop a high titre antibody with a Gm(a) specificity. In an examination of 130 pairs of maternal and cord blood, Vyas et al. (1970) found an anti-IgA antibody with limited specificity in one specimen of cord blood which was not present in the corresponding maternal blood. It was postulated that this antibody must have been produced by the foetus, probably as a result of sensitisation by maternal IgA. This foetal sensitisation may persist into adulthood. The data of McKay and Thom (1971) suggest that in many instances where maternal sera contain anti-allotype antibodies, the source of sensitisation is not the foetus but the maternal grandmother. A similar idea was entertained by Steinberg and Wilson (1963) who observed that antibodies against a hereditary γ-globulin factor was present in eight non-transfused patients who themselves were lacking the factor but each patient's mother had it. The probability that this was due to chance was calculated to be very low, so it was concluded that these antibodies could have been formed against the allotype of their mothers' γ-globulin in utero.

The presence of maternal anti-allotype antibodies does not appear to be associated with any clinically obvious symptoms in the foetus. Nathenson et al. (1971) examined the sera of 1,763 normal pregnant women for antibodies against Gm(a), Gm(b) and Gm(f) and found them to be present in 28 (1.59%). All, but one, of these 28 mothers delivered normal infants. The one case of foetal death was a pair of premature twins. Four infants were found to be incompatible with their mothers for Gm groups while seven infants were compatible out of 11 families which were followed up. The IgG levels in all these infants monitored serially over a period were within normal limits so it would appear that foetal-maternal incompatibility for Gm factors does not result in any clearly definable deficiencies of immunoglobulin synthesis. However, the possibility that there might have been some suppression of one allotype with the compensatory production of another allele cannot be entirely excluded. Thom and McKay (1971) similarly found no relationship between the presence of anti-globulin antibodies in pregnant women and occurrence of pregnancy complications, neonatal illness or neonatal deaths. These antiglobulin antibodies in pregnant women also had no demonstrable effects on total IgG concentration or proportion of IgG sub-classes in their infants when measured at six months of age.

The overall conclusion would seem to be that, although both the mother and the foetus can be sensitised to each other's immunoglobulin allotype and the potential for allotype suppression exists, the net effect of anti-allotype antibodies in human foetal-maternal interaction appears to be small, unlike in experiments on pregnant mice where antibodies directed against genetic groups of γ-globulin are associated with an increased incidence of congenital malformation and foetal deaths (Lieberman and Dray 1964). In relation to anti-Gm allotypes, at least one explanation may be that much of this antibody in maternal serum is found in the 19S globulins and only a small proportion is of 7S class (Nathenson et al. 1971), so very little of this antibody will be transmitted to the foetus. There has been one report of an anti-Gm(a) antibody with characteristics of IgA (Allen 1967) but this immunoglobulin also does not cross the placenta in any appreciable quantity, so its effects on the foetus would be minimal. It is an interesting speculation that suppression by maternal antibodies on the part of the foetus to synthesise paternally inherited molecules may not necessarily be confined to immunoglobulin allotypes. Such a mechanism could be involved in other allelic systems like HL-A or other antigens, whereby it may be postulated that preventing the expression of paternally derived antigens in the foetus by maternal antibody may be another way the foetus is protected against maternal cell-mediated immunity (Tuffrey et al. 1976).

10

Effects of antigenic disparity on foetal-maternal interaction

10.1 Effects on placental weight and size

Billington (1964), using A_2G and C57BL inbred mice, found that placental weight was increased when females of either strain were mated to males of the opposite strain. A_2G embryos also produced heavier placentae than C57BL embryos when both were transplanted to C57BL foster mothers. It was proposed that increased antigenic disparity between mother and foetus could result in increased placental weight. Similar effects on placental weight could be achieved by prior sensitisation of female mice to paternal strain antigens (James 1965, 1967). Female C57BL mice were divided into three groups. The first group consisted of untreated controls. The second 'immune' group had recently received skin grafts and/or spleen cell injections from A_2G mice, while a third 'tolerant' group had received spleen cell injections from A_2G mice at birth. On mating to A_2G males, it was found that the embryos in 'immune' females had heavier placentae than the controls, while those in 'tolerant' females had lighter placentae. From these observations, Clarke and Kirby (1966) formulated their hypothesis that foetal-maternal antigenic disparity was beneficial to the development of the embryo and it was because of this selective system that a balanced polymorphism for transplantation antigens was maintained in mammals.

Human data, however, are sparse and conflicting. Warburton and Naylor (1971) reported that placental weight and birth weight showed a tendency to increase with parity, the greatest increment occurring between parities 1 and 2. The effects of successive pregnancies by the same or by different fathers were also compared and it was found that the increments in placental and birth weight were usually smaller when the fathers changed between pregnancies. These results were interpreted as supporting Clarke and Kirby's (1966) hypothesis in that the increase in placental weight with parity if the father remained the same was thought to be due to a greater degree of maternal sensitisation to paternal antigens.

In an analysis of maternal blood groups and placental weight, Jones (1968a) reported that the mean placental weight for group 'O' mothers was 629 ± 3.1 g compared to 639 ± 3.1 g for groups 'A', 'B', and 'AB' combined. The mothers were not divided according to parity. No foetal blood groups were studied but it was assumed from ABO gene frequency calculations that group 'O' mothers would be expected to be incompatible with their foetuses more often than mothers of the other blood groups. The conclusion was that disparity between mother and foetus for ABO antigens resulted in a smaller placenta, a finding which was, therefore, the reverse of that observed in animal studies. Subsequent studies, when ABO groups of mother and child pairs were analysed, revealed no difference at all in placental weights in compatible and incompatible pregnancies. Seppälä and Tolonen (1970) studied the ABO blood groups of 3,045 mother/child pairs but excluding Rh immunised mothers. The mother/child pairs were divided into three groups of compatible (O/O, A/A, B/B, AB/AB), pseudocompatible (A/O, B/O, AB/A, AB/B), and incompatible (O/A, O/B, A/B, B/A, A/AB, B/AB). These were further subdivided into primiparous and multiparous. No significant differences were observed in the three groups as regards placental weight, birth weight and length of gestation. Furthermore, contrary to the observations of Jones (1968a), the mean placental weight in group 'O' mothers was found not to be lower than that of combined 'A', 'B' and 'AB' mothers in both primiparous and multiparous cases. Hohler et al. (1972) examined 727 normal placentae for total weight, dry weight and water content. These data were then related to maternal and foetal ABO and Rh blood groups. Again, no association was found between foetal-maternal blood group incompatibility and placental weight.

Foetal-maternal incompatibility for leucocyte antigens also appears to have no clear-cut effects on placental weight or birth weight. Brain (1968) compared a group of 86 pregnant women with leucocyte agglutinins in their sera with a control group of 86 subjects, matched for parity and duration of pregnancy who had no demonstrable agglutinins. He found no difference in the mean birth weights in the two groups.

Tait et al. (1974), using a leucocyte migration inhibition assay as a measure of maternal cell-mediated immunity towards foetal antigens, found that a positive reaction correlated with a smaller placenta but birth weight was not affected. On the other hand, Jenkins and Good (1972), using a two-way MLR between 72 pairs of maternal/foetal cells as a measure of antigenic disparity, found that those pairs showing an increased degree of transformation and DNA synthesis compared with single dose cultures were associated with larger placentae. It does seem strange, however, that almost half the MLR between mother-infant pairs in this study should show no more reactivity than in single dose cultures.

It is clear from the above review that antigenic disparity between mother and foetus does not seem to influence placental weight or birth weight to any great extent in human reproduction. Even the results and conclusions from original animal studies are now increasingly being questioned, as more and more recent evidence points in the opposite direction (McLaren 1975). It would seem that the hypothesis of antigenic disparity between mother and foetus being beneficial to the development of the latter and thereby contributing to the maintenance of histocompatibility antigen polymorphism is probably no longer tenable.

10.2 Influence of sex-linked antigens

The human sex ratio (M:F) at birth is approximately 109:100 with a slight variation in different population groups. Serr and Ismajovich (1963) reported a figure of 165.9:100 among 125 therapeutic abortions (i.e. where the foetuses were not abnormal) between the 5—8th week of gestation. If this ratio were to be projected further back to conception, it may well be very much higher. This preponderance of males has been cited as further support for the hypothesis that genetic disparity between mother and foetus is beneficial to the development of the foetus (Kirby et al. 1967; Kirby 1970), since the male zygote has an additional Y-antigen which is not possessed by the mother. As we have discussed in the preceding section, this hypothesis appears unlikely. In fact, male conceptuses have been observed to be spontaneously aborted more frequently than females (Serr and Ismajovich 1963) and more male foetuses are associated with ante-partum and accidental haemorrhages (Rhodes 1965), so there appears to be a greater differential loss of male foetuses between conception and birth. When viewed in conjunction with the observation that female placentae are more prone to undergo neoplastic transformation (see Chapter 12), the combined data would seem to indicate that the female conceptus is better adapted to survive in the maternal uterine environment than the male.

In terms of transplantation biology, this differential viability may be due to the presence of an histocompatibility antigen controlled directly or indirectly by genes on the Y chromosome. There is already considerable evidence for the existence of such a system in animal species. In inbred mice, for example, female to male isografts are usually accepted but similar grafts from male to virgin females are rejected (Eichwald and Silmser 1955). Tolerance to these male skin grafts can be induced in the females by successive matings, the degree of tolerance being roughly proportional to the number of previous pregnancies (Prehn 1960). While virgin females rejected all male skin grafts, 60% of similar grafts survived in females who have had 1—3 litters increasing to 90% graft survival in females who have had 4—6 litters.

Although many investigators found no significant difference in survival rates between male and female recipients in human transplantation (Beleil et al. 1972; Gerhard and Terasaki 1977), a survey by Oliver (1974) showed a significantly better survival of female recipients of male renal allografts compared to female recipients of female allografts. This was observed particularly in multiparous and not in nulliparous recipients suggesting the possibility of development of tolerance to male antigens as a result of previous pregnancies. This tolerance may be mediated by 'blocking' factors, perhaps anti-Y antibodies, for certain sera from multiparous women have been observed to inhibit the MLR of female lymphocytes when stimulated by male HL-A incompatible lymphocytes but not when similarly stimulated by female HL-A incompatible lymphocytes (Brochier et al. 1974).

In contrast, other data on the human sex ratio seem to indicate that successive pregnancies result, not in tolerance, but in increased sensitisation to male antigen. Renkonen et al. (1962) found that the sex ratio at birth became progressively lower the greater the number of previous male pregnancies. This finding suggested that previous male pregnancies could immunise some mothers against the male (Y) antigen. This resulted in a greater differential loss of male foetuses and, in turn, would reduce the sex ratio at birth. However, McLaren (1962) failed in an attempt to test this hypothesis experimentally by sensitising inbred strains of C57BL female mice with male spleen cells and spermatozoa, and also by grafting male skin to female recipients. These sensitised females were then mated and the sex ratio of the first litter was determined. No deviation from the normal sex ratio was observed. It must, however, be remembered that experiments on isogeneic strains of mice may not be directly comparable with the situation in man. In human outbred populations, the expression of a weak antigenic system like the Y-linked system is likely to be complex and may be dependent on the degree of interaction with other stronger histocompatibility systems.

An association between a Y-linked antigenic system and ABO blood groups is supported by the findings of Allan (1959) who collected a large number of cases of his own and also analysed other series from the literature. It was found that the sex ratio at birth of 'AB' mothers was significantly higher than that of 'O', 'A', and 'B' mothers combined. The sex ratio of group 'O' babies as a whole, regardless of the blood group of the mother, was also significantly greater than that of group 'A' babies as a whole. These results indicate that the Y-linked antigen is hardly expressed in the absence of ABO incompatibility. That the Y antigen may only manifest itself through the cumulative effects with ABO incompatibility is supported by the studies of Toivanen and Hirvonen (1970a) on placental weight. They found that only male placentae from the foetuses who were ABO incompatible with their mothers were heavier than those who were compatible, and male placentae were heavier than female placentae only in ABO incompatible cases. A similar synergistic action of Rh and Y-linked antigens may also occur. Scott and Beer (1973) reported that all eight of their patients who developed anti-D before delivery of their first child gave birth to male infants. The series was subsequently enlarged to 22 cases where 19 gave birth to male infants and only three had female infants (Scott et al. 1977). Renkonen and Timonen (1967) have also observed that among the first-born children of Rh negative mothers who developed erythroblastosis, there were more boys than expected, the male to female ratio being 1.74 compared to 1.062 in normal controls in Finland. These observations, therefore, indicate that there is a greater risk of maternal sensitisation when the foetus is incompatible for both the Rh and Y antigens.

A similar association between the Y-linked and the HL-A system may also be operative in human reproduction. Johansen et al. (1974) found the sex ratio at birth was 1.82 among 61 primigravidae who developed HL-A antibodies compared to a ratio of 0.99 among 384 mothers who did not, suggesting the male foetus was more strongly immunogenic than the female. There was also a tendency among the group of women with antibodies for the sex ratio to fall, as parity increased, from 1.82 in primigravidae to 1.26 after one previous birth and to 1.10 after two or more births. This implies that increasing sensitisation with successive pregnancies can operate selectively against the male foetus which is in agreement with the data of Renkonen et al. (1962). Recently, Goulmy et al. (1977) presented results that human cell-mediated cytotoxic reactions against Y antigens were restricted by an HL-A product in that only targets carrying HL-A2 were lysed. The disparate results obtained about the presence of Y-linked antigens in man may, therefore, be due to some series not having included any HL-A2 positive combinations.

There is evidence to suggest that an X-linked antigenic system can similarly influence the interaction between a female foetus and its mother. An example of this is provided by the Xg^a blood group which is inherited via the X chromosome so that only the daughter of an Xg^a positive father and Xg^a negative mother would be incompatible with the mother but not the son. If this incompatibility is detected by the mother early in gestation, it is conceivable that this may lead to a preferential loss of daughter conceptuses, resulting in a high sex ratio at birth. This has been observed by Jackson et al. (1969) who reported that among the four possible different presentations of Xg^a matings, the one where an Xg^a positive father was married to an Xg^a negative mother had the highest sex ratio at birth with 113 males to 82 females (60.3% males). This sex ratio became even higher with a figure of 63:26 (70.8% males) after the birth of one previous daughter, the hypothesis being that preceding maternal sensitisation to the Xg^a antigen had a detrimental effect on subsequent female pregnancies.

The overall conclusion would seem to be that sex-linked antigens do have some influence on the human foetal-maternal interaction but the exact consequence to the foetus is, at present, unclear. Some data may be interpreted as indicating a detrimental effect on the foetus of appropriate sex with increasing maternal sensitisation, while others seem to suggest that tolerance develops with increasing parity. Finally, it must be pointed out that there may be other factors involved in the differential survival of male and female conceptuses. It has been reported, for example, that serum HCG levels close to term are higher in women bearing female foetuses, indicating that either the sex of the foetus can exert control of HCG production by the placenta or there is a primary genetic difference in placental function between male and female (Boroditsky et al. 1975). Since HCG plays an important immunoregulatory role in pregnancy, this differential production of hormone may influence the survival and growth of male and female placentae in utero. Such a differential survival of trophoblast cells has been observed in guinea pigs where allografts of separated cells from female trophoblast survived considerably longer than cells from male trophoblast (Borland et al. 1970).

10.3 Influence of allo-antigens

10.3.1 Blood group antigenic system

Early reports, mainly of a statistical nature, have indicated that foetal-maternal incompatibility for ABO blood groups may have a detrimental effect on foetal survival, manifested either as infertility or increased rate of abortions. Waterhouse and Hogben (1947), by assembling data from the literature, found a highly significant shortage of group 'A' children from matings of group 'O' mothers with group 'A' fathers. This deficit increased with increasing birth order. It was inferred that there was an intense selection against group 'A' foetuses by group 'O' mothers which might have an immunological basis. In an analysis of 7,856 consecutive mother-child pairs of known blood group, Bryce et al. (1950), in Australia, provided evidence of a relative deficiency of group 'AB' infants and irregularities in the distribution of blood groups among the children of group 'A' and 'B' mothers. These observations were considered tc be suggestive of differential fertility or foetal viability or both. Further data were subsequently provided which confirmed these earlier findings. It was found in Melborne and Perth that group 'A' women had a higher average number of pregnancies than group 'O' women. In addition, a comparison of a calculated and observed number of children in different mother-child blood group combinations for 16,179 single births revealed a significant deficiency of group 'A' children born to group 'O' mothers and of group 'AB' children born to group 'A' and 'B' mothers. This deficiency was not apparent for first-born children, was present for second-born children, and was greatest for third-born children (Kirk et al. 1955). The results of Matsunaga and Itoh (1958) from Japan also implied a deficiency of group 'A' children of group 'O' women married to group 'A' men, and of group 'B' children of group 'O' women married to group 'B' men.

The above statistical studies, therefore, indicate that foetal-maternal ABO incompatibility can exert strong selective pressures and may have adverse effects on human reproductive performance (Brit. med. J. 1954). There are, however, many criticisms of these data. Bennett and Brandt (1954) rejected the primary hypothesis of progressive maternal inhospitality to group 'A' foetuses by group 'O' mothers and criticised the conclusions of Waterhouse and Hogben (1947) on the grounds of heterogeneity of data. Edwards (1957) made a critical evaluation of the data presented and found that grouping errors (over 10% of group 'AB' infants being grouped as 'B' in two series) and paternity errors (over 5% of children were not fathered by their mother's husband in one series) had so complicated the analyses that he had to conclude that any difference in fertility related to ABO blood groups had not yet been satisfactorily demonstrated at the statistical level. Direct investigations on the ABO blood groups of sterile couples (Sjöstedt et al. 1951) have since revealed no significant deviations from control couples and this applied also to the MN and Lewis blood groups (Grubb and Sjöstedt 1955). The corollary to this is the investigation by Wren and Vos (1961) who found that ABO incompatible partners had just as many children as compatible partners. At the present time, therefore, evidence concerning the association between ABO incompatibility and infertility must be regarded as inconclusive.

There have also been many studies on the part played by ABO incompatibility in the induction of spontaneous abortions and early foetal wastage. A positive correlation was reported by Levine (1946) and this was confirmed by McNeil et al. (1954) who found a significantly higher percentage of aborters among ABO incompatible matings (Table 10.1). The group of aborters consisted of women who had aborted twice or more times during the first twenty weeks of gestation. On further analysis of the group of aborters, it was found that when the father was group 'O', the rate of abortion ranged from 11—15%, regardless of the blood group of the wife. If the mother was group 'O' and the father was group 'A' or 'B', these matings resulted in abortion rates of 24.2% for group 'A' husbands to 45.1% for group 'B' husbands. Wren and Vos (1961) had similar findings with 45% of 122 cases of spontaneous abortions having incompatible ABO groups between husband and wife compared to 30% for a control series. In contrast, Sjöstedt et al. (1951), in

Table 10.1 Number of aborters and non-aborters in ABO compatible and incompatible matings.

	Aborters	Non-aborters	Total
ABO incompatible matings	49	122	171
ABO compatible matings	36	197	233

With kind permission from McNeil, C. et al. (1954) *Amer. J. clin. Path.* 24, 767–773.

a study of 242 marriages in which at least two abortions or foetal deaths of unknown cause had occurred, found no increase in the frequency of ABO incompatibility between husband and wife compared to controls. This lack of correlation was confirmed in a later series (Grubb and Sjöstedt 1955) but it was now observed that there might be a slightly higher frequency of ABO incompatible matings in cases of late foetal death. Vos (1965), on the basis of the presence of anti-A or anti-B haemolysins in maternal blood, also formed the opinion that ABO incompatibility might be associated more often with the later stages of obstetric complications like stillbirths and neonatal deaths rather than with early abortions. It is possible that these cases of foetal mortality in the later stages of gestation may have been secondary to ABO haemolytic disease.

Blood group analyses of husband and wife pairs can only provide an indirect measure of foetal-maternal incompatibility and this may be responsible to a large extent for the conflicting results in the literature. More exact information can be obtained if the blood groups of the mothers are directly correlated with those of their aborted foetuses. Several studies of this nature have now been done. Allen (1964) determined the blood groups in spontaneously expelled foetuses or their placentae of 6—18 weeks gestation age and compared the results with the blood groups of the mothers in a series of 40 cases. A distinct difference was noted, with an unusually large proportion of abortuses being group 'B'. In addition, an analysis of 27 mother-abortus pairs showed 10 (37%) to be incompatible. Again the most striking feature was that seven of the 10 incompatibilities were due to antigen 'B'. The results of a larger study of spontaneous abortions not exceeding 20 weeks gestation age were presented by Takano and Miller (1972). They grouped spontaneously aborted foetuses by employing the mixed-agglutination method on foetal red cells or, if these were not available, on tendinous fibres of the foetal abdominal wall. Of 78 abortuses examined, 33 (44.7%) were incompatible with the mother. This was significantly higher ($p < 0.01$) than the expected figure calculated from the ABO phenotype distribution in the general population.

An important cause of spontaneous abortion is chromosomal anomalies, so that ideally these cases should be excluded by karyotyping the abortuses before any blood group analyses are attempted. This was done in a recent study by Lauritsen et al. (1975) who only grouped those foetuses aborted during the first 16 weeks of gestation which were karyotypically normal. The results were then compared with the blood groups of the parents. The findings were as follows:

(1) there was a significantly higher frequency of ABO incompatibility between mother and abortus than in controls;

(2) there was a significantly higher frequency of ABO incompatibility between mother and father than in controls; and

(3) the ABO phenotypes of the abortuses deviated significantly from the general population, there being more group 'A' and group 'B'.

The balance of evidence, therefore, would seem to indicate that foetal-maternal ABO incompatibility can result in early foetal wastage, but the extent to which this occurs appears to be insufficient to have any significant effects on ABO gene frequencies (Cohen 1970). This effect on the foetus seems to be confined to ABO incompatibility, for the other red cell antigens have not been shown to influence foetal well-being. No difference was found by Grubb and Sjöstedt (1955) between aborters and controls with respect to the frequency of Rh incompatibility, nor did the observed distribution of mating classes for MN, Lewis blood groups, secretor and non-secretor characteristics deviate from that expected. Lauritsen et al. (1976a) studied the frequency of antigen incompatible matings with respect to Rh, Lutheran, MN, S, Lewis, Kell, P, and Duffy systems in 481 parents of early spontaneous abortions. No significant differences were observed when the results were compared with the calculated mating frequencies in control samples. Thus, incompatibility for all these other red cell antigenic systems appears unimportant in the aetiology of early spontaneous abortions.

10.3.2 Major histocompatibility antigenic system

Maternal sensitisation to foetal HL-A antigens as evidenced by the production of allo-antibodies does not appear to have any detrimental effects on foetal survival. Jensen (1962) found no relationship between frequency of abortions and women with leucocyte antibodies in their sera. Similarly, Ahrons (1971a), in a survey of 1,726 pregnant women for cytotoxic antibodies also did not find any correlation between the presence of antibodies and the outcome of pregnancy as manifested by abortions, stillbirths, prematurity and congenital malformations. Zmijewski et al. (1967) were perhaps the only investigators to have reported that women who were habitual aborters had a higher incidence (35.29%) of leucoagglutinins in their sera compared to normal fertile women where antibodies were detected in 25.06%.

In a preliminary study, Terasaki et al. (1970) thought they could just discern an association between the presence of leucocyte antibodies in the mother and the incidence of congenital anomalies, but when the series was subsequently enlarged, the correlation was no longer apparent (Sever and Terasaki 1970). On the basis that maternal leucocyte antibodies might not result in any one particular kind of foetal damage, Harris and Lordon (1976) compared the course of pregnancy in 28 patients with lymphocytotoxic antibodies with 101 patients without antibodies, with respect to a group of obstetric complications which included pre-eclampsia, foetal distress, carbohydrate intolerance, unexplained foetal death, intrauterine growth retardation, congenital anomaly and premature labour. Although no difference in any of these complications was found when tested individually, as a group they tended to occur more often in mothers with cytotoxic antibodies.

In an analysis of the frequency of HL-A incompatible matings in 481 patients with early spontaneous abortions, Lauritsen et al. (1976a) observed no significant difference from the calculated mating frequencies in control samples. There was also no deviation of husband/wife pairs for HL-A phenotypes compared to controls, regardless of whether the abortuses were karyotypically normal or abnormal, so it seems that HL-A incompatibility is also not responsible for foetal chromosomal abnormalities.

Bardawil et al. (1962) observed that in a group of 20 pregnant women whose last three or more pregnancies had terminated in spontaneous abortions, all manifested rapid rejection of skin grafts from husbands four times more frequently than with grafts from unrelated donors. It was concluded that an increased degree of maternal sensitivity towards husband's antigens might have been responsible for the recurrent abortions. That a high degree of husband-wife incompatibility may be

a factor in the aetiology of spontaneous abortions is supported by in vitro data. Using a two-way MLR between husband and wife pairs, Halbrecht and Komlos (1968) found the mean percentage of transformed cells was 5.7% in a group of normal fertile couples but, among a group of 22 women who had had repeated abortions, the mean percentage was 14%, 17.1%, and 19.8% for those having had one, two and three abortions respectively. The results obtained by Ohama and Kadotani (1971) showed a similar trend. The mean percentage of transformed cells in a two-way MLR between different groups of husband and wife pairs were found to be as follows:
(1) sterile couples (i.e. those with no children after three years of marriage) had a mean transformation percentage of 10.1 ± 6.8;
(2) those couples who have had two or more previous abortions had a mean transformation percentage of 9.2 ± 6.5; and
(3) the mean transformation for control normal fertile couples was 4.7 ± 6.5. The difference between aborters and controls did not reach statistical significance but the degree of transformation in sterile couples was significantly different ($p < 0.05$) from controls. The cause of the sterility might be due to early embryonic loss or it could be a result of pre-zygotic selection against incompatible spermatozoa.

Recent MLR studies, however, have resulted in contrary findings. Lauritsen et al. (1976b) studied 29 couples with recurrent spontaneous abortions by the one-way MLR. Only those cases where the abortuses were shown to be karyotypically normal were included. They found a significantly depressed MLR in these mothers when stimulated by the respective fathers' lymphocytes but not when stimulated by unrelated lymphocytes. The fathers' lymphocytes stimulated unrelated responders normally so they were not poor stimulators. These results suggest that a depressed maternal cellular recognition of paternal histocompatibility antigens may be related to increased foetal wastage. This conclusion, therefore, is the reverse of what is expected from earlier studies and may be an example of homozygote disadvantage in human reproduction (Beer and Billingham 1977). It has been reported that a significantly higher percentage of women with repeated abortions shared common HL-A antigens with their husbands compared to control groups (Komlos et al. 1977), suggesting there is an increased incidence of homozygotic foetuses in these cases of disturbed pregnancy. This may be interpreted as being in support of the conclusion that genetic compatibility between mother and conceptus tends to reduce reproductive efficiency. Alternatively, it is possible that certain HL-A haplotype associations may lead to functional disturbances in pregnancy. The observations of Lindblom et al. (1972) are in accord with this hypothesis. They studied the HL-A types of eight couples with unexplained infertility and found that haplotypes which, in a control group of fertile couples showed negative associations between 1st and 2nd locus alleles, seemed to occur more frequently among the infertile couples. It was postulated that union of two gametes with certain haplotypes may prevent proper development of a viable foetus.

10.4 Pre-zygotic selection

It must not be thought that selective pressures due to foetal-maternal incompatibility are only exerted through abortions and early foetal wastage. The possibility that this selection may take place at an even earlier stage of the reproductive process before fertilisation should be considered (Clarke 1968). Behrman et al. (1960) postulated that infertility might be due to anti-A or anti-B iso-antibodies in cervical secretions acting on incompatible sperms. For example, if the husband was heterozygous 'AO' and the mother was 'O', her cervical iso-antibodies would select against 'A'-bearing sperms, thereby resulting in the observed excess of group 'O' children born to A♂ x O♀ matings. In support of this hypothesis, they described seven ABO incompatible couples who had tried and failed to have children over the past 10 years. Subsequently, nine offsprings were born and all were group 'O'.

The concept of pre-zygotic selection makes the assumption that human spermatozoa possess allo-antigens and that these antigens are expressed in an haploid manner, so that spermatozoa from an heterozygous male will consist of two populations, of which one will be selected against. In addition, an effective immune response must be available in the female genital tract. Present evidence would seem to indicate that these conditions may be fulfilled.

10.4.1 Allo-antigens of human spermatozoa

As early as 1926, Landsteiner and Levine suggested that human spermatozoa contained substances identical with or similar to the blood group factors A and B of human red cells. Since then, the presence of blood group antigens on human spermatozoa has been confirmed by Gullbring (1957) using a mixed agglutination technique, and by Shahani and Southam (1962) by immunofluorescence, although Holborow et al. (1960) were unsuccessful with the latter method. This disparity in results may be because the period of staining required for spermatozoa is much longer than that usually employed for this type of procedure, for Shahani and Southam (1962) stained their preparations for one hour at 37°C and then left them overnight. It has been suggested that the blood group antigens detected may not be true spermatozoal membrane antigens but are blood group substances from seminal fluid adsorbed on the surface (Parish et al. 1967). Both Gullbring (1957) and Shahani and Southam (1962) provided evidence that spermatozoa from AB donors appeared to be made up of two populations, those staining with anti-A and those staining with anti-B, indicating the possible haploid expression of these antigens. The absence of double staining would seem to be against the random adsorption of blood group substances from seminal fluid. The D antigen, on the other hand, cannot be demonstrated conclusively by either mixed agglutination, absorption, or elution techniques (Levine and Celano 1961). This may be a reflection of relative deficiency of these antigens rather than total absence.

The actual importance of these spermatozoal blood group antigens in pre-zygotic selection is not clear. Although absorption studies have shown that spermatozoa have eight times more blood group substances per spermatozoon than are present per red cell, surprisingly, spermatozoa do not appear to be immobilised either by 'natural' or 'immune' blood group antibodies (Isojima and Tsuzuku 1968), so it is difficult to visualise how selection is mediated in vivo. Ackerman (1967) suggested that the mode of action might be on the metabolism of the spermatozoa. Specific antibody reacting with spermatozoal antigens could change the metabolism from a primary glycolytic pathway to a secondary oxidative pathway. Such a change might be expected to decrease the viability of the affected spermatozoa and consequently their fertilising capacity. It is interesting to note that this diminution in anaerobic glycolysis only occurred when spermatozoa from secretors, but not from non-secretors, were incubated with specific antiserum, which seemed to support the view that the antigens on the surface of spermatozoa taking part in the reaction with antibody might represent adsorbed blood group substances.

The presence of HL-A antigens on human spermatozoa has also been reported. Fellous and Dausset (1970) found that when spermatozoa from heterozygous donors were tested with the appropriate anti-HL-A antisera, lysis of approximately half the population occurred, whereas 70—80% of spermatozoa from homozygous donors were lysed under similar conditions. This difference in cytotoxicity suggests the possible existence of two populations of spermatozoa in heterozygous donors, with each sperm expressing one HL-A haplotype. Arnaiz-Villena and Festenstein (1976) also presented evidence for the haploid expression of HL-A antigens by human spermatozoa, although their results appear to be open to alternative interpretations (Boettcher 1977). Like the situation with blood group antigens, the possibility that spermatozoal HL-A antigens may also be adsorbed from seminal plasma has been suggested (Singal et al. 1971). These investigators demonstrated the presence of substances in human seminal plasma that inhibited specific anti-HL-A antibodies conforming to the HL-A phenotype of the specimen donor.

From the data presented, it may be concluded that human spermatozoa probably do exhibit surface allo-antigens but it is still not certain whether these are true membrane antigens or are soluble substances adsorbed from seminal plasma. Perhaps in practice this distinction may not be too important if interaction of these surface antigens with appropriate maternal antibody can result in a decreased viability of the affected spermatozoa. Either kind of antigens would explain the relative infertility in incompatible matings. However, only the true haploid expression of allo-antigens would permit selection to occur.

10.4.2 Immunological response in the female genital tract

There is much evidence to suggest that the human cervix is capable of mounting a local secretory immune response. Plasma cells are abundant in cervical epithelium and cervical secretions contain immunoglobulins. Although IgG, IgM, and IgA are all present (Tourville et al. 1970), IgA appears to be the predominant immunoglobulin class, making up about 65% of the total (Rebello et al. 1975). In an evaluation of the results from several studies, Vaerman and Férin (1974) came to a similar conclusion that the IgA/IgG ratio in cervical secretions seemed much higher than that found in serum. The low ratios in some earlier data were probably due to the use of 7S serum IgA as a standard against which 11S SIgA of cervical secretions was compared, for it has been demonstrated that equal amounts of the two types of IgA, when measured by radial immunodiffusion, could differ by a factor of three to four. The secretory component has also been identified in cervical secretions (Hulka and Omran 1969), some of this being bound to IgA (Waldman et al. 1972a).

Infections of the female genital tract by N. gonorrhoeae, T. vaginalis or C. albicans have been reported to be associated with an increase in numbers of plasma cells containing all three classes of immunoglobulins, but particularly of IgA, in the lamina propria of the endocervix (Chipperfield and Evans 1972). Specific IgA antibody to Candida with 90% of the antigen-binding capacity present in this immunoglobulin class has been found in cervical secretions (Waldman et al. 1972a). Artificial local immunisation of the female genital tract with typhoid vaccine (Straus 1961), Candida vaccine (Waldman et al. 1972b), and polio vaccine (Ogra and Ogra 1973) have all resulted in the appearance of specific antibodies in cervical secretions. The antibody activity was largely associated with IgA and the response in the genital tract was elicited in the absence of any coincidental response in serum. Parenteral immunisation also resulted in the appearance of specific antibodies in cervical secretions but, in this case, the response was limited to IgG. These antibodies were detected in cervical secretions at the same time as the attainment of the highest titre of similar antibody in serum.

All these observations indicate that the female genital tract can act as a local secretory immune system with the production of specific IgA antibodies, when faced with antigenic challenge. In addition, serum IgG antibodies may also make some contribution to the immunological content of cervical secretions. The ABO haemagglutinins detected in cervical mucus (Gershowitz et al. 1958) may be examples of serum-derived antibodies. An examination of cervical mucus from 182 randomly selected women by Solish et al. (1961) revealed 23.7% to contain iso-agglutinins, this percentage rising to 63.4% if more than one specimen was examined per patient. Group 'O' women had agglutinins more often than group 'A' or 'B' together. This observation, therefore, conforms to a similar pattern found for the appearance of 'immune' anti-A and anti-B in maternal sera following incompatible pregnancies where there is also an excess frequency in group 'O' mothers. Regardless of their origin, the presence of these iso-antibodies in cervical secretions together with the expression of relevant antigens by human spermatozoa would seem to fulfil the necessary conditions for gametic selection in the female genital tract.

11

Immunological factors in pre-eclampsia and eclampsia

The cause of pre-eclampsia is not known but theories abound as to its aetiology. Indeed, it has been described as the disease of theories (Jeffcoate 1966). One theory which has received varying degrees of support over the years is that the disease may have an immunological basis with some defects in immunoregulation leading to widespread systemic pathology (Brit. med. J. 1976; Jenkins 1976; Scott and Jenkins 1976).

11.1 Foetal-maternal interaction at a single gene locus

A theoretical possibility which has been suggested (Kalmus 1946; Penrose 1946) is that incompatibility for a single hypothetical antigen 'A' may be responsible for the disease. This will occur when an aa mother conceives and reacts against an Aa foetus, a situation which is analogous to Rh incompatibility. An essentially similar mechanism, but operating in a reverse manner was put forward by Platt et al. (1958), where the mother possessed the offending antigen and the disease is due to reaction of an aa foetus against an Aa mother.

It is clear from genetic considerations that in both these situations, it would be impossible for either the mothers of affected patients to have pre-eclampsia during the relevant pregnancy or for the daughters of affected patients to develop the disease. For example, with reference to the hypothesis of Platt et al. (1958), the woman with pre-eclampsia must be a heterozygote Aa who has conceived a foetus with a genetic constitution of aa. Since she is Aa, her mother could not possibly have developed pre-eclampsia during that pregnancy, no matter what her genetic constitution. Similarly, a daughter arising from a pre-eclamptic pregnancy cannot later develop the disease because she herself is aa. Yet these cases do occur. In the survey by Platt et al. (1958), it was found that of the 100 women with pre-eclampsia, there were three cases in which the mother had pre-eclampsia during the pregnancy from which the proband arose. This was confirmed by other reports of occurrence of eclampsia in mother-daughter pairs (Humphries 1960). Not only can daughters from toxaemic pregnancies suffer from the disease, they appear to be affected more often than those from control groups, as is shown by the careful study of Chesley et al. (1968) on the incidence of eclampsia among daughters of 260 surviving eclamptic women over a period of 20 years. Thus, it would seem that the theoretical genetic models proposed for the causation of pre-eclampsia or eclampsia are probably too simple and, if indeed the disease were to be due to foetal-maternal genetic incompatibility, then it is likely to be over a series of alleles at different loci.

11.2 Foetal-maternal incompatibility

Since the participation of a single gene in the pathogenesis of pre-eclampsia appears unconvincing on present evidence, investigators have explored the general concept that the greater the degree of foetal-maternal antigenic incompatibility, the more frequently the disease will develop.

11.2.1 Population studies

This concept appears to be supported by the studies of Stevenson et al. (1971, 1976) in Turkey where there is a high frequency of consanguineous marriages. Their data strongly suggested that consanguinity with their husbands was less frequent in women who developed pre-eclampsia than in those who did not have the disease. A conceptus from a consanguineous marriage will, on average, have more compatible genes with the mother than a conceptus from two unrelated parents, so these results may be interpreted as showing a greater predisposition to develop pre-eclampsia with increased foetal-maternal genetic incompatibility.

11.2.2 *Twin studies*

It is well documented that pre-eclampsia occurs more frequently in twin pregnancies than in single pregnancies (McFarlane and Scott 1976). If there is foetal-maternal incompatibility, then monozygotic twins will express a double dose of this incompatible antigen and the resulting pre-eclampsia would be expected to be more severe. In dizygotic twins, there will be a double chance for an incompatible antigen from a heterozygote father to be inherited by at least one conceptus and thereby increasing the frequency of developing pre-eclampsia. The findings of Stevenson et al. (1976) from five different twin studies that pre-eclampsia was more common in unlike-sex pairs (must be all dizygotic) than in like-sex pairs (may be monozygotic or dizygotic) are consistent with this hypothesis (Table 11.1). Although the differences observed were only of borderline significance, the consistency of the five sets of data was considered impressive by the authors. However, a later study of 1,045 twin gestations in Leeds by McFarlane and Scott (1976) failed to reveal any difference in the incidence of pre-eclampsia between dizygotic twins and like-sex 'presumed' monozygotic twins. Campbell et al. (1977), defining zygosity by sex, blood groups, red cell enzymes and placental enzymes, also found no difference in the frequency of severe or mild pre-eclampsia in monozygotic and dizygotic twins, nor was there any association when gravidity was taken into account. A serious difficulty with twin studies is that it is not possible to entirely confirm monozygosity unless the placenta is available for examination. Without this criterion, a group of apparent monozygotic twins are bound to include a few dizygotic pairs which, by chance, are

Table 11.1 Frequency of pre-eclampsia in twin pregnancies.

	Like-sex twins		Unlike-sex twins	
Centre	All	Pre-eclampsia (%)	All	Pre-eclampsia (%)
Alexandria	204	24 (11.8)	143	21 (14.7)
U.K.	142	54 (38.0)	54	28 (51.9)
Belfast	337	59 (17.5)	208	53 (25.5)
Oxford	314	128 (40.8)	185	93 (50.3)
Ankara	159	14 (8.8)	112	13 (11.6)

With kind permission from Stevenson, A. C. et al. (1976) *J. med. Genet.* 13, 1–8.

similar for many characteristics. This will dilute any true differences in the incidence of pre-eclampsia which may exist between monozygotic and dizygotic twin gestations.

11.2.3 Sex ratio

In an earlier chapter, we have discussed the possible effects of a Y-linked transplantation antigen in human placentation. The conclusion was that this antigen might act in association with antigens of the HL-A or ABO systems resulting in potentiating foetal-maternal antigenic incompatibility. If a high degree of incompatibility does predispose to pre-eclampsia, then one would expect to find the disease associated more frequently with a male conceptus. Such an observation was first made by Salzmann (1955) who noticed that, while there were about 5% more boys born than girls in normal pregnancies (i.e. a sex ratio of 105:100), this was increased to 14.4% more boys in eclamptic pregnancies. This increase in the sex ratio was particularly marked in primiparous eclamptics where there were 29.9% more boys born. A later study by Toivanen and Hirvonen (1970b) confirmed these findings. Of 1,061 babies born to toxaemic mothers, the sex ratio was found to be 1.24 compared to 1.03 in control non-toxaemic mothers. This sex ratio was even higher (1.71) in those with severe toxaemia with urine proteins of more than 3 g/24 hours. No difference in ABO and Rh blood groups between toxaemic and control mothers was detected, so the increased sex ratio was unlikely to be due to these factors. Scott et al. (1976) also found a similar trend for a higher sex ratio in pre-eclampsia with a figure of 1.13 among babies born to 46 pre-eclamptic mothers compared to 1.06 in a control group.

Toivanen and Hirvonen (1970b) postulated that the presence of a Y-linked antigen increased the histoincompatibility between a male foetus and his mother and thereby potentiated the immunogenicity of other placental antigens which might be important in inducing pre-eclampsia. Salzmann (1955), on the other hand, favoured a sex-associated explanation in that pre-eclampsia was due to maternal reaction against foetal hormones, especially those produced by a male foetus.

11.2.4 Blood group antigens

Attempts to confirm the association of pre-eclampsia with foetal-maternal incompatibility by analysing more specific antigens like blood groups have produced conflicting results. The initial reports by Pike and Dickens (1954) on 541 toxaemic cases did show an 18% increase in group 'O' among toxaemic patients over non-toxaemic mothers. This supported the foetal-maternal incompatibility hypothesis in that a group 'O' mother had a greater chance of bearing a heterospecific foetus and, therefore, maternal iso-immunisation would occur with a greater frequency. However, they were unable to confirm these findings in a later series (Dickens et al. 1956) so they had to conclude that the results from the first series might have been due to chance. In a survey of 149 toxaemic patients out of 1,087 pregnancies, Andrews (1959) did not find any preponderance of group 'O' among toxaemic patients. He also compared foetal ABO and Rh blood groups with those of the mothers but he found no difference in the incidence of homospecific and heterospecific pregnancies between toxaemic and non-toxaemic groups. Pearson and Pinker (1956), in a series of 675 toxaemic patients, similarly found no detectable association with blood groups. From these studies, it is clear that foetal-maternal iso-immunisation for blood group antigens appears to be unimportant in the pathogenesis of pre-eclampsia.

Viewing maternal blood group data as possible indicators of susceptibility rather than as potential foetal-maternal incompatibility, the results of May (1973) seem to point to an increased risk of pre-eclampsia in group 'A' women. It was noted that among a group of primigravidae, 35 out of 103 group 'A' mothers developed pre-eclampsia, compared to 18 out of 101 group 'O', giving a relative risk of A:O of 2.7:1. It was pointed out that this relative risk was about the same as that for developing venous thrombosis while on oral contraceptives, where the A:O ratio was 2.8:1. It was, therefore, postulated that the increased risk of group 'A' women to develop pre-eclampsia could be another manifestation of an increased tendency to intravascular coagulation. Other surveys, however, have been unable to confirm any association between toxaemia and blood group 'A' (Hurst et al. 1946; Harlap and Davies 1974; Scott et al. 1976), so the evidence for any blood group-associated genetic susceptibility to pre-eclampsia must be regarded at the moment as inconclusive.

11.2.5 Histocompatibility antigens

To date, there is very little in the literature on the association between pre-eclampsia and antigens of the histocompatibility complex. Perhaps the report by Need (1975) may be viewed in this context. A woman with two husbands had a normal delivery of twins with husband one but developed severe pre-eclampsia during a singleton pregnancy with husband two. This is the reverse of what may be expected, for the incidence of pre-eclampsia in a first pregnancy carrying twins is usually high, while the incidence in a second pregnancy after a normal first confinement is usually low. On serotyping of both spouses, it was found that husband one possessed no HL-A specificities which were not also present in the wife, indicating the possibility of complete HL-A compatibility. Husband two, on the other hand, possessed four HL-A specificities not possessed by the wife. In addition, one-way MLR between the spouses showed an eight-fold increase in transformation when wife's cells were cultured with cells from husband two compared to cells from husband one, indicating a greater degree of incompatibility for antigens coded by the MLR locus between wife and husband two. Blood group analyses for ABO and Rh antigens of foetal blood showed complete identity between the twins of the first pregnancy and the mother, but the conceptus from the second pregnancy was group 'O', Dd while the mother was group 'A', dd. The conceptus in the second pre-eclamptic pregnancy was, therefore, incompatible to the mother for ABO as well as Rh antigens and could possibly also be incompatible for some HL-A and MLR specificities. Thus, the results are consistent with the hypothesis that a greater degree of foetal-maternal incompatibility may be an important factor in pre-eclampsia. This report was based on only one case and it would be interesting to see if other studies in the future will arrive at similar conclusions.

Data on maternal HL-A antigen frequencies in pre-eclamptic patients revealed no unusual distribution compared to controls (Scott et al. 1976) so, like ABO blood groups, there does not appear to be any association between HL-A specificities and susceptibility to pre-eclampsia. In an outbred population like man, it is clear that foetal-maternal incompatibility for major transplantation antigens will be the rule rather than the exception. It is, therefore, difficult to quantitate any slight differences that may exist in pre-eclamptic cases and normal controls. In the analysis of individual antigens, the situation is further influenced by the known interaction between genes from one locus with those of another, like the protection afforded by ABO incompatibility against Rh iso-immunisation. This makes attempts to correlate aspects of blood group or HL-A antigens with the incidence of pre-eclampsia highly complicated.

11.3 Maternal immunological response

It may be that, rather than just foetal-maternal incompatibility, it is the ability or otherwise of the mother to mount an effective immune response in the face of foetal antigenic challenge which is important in pre-eclampsia. In mice, the capacity to mount a T-cell response to certain well-defined antigens is controlled genetically (McDevitt and Benacerraf 1969) and these genes have been named immune-response (IR) genes. Many of these IR genes are linked to the principal transplantation locus. In man, specific IR genes have not yet been identified but the reported association of particular diseases with individual HL-A antigens, like the highly significant association of HL-A27 with ankylosing spondylitis (Caffrey and James 1973) may reflect the presence of a particular IR gene linked to an HL-A specificity. The lack of any unusual distribution of HL-A antigens among 46 cases of pre-eclampsia reported by Scott and Beer (1976) appears discouraging in this respect, but their series is small, and it would be wise to reserve judgement until further data are available.

11.3.1 Humoral immune response

An alternative approach is to look at the production of antibodies by pre-eclamptic women as a measure of their immune response capacity. Hulka and Brinton (1963) collected sera from patients with eclampsia at various stages of pregnancy, during labour, and immediately post-partum. By fluorescein labelling and localisation to placental sections, they found that anti-trophoblast antibodies appeared in the sera of these women very early during the puerperium and in some cases even during labour. This was in marked contrast to normal pregnancy where anti-bodies were not detected until at least the 4th post partum day (Hulka et al. 1963). This early appearance of antibodies may be a manifestation of a breakdown in maternal tolerance to trophoblast antigens and the immune response thus mounted could initiate the systemic lesions of pre-eclampsia.

In a retrospective survey of 78 women whose sera had been shown to contain leucocytotoxic antibodies during pregnancy, the incidence of pre-eclampsia in this group was found to be no different from a control group where similar antibodies were not detected (Fingleton 1971), so maternal humoral response to foetal HL-A antigens appears to be unimportant in the genesis of pre-eclampsia. If anything, maternal hyporesponsiveness seems to occur in pre-eclamptic patients. Jenkins et al. (1977) collected a total of 70 sera samples from 37 cases of severe pre-eclampsia and found no cytotoxic antibodies in any of these samples when tested against husbands' lymphocytes and also against lymphocytes from a panel of 20 unrelated donors. In a control group, cytotoxic antibodies against husbands' HL-A specificities were demonstrable in seven out of 72 sera samples. The possibility that pre-eclampsia is an immune-complex disease will be discussed in a later section. If this is so, then it must be pointed out that failure to detect circulating antibody in pre-eclamptic patients may be because most of the antibody has been deposited as immune complexes and is, therefore, not an indication of maternal hyporesponsiveness. Against these negative findings is the report of Tiilikainen and Kauranen (1969) who observed that cytotoxic antibodies against a panel of 20 lymphocyte preparations were detected more frequently in toxaemic patients than in normal pregnant controls, this being particularly evident in the primiparous group.

11.3.2 Cell-mediated immune response

Gaugas et al. (1975) examined the degree of spontaneous lymphocyte transformation over 2 hours and 24 hours in a group of 15 patients with mild pre-eclampsia and 19 with severe pre-eclampsia in comparison with a group of non-toxaemic mothers. No differences were detected. This study was prompted by the observation that patients just prior to graft rejection exhibit a 6—7 fold increase in spontaneous lymphocyte transformation. Petrucco et al. (1976), on the other hand, found spontaneous lymphocyte DNA synthesis to be significantly reduced in mild pre-eclampsia but this was not observed in cases of severe pre-eclampsia. The explanation for this is not immediately apparent. The lymphocyte response to PHA in 45 women with severe pre-eclampsia was found by Need et al. (1976) to be significantly lower than in normal controls, both during and after pregnancy. This occurred in the presence or absence of autologous serum, so it was concluded that this indicated an inherent depressed T-cell function in pre-eclamptic women.

The balance of evidence seems to slightly favour a possible association between pre-eclampsia and maternal hyporesponsiveness. The preponderance of this disease in primigravidae offers further support for this conclusion. Maternal hyporesponsiveness may be important in relation to pre-eclampsia as an immune-complex disease.

As pointed out by Peters and Lachmann (1974), for chronic immune-complex nephritis to develop, there must be a persistent source of antigen and an antibody response to it. The immune response must provide sufficient antibody to generate the immune complexes but not so much as to result in the over-rapid elimination of antigen. Pregnancy provides a persistent source of foetal antigenic challenge, so it can be envisaged that an abnormally low maternal immune response may provide just the right conditions for the formation of immune complexes.

11.4 The utero-placental unit

At least two organs are invariably involved in pre-eclampsia, the utero-placental unit and the kidney, but it is still hotly debated how one influences the other (Lancet 1975).

Pre-eclampsia occurs during normal pregnancy and also with hydatidiform moles and choriocarcinomas where there are no co-existing foetuses. The disease has been reported in ectopic gestations (Paterson 1976). From these observations, the presence of placental tissue alone appears to be a pre-requisite for the development of pre-eclampsia without the necessary involvement of the foetus or uterus. The occurrence of the disease is also closely linked to placental size, as indicated by the onset of the disease in the latter stages of pregnancy and the association with multiple births and molar pregnancies, conditions where there is a great increase in placental mass. This seems to be a function of placental mass alone as other conditions producing uterine distention, like hydramnios, are not similarly correlated with the disease (Scott 1958).

It is possible that the basic predisposing factor is placental ischaemia, resulting from an inadequacy of the uterine vasculature to bear the increased demands of pregnancy, especially those with a large placenta. This ischaemia could arise in one of two ways. Either the growth of the placenta somehow outstrips its blood supply or there is some obstruction or abnormality of the vascular tree. It has indeed been observed that placental blood flow is considerably reduced in pre-eclampsia (Browne and Veal 1953). Radio-isotope sodium clearance measurements have shown that the blood flow through the uterine wall was reduced to half the normal rate in pre-eclampsia and to one quarter in eclampsia (Morris et al. 1955). Indirect evidence that this may be an initiating rather than a secondary effect comes from the study of Becker (1948) who, noticing that a large proportion of pre-eclamptic cases occurred in primigravidae, measured the blood flow through the uterine arteries of normal women and found that it was, on average, considerably less in first than in subsequent pregnancies. In animal experiments constricting the uterine arteries of pregnant dogs led to progressive hypertension and proteinuria which disappeared immediately on termination of pregnancy (Hodari 1967).

Histological studies have revealed abnormalities in the myometrial blood vessels in pre-eclampsia (Zeek and Assali 1950; Robertson et al. 1967). These vascular lesions, described as 'acute atherosis' were characterised by fibrinoid necrosis and inflammatory infiltration of the vessel wall, an appearance very similar to that found in the blood vessels of rejected kidney transplants. In rejected kidneys, the lesions are due to host immune response to allo-antigens of endothelial cells lining the blood vessels. A similar immunological mechanism may be operative in pre-eclampsia. This is supported by the study of Kitzmiller and Benirschke (1973) who observed fluorescent staining with anti-Ig and anti-C3 in the decidual vessels from four women with pre-eclampsia. The decidual vessels from four women with hypertension and in seven women with normal pregnancies were all negative. On the basis of extensive human and primate studies, Hamilton and Boyde (1966) concluded that placental syncytiotrophoblast cells invaded maternal spiral arteries during early placentation and formed the lining of these vessels. The findings of Kitzmiller and Benirschke (1973), therefore, may indicate the presence of maternal immunological reaction to these trophoblast cells in decidual vessels, leading to impairment of placental blood flow and placental damage. Placental infarcts have been observed by Zeek and Assali (1950) to be more frequently associated with toxaemic (34 out of 71) than with non-toxaemic pregnancies (3 out of 143).

An important sequel to placental infarction could be trophoblast emboli into the maternal circulation, leading to increased load of trophoblast antigens. It has been observed that while trophoblast emboli are not uncommon findings in normal pregnancy (Douglas et al. 1959; Attwood and Park 1961), in toxaemic pregnancy the amount of circulating trophoblast material is substantially increased. Jäämeri et al. (1965) found, on average, about 20 times more trophoblast cells in the uterine veins of toxaemic women during caesarian section than in normal controls. Roffman and Simons (1969) observed a woman with pre-eclampsia and placenta increta who died of widespread pulmonary trophoblastic embolism. They quoted Schmorl who, in 1893, reported trophoblastic emboli in the lungs of 14 out of 17 women who died from toxaemia. However, it had not been established whether the increased trophoblastic deportation, in fact, preceded the disease or was a result of eclamptic seizures.

11.5 The kidney

11.5.1 Intravascular coagulation

The occurrence of proteinuria in pre-eclampsia focuses attention on the kidney as an important organ of involvement (Brit. med. J. 1974). This proteinuria appears to be of glomerular origin. Both light and electron microscopic studies have shown glomerular changes, described as swelling and proliferation of endothelial cells, increase in mesangial cells and matrix, and abnormal granular deposits between and within endothelial cells and on the endothelial aspect of the basement membrane (Thomson et al. 1972). Immunofluorescent studies of renal biopsies from toxaemic patients have demonstrated the consistent presence of fibrin-like material in the glomeruli, but no γ-globulin or complement was detected (Vassalli et al. 1963a; Morris et al. 1964). The presence of this fibrin-like material suggests that some kind of thrombotic mechanism leading to slow intravascular coagulation may be involved. This is supported by the observations of Bonnar et al. (1971) on pre-eclamptic and eclamptic women. They found raised levels of fibrin degradation products which could reflect fibrinolysis of intravascular fibrin and also a low platelet count which could be a result of increased consumption due to intravascular coagulation. Significantly higher levels of fibrin degradation products in pre-eclampsia and eclampsia than in normal pregnancy was also observed by Henderson et al. (1970), in a study of African women. The level of these products in the sera of normal non-pregnant women was found to be 1—2 μg/ml, while that for normal pregnant women was 4—8 μg/ml. In pre-eclamptic women, the level of fibrin degradation products rose to 20—30 μg/ml, and was even higher in cases of eclampsia. In contrast, no appreciable changes were seen in cases of essential hypertension, so the effect was not secondary to a rise in blood pressure. Studies by Wardle and Mennon (1969) and Howie et al. (1971) also indicated that intravascular coagulation occurred in pre-eclampsia. Preston et al.

(1972) reported that urinary levels of fibrin degradation products were higher than would be expected from plasma levels, suggesting that a local fibrinolytic activity in the glomeruli could also be taking place.

Experimentally, thromboplastic infusion into rabbits can produce ultrastructural glomerular lesions resembling those of toxaemia of pregnancy (Vassalli et al. 1963b). All these observations, therefore, strongly suggest that intravascular coagulation is an important and perhaps even a primary event responsible for the pathological lesions found in toxaemia. Pregnancy seems to be associated with an alteration in the fibrinolytic enzyme system of the blood (Bonnar et al. 1969) with an enhanced capacity to form fibrin but a diminished ability to lyse fibrin. This alteration has undoubted advantage in haemostasis and in maintaining the integrity of maternal and foetal circulations during pregnancy, but it will also mean that pregnant women are highly susceptible to intravascular clotting.

If indeed intravascular coagulation is a primary event in pre-eclampsia, it is pertinent to ask what triggers it off. Trophoblast has a higher thromboplastic activity than any other tissue (Chargaff 1945) and it is possible that an infarcted placenta together with the resultant increase in trophoblastic emboli may release sufficient thromboplastic material to initiate the series of events leading to intravascular thrombosis (Vassalli and McCluskey 1965). The manifestations of intravascular coagulation in toxaemia of pregnancy are very similar to those seen in rabbits which develop the generalised Shwartzman reaction after intravenous injection of bacterial endotoxin (McKay et al. 1953). The fibrin deposition in the glomerular capillaries and hepatic arterioles, resulting in congestion and occasionally haemorrhage and necrosis, are lesions seen in both conditions, which led to the suggestion that some material released from the placenta may have precipitated a similar state of intravascular coagulation in pre-eclampsia (McKay 1962). The actual mechanism of the Shwartzman reaction, however, has never been satisfactorily explained. The fact that it only occurs after the second dose of bacterial endotoxin suggests an immunological basis so that at least it bears a superficial resemblance to hypersensitivity reactions, perhaps analogous to a generalised Arthus reaction.

11.5.2 Type III hypersensitivity

Much evidence has now accumulated that many human glomerulonephritides are caused by the glomerular deposition of antigen-antibody complexes (Peters 1975). The concept that immune complexes can lead to renal lesions is also well established from animal experiments where these lesions occur as part of a general syndrome of serum sickness after the administration of large doses of foreign protein (Germuth 1953; Dixon et al. 1958). It is, therefore, possible that a similar serum sickness-like reaction to placental proteins may lead to glomerular lesions in pre-eclampsia. However, the inability to demonstrate γ-globulins and complement in the kidney of toxaemic patients in earlier studies was against such an immunological mechanism but recently, Petrucco et al. (1974), in an immunofluorescent study of renal biopsies on 11 patients with pre-eclampsia, detected large amounts of IgM with lesser amounts of IgG in the glomeruli. These occurred as patchy deposits in the capillary loops. Complement was constantly found within the afferent and efferent arterioles and, in severe cases, also seen within the glomeruli. In four cases, repeat biopsies three months post partum showed disappearance of all traces of immunoglobulins. These findings are consistent with the deposition of immune complexes, so the pathogenesis of the renal lesions in pre-eclampsia could be due to a Type III immunopathological mechanism. Since IgM is the predominant immunoglobulin found, it is possible that the negative findings in earlier studies were due to the use of anti-whole immunoglobulin which might not have contained sufficient anti-IgM activity.

Serum IgG and IgM levels have been reported to be significantly lower in toxaemic patients than in normal pregnant controls (Yang et al. 1975). While both IgG and IgM were found in the urine of these toxaemic patients, the amount of urine IgG decreased as the disease improved, but the amount of urine IgM did not correlate with the course of the disease. It was thought that the low level of serum IgG in pre-eclampsia could be due to leakage into the urine from glomerular damage, while the low level of serum IgM could have resulted from deposition of this immunoglobulin as immune complexes. However, cord blood IgM was found to be significantly higher in toxaemic pregnancies, so the alternative explanation must be entertained that the low serum IgM level in toxaemic patients could be due to leakage of maternal IgM into the foetal circulation across a damaged placenta.

If pre-eclampsia is an immune complex disease, one would expect to find increased complement consumption, but available evidence would seem to indicate that this is not so. Using a sheep red cell haemolysis assay, serum complement activity was found to be the same in toxaemic and normal pregnant women controls (Prall and Kantor 1966; Kitzmiller et al. 1973), although patients with acute glomerulonephritis showed reduced complement activity (Thomson et al. 1939). Quantitative immunodiffusion analyses of individual complement components like C3 in sera of toxaemic patients also failed to reveal any significant deviation from normal pregnant controls (Millar and Mills 1972). A recent study confirmed no changes in the serum concentration of Clq, C3 and C4 in toxaemic patients (Thomson et al. 1976). Although these investigators found increased anticomplementary activity in the sera of toxaemic patients, there was no evidence of increased complement activation as measured by C3 and C3 proactivator conversion, indicating that the anticomplementary activity was probably not due to circulating immune complexes.

The presently available results on serum complement levels and activity in toxaemic patients, therefore, do not support the immune complex aetiology of this disease. It should be pointed out, however, that serum complement activity in normal pregnancy varies during different stages of gestation (Soliman et al. 1971; Baines et al. 1974), so that any comparisons made with toxaemic patients must be carefully matched for this variable. There also appears to be a gradually increasing complement activity as pregnancy progresses when compared to non-pregnant controls (Baines et al. 1974), which may reflect an increased production of complement components by the liver occasioned by pregnancy. Any increased utilisation in toxaemia could be masked by this increased production. Finally it is, of course, possible that the consumption of complement by toxaemic patients is insufficient to affect the serum levels significantly.

11.5.3 Type II hypersensitivity

Antigenic similarity between the human placenta and kidney is well documented (Steblay 1962; Boss 1965; Curzen 1968) and it is possible that immunological cross reactivity by maternal anti-placental antibodies on the kidney could form the basis of a Type II immunopathological mechanism for the renal lesions in pre-eclampsia. Animal experimental studies have suggested that this may be so. Beveans et al. (1955) found that intravenous infusion of rabbit anti-dog placental antibodies would produce nephritis in both pregnant and non-pregnant dogs. Similar cross reactivity has also been observed with antibodies raised to heterologous placenta. Gang et al. (1974) produced antibodies towards human and rat trophoblast basement membrane. When injected intravenously into virgin, male, or pregnant rats, both antibodies localised exclusively to glomerular basement membrane of rat kidney.

In an immunofluorescent study of six biopsy specimens from toxaemic patients, Tribe et al. (1974) confirmed the findings of Petrucco et al. (1974) of the presence of immunoglobulins, especially IgM, in the renal glomeruli. In contrast to the patchy distribution of immunoglobulins described by Petrucco, a more linear distribution within the capillary loops was observed, an appearance more in line with a Type II immunopathological mechanism with cross reaction against glomerular basement membrane.

11.5.4 Source of antigens

Although available evidence points to placental tissue as the most likely antigenic source for the initiation of immunopathological lesions in pre-eclampsia, it is not yet clear what placental antigens are involved. In the experimental glomerular lesions produced in rats by Gang et al. (1974), the antibodies used were raised against a purified human chorionic glycoprotein from trophoblast basement membrane. Human placental polysaccharide has also been observed to cause lesions similar to those found in toxaemic patients when injected intravenously into pregnant rabbits and in rabbits previously sensitised to the polysaccharide, but not in normal non-pregnant rabbits (Kaku 1953). The presence of antibodies to this placental polysaccharide was detected in the sera of 20 out of 119 (17%) toxaemic patients by a precipitation reaction, with titres ranging from 100—800. This reaction was positive in only one out of 39 normal pregnant women. When a complement-fixation assay was used, a positive reaction was observed in 30 out of 142 (21%) toxaemic patients while only two out of 81 normal pregnant women had detectable antibodies. These observations, therefore, indicate that placental polysaccharide may play an important role in the aetiology of toxaemia.

11.6 Proposed pathogenic mechanism for pre-eclampsia

From the foregoing discussion, it can be seen that the aetiology of pre-eclampsia is highly complex and is likely to involve many interrelating factors. Although the pathological lesions in the disease are well recognised, there is still a great deal of controversy regarding the sequence in which they appear and how they are caused. Immunological factors may have an important part to play in the pathogenesis. A working hypothesis is proposed as follows.

The initiating lesion is placental ischaemia with resultant infarction and deportation of trophoblast emboli into the maternal circulation. Ischaemia is due to vascular damage, possibly as a result of maternal immunological reaction against foetal antigens in decidual vessels, a situation analogous to rejection of transplanted organ. Foetal-maternal antigenic disparity would be expected to have an effect on the intensity of this reaction, as would the genetic ability of the mother to mount an immunological response to foetal antigens. The possibility that foetal-maternal incompatibility may also increase placental mass is relevant as this will place an additional burden on the blood supply.

The infarcted placenta and trophoblast emboli may then affect other organs. One possible mechanism is by the production of disseminated intravascular coagulation leading to ischaemia or congestion of organs like the liver or kidney, changes which are frequently seen in toxaemia. This intravascular coagulation could be precipitated by the widespread formation of immune complexes between maternal antibodies and trophoblast antigens and the fixation of complement in a kind of generalised Arthus phenomenon. The depression of the fibrinolytic enzyme system during pregnancy further predisposes to this condition. In addition, maternal antibodies against trophoblast antigens may cross react with her own kidney glomerular basement membrane, leading to further damage to this organ, thereby producing the characteristic symptoms of proteinuria and hypertension of renal origin.

12

Immunological factors in trophoblast neoplasia

During normal pregnancy, the placenta consists of a mass of trophoblast cells, many of which are bizarre in shape and size, invading the uterine decidua to varying depths. Frequently, pieces of trophoblast tissue are deported via the maternal circulation to lodge in the lungs of the mother. This is normal physiological behaviour of implantation, but in other situations these characteristics — lack of cellular differentiation, invasiveness and metastatic potential — would be descriptive of a malignant neoplasm. The dividing line between normal and malignant trophoblast, therefore, is not a clear one and the behaviour of trophoblast neoplasms may be said to represent a breakdown in the normal immunological equilibrium maintained between the placenta and mother (Loke 1975). It would be logical to suppose that the factors responsible for this breakdown are likely to be related to those properties which have aided normal trophoblast to circumvent maternal rejection during normal human pregnancy. With its genetic endowment from both parents, trophoblast neoplasm is the only documented example of a naturally occurring human allogeneic tumour and is thus ideal for a study of the tumour-host relationship.

There are two main varieties of trophoblast neoplasms:

(1) hydatidiform mole, and
(2) choriocarcinoma.

In hydatidiform mole, the central core of the chorionic villus is markedly distended, giving rise to the typical grape-like macroscopical appearance of these tumours (Fig. 12.1). These structures might have

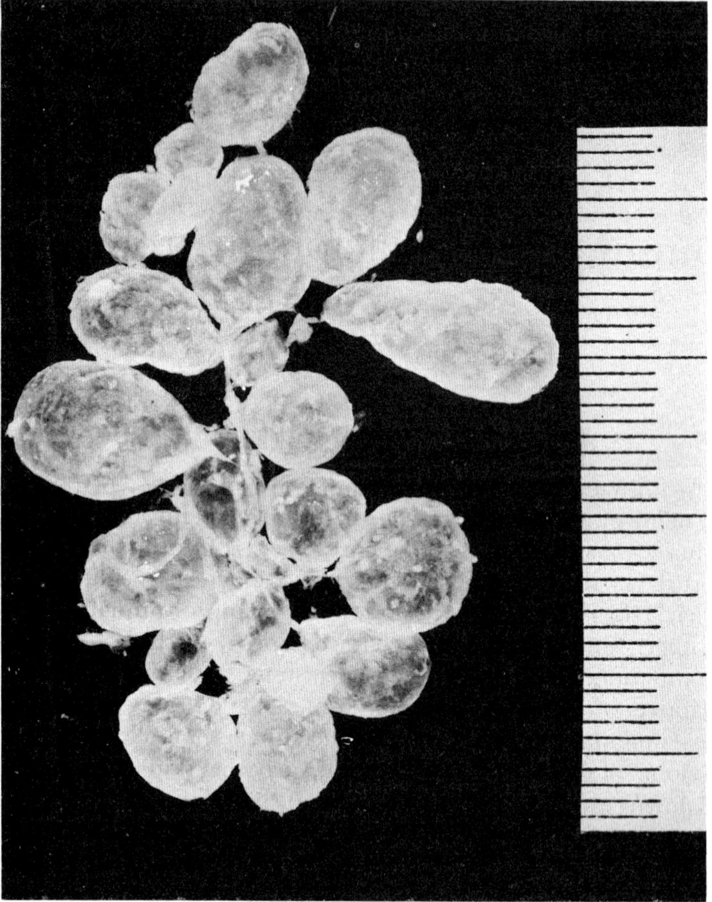

Fig. 12.1 Grape-like distention of chorionic villi in hydatidiform mole. From Loke, Y. W. (1975) In: *Comparative Placentation. Essays in Structure and Function*, Ed.: Steven. Academic Press, pp. 282—293.

been mistaken for individual embryos in the 13th century story of the Countess Margaret who was described as bringing forth 365 infants at one birth (Rather 1971).

Histologically, varying degrees of trophoblastic proliferation can be seen (Fig. 12.2). In choriocarcinoma, all villous structure is lost and the tumour consists entirely of closely packed, highly proliferative trophoblast cells infiltrating uterine and other tissues. There is no doubt that

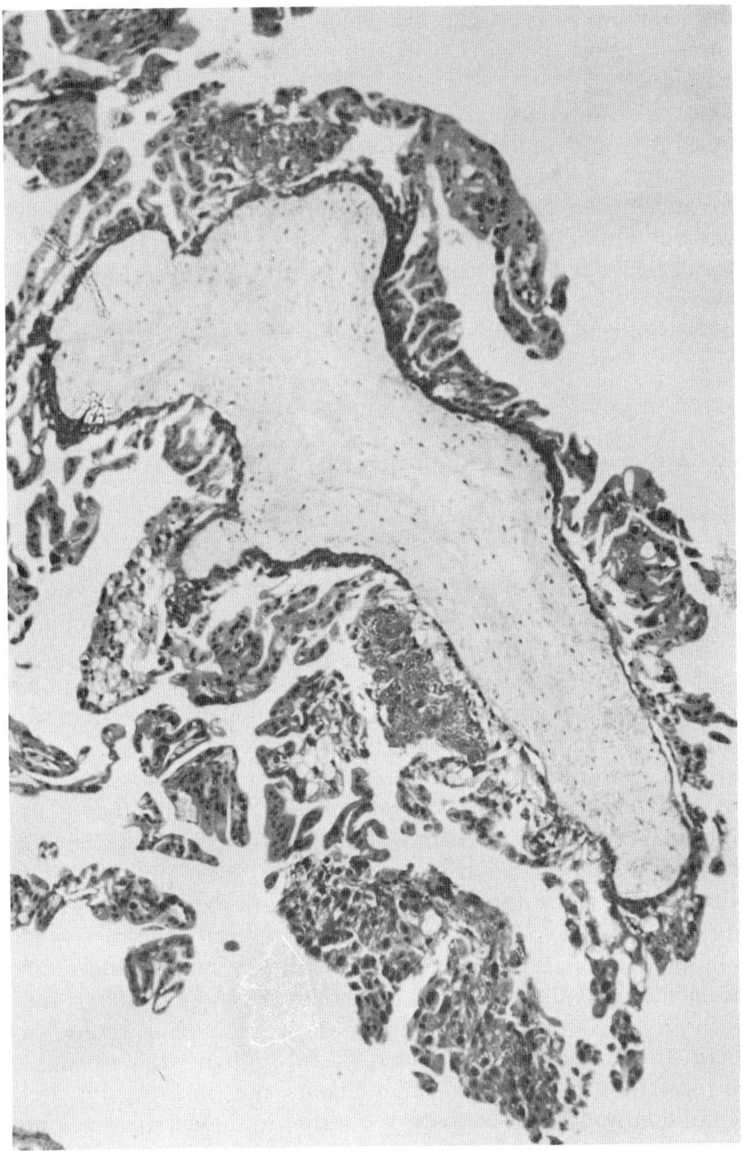

Fig. 12.2 Section through a hydatidiform mole villus showing marked proliferation of the trophoblast. From Loke, Y. W. (1975) In: *Comparative Placentation. Essays in Structure and Function*, Ed.: Steven. Academic Press, pp. 282—293.

choriocarcinoma is a highly malignant tumour and, without treatment, most patients will eventually succumb to generalised metastases.

The clinical course followed by a hydatidiform mole is more uncertain. Some are benign and are spontaneously expelled from the uterus after a varying period but others may invade deeply into the myometrium or even penetrate the uterus to involve pelvic viscera. These 'invasive moles', although locally destructive, do not usually metastasise. The most important feature of hydatidiform mole, however, is that some of them may become choriocarcinomas and it is generally agreed that 40—50% of all choriocarcinomas are preceded by moles.

12.1 Antigenicity and immunogenicity of trophoblast neoplasms

12.1.1 Clinical observations

The spontaneous regression rate of choriocarcinoma is said to be relatively high compared to other malignant growths and it is suggested that this may be due to host recognition of the allogeneic nature of the neoplasm. Further support for this suggestion is the observation that, in contrast, spontaneous regression is extremely rare in testicular choriocarcinoma, a tumour which originates from the pluripotential testicular germ cells with, therefore, complete genetic identity between host and tumour. It must be remembered, however, that placental trophoblast cells have a definite life-span which is sufficient for the period of gestation, so this natural death, even in the malignant equivalent, could be responsible for the cases of spontaneous remissions rather than any host immunological intervention. The success rate of chemotherapy is also relatively high with placental choriocarcinoma compared with other malignant tumours (Hertz et al. 1961), and this has been considered as due to a weak immune response acting synergistically with chemotherapy (Billingham 1967). Testicular choriocarcinomas, on the other hand, do not respond well to chemotherapy. It must be pointed out that in these testicular tumours, the choriocarcinomatous elements are but one part of a teratocarcinoma and it is possible that it is these other tissues which are relatively insusceptible to treatment. In the interpretation of these observations, it is also well to remember that the diagnosis of choriocarcinoma from some of the more florid forms of hydatidiform moles may prove difficult both histologically and clinically (Park 1971). The behaviour of hydatidiform moles follows a generally more benign course, so their mistaken designation as choriocarcinomas will introduce a favourable bias into the follow-up statistics of the latter.

12.1.2 In vitro demonstration of choriocarcinoma antigens

In the same type of experiment as they used for normal trophoblast cells, Currie and Bagshawe (1967a) reported that cultured choriocarcinoma cells were killed by lymphocytes from the patient and also by allogeneic lymphocytes after four days incubation. The indiscriminate killing by both patient's and allogeneic lymphocytes, the delay in onset of lysis, and the absence of antibody in the culture, indicated that the reaction was unlikely to be mediated by sensitised lymphocytes or by K-cells. The authors concluded this was a form of 'allogeneic inhibition' due to choriocarcinoma cells expressing antigenic groupings foreign to and detectable by allogeneic lymphocytes. It may be analogous to a mixed lymphocyte reaction with choriocarcinoma cells functioning as stimulators.

Srivannaboon (1971) managed to raise antibodies in rabbits against choriocarcinoma cells grown in hamster cheek pouch. After absorption with human placenta, kidney, HCG, hamster serum, and hamster placenta, the antibody still reacted with a single precipitin line in immunoelectrophoresis and immunodiffusion against choriocarcinoma cell extracts. This was taken to indicate the presence of an antigen in choriocarcinoma which was absent in normal human placenta. In addition, this antiserum was cytotoxic to cultured choriocarcinoma cells in vitro. It is, however, difficult to judge the clinical relevance of the expression of an apparent tumour-specific antigen by cells derived from a cell-line.

12.1.3 Histological evidence for maternal immune response

In a histological examination of 43 invasive moles, Park (1971) reported abundant lymphocytes and plasma cells in immediate or close proximity to the hyperplastic trophoblast. There was a corresponding lack of polymorphonuclear neutrophils, a cell type which one would expect to find if the reaction was a non-specific one in response to products of tissue destruction. A similar lymphocytic infiltration was found by Elston (1969) around tumour deposits in 35 out of 38 cases of choriocarcinoma. Since this is the kind of histological picture associated with allograft rejection, it was thought that a similar host rejection response might be operative in trophoblast tumours.

Elston (1969) attempted a correlation between degree of cellular infiltration and subsequent response to treatment. He found that 10 out of 13 patients with 'severe' lymphocytic infiltration were free from recurrence a year after treatment as against only seven out of 20 patients with 'mild' infiltration. It is not clear if the histological material for these studies was all obtained before any form of treatment was instituted. If it was, then one may interpret the results as further supporting evidence for the synergistic effects of host immunological reaction and therapy. The study of Mogensen and Olsen (1973) of histological material from 31 patients who had not yet received treatment did show a significant correlation between intensity of lymphocytic infiltration and subsequent recovery.

12.1.4 Leucocyte antibodies in sera of patients with trophoblast neoplasms

It was observed by Ivavkova et al. (1968) that 12 out of 13 choriocarcinoma patients had cytotoxic antibodies against husbands' leucocytes. Similarly, Mathé et al. (1964) reported the presence of agglutinins against husbands' leucocytes and thrombocytes in the sera of all their five patients with metastatic choriocarcinoma. Although these observations suggest that choriocarcinoma can sensitise the mother towards paternally derived antigens, it is not possible to be certain that some of the antibodies present may not have been made during a previous pregnancy. In a later study, Lawler et al. (1974) investigated 11 patients with hydatidiform mole at their first pregnancy. None of these patients have had a previous blood transfusion. Four of these 11 patients (36%) had demonstrable HL-A antibodies specific for an antigen present on the husband's leucocytes. Since there are no foetal blood vessels traversing the mesenchymal core in hydatidiform moles, it is unlikely that foetal blood cells are the source of sensitisation. It would appear, therefore, that the molar tissue itself may express HL-A allo-antigenic specificities.

12.2 Maternal tolerance

The effective rejection response by an allogeneic host to choriocarcinoma is well illustrated by the report of a case where this neoplasm was accidentally transplanted to a renal graft recipient via an affected kidney (Gokel et al. 1977). This patient developed a high serum HCG level but after removal of the kidney and stopping immunosuppression, the hormone level fell gradually in the same pattern as that seen after treatment of choriocarcinoma with methotrexate and not abruptly as in parturition. It was concluded that this indicated that residual tumour cells in the recipient were slowly destroyed by the returning immunological reactivity after cessation of immunosuppression. This case, therefore, provides an example where an homologous transplant of choriocarcinoma which has survived in an immunosuppressed host, will subsequently regress with the return of immunocompetence. Can it be that some form of immunosuppression is responsible for the highly invasive nature of choriocarcinoma in pregnant women?

There are a number of observations that patients with choriocarcinoma have an impaired rejection reaction against husbands' skin grafts but not against grafts from unrelated donors. Robinson et al. (1963) initially reported two choriocarcinoma patients who rejected grafts from unrelated donors in 14 and seven days respectively, while husbands' grafts were still surviving after three and two months. These studies were subsequently extended to five patients with choriocarcinoma and two patients with hydatidiform mole (Robinson et al. 1967). In four patients with choriocarcinoma, husbands' skin grafts survived beyond 21, 28, 63 and 90 days, while grafts from unrelated donors were rejected within 10—15 days. In the remaining one patient who survived choriocarcinoma seven years ago, husband's graft survived only 14 days and in the two patients with hydatidiform mole, husbands' grafts survived 10 and 14 days respectively. No compatibility in leucocyte antigens was found between husband and patient in these cases. These data seem to indicate that the impaired graft rejection observed in women with disseminated choriocarcinoma is a specific tolerance towards husbands' tissue and not a generalised immune paralysis created by the neoplasm or by treatment. The lack of tolerance observed in the two patients with hydatidiform mole and in the one who survived choriocarcinoma for seven years may be interpreted equally as either the cause of the relatively benign nature of the tumour in these three cases or the result of a deficiency of tolerogenic tumour material.

The main reason why it is difficult to decide whether maternal tolerance is the cause or the result of trophoblast neoplasia is the lack of appropriate control data concerning the survival of husbands' skin grafts to normal pregnant and non-pregnant women. At least, animal studies have shown that tolerance to male skin grafts in isogeneic female mice can be induced by successive matings, the degree of tolerance being roughly proportional to the number of prior pregnancies (Prehn 1960). From this, one would expect choriocarcinoma to develop more frequently in multiparous women, if tolerance were to be an important predisposing factor. The data from Singapore do show a higher frequency of choriocarcinoma among multiparous women (Chan 1967). On the other hand, there is evidence to indicate that tolerance has developed as a result of a rapidly growing tumour. The observation that, occasionally, metastatic deposits of choriocarcinoma will regress after surgical removal of the primary growth in the uterus may be explained by a breaking of tolerance due to reduction of antigenic load.

Rudolf and Thomas (1970) reported that lymphocytes from two women with choriocarcinoma and one with invasive mole all responded to stimulation by lymphocytes from their children in a one-way MLR, indicating there was no inherent impairment of lymphocyte function towards paternally derived antigens. Other T-cell functions also appear to be unimpaired as demonstrated by marked skin reactions to PPD in choriocarcinoma patients (Walden et al. 1976). Perhaps the defective graft rejection observed in choriocarcinoma patients is mediated by the development of 'enhancing' or 'blocking' antibodies. This is supported by the observations of Mathé et al. (1964) of an inverse relationship between antibody titre and skin rejection, so that those choriocarcinoma patients with the highest titre of anti-husband leucocyte agglutinins rejected husbands' skin grafts slowest.

The potential danger of tumour enhancement, therefore, is a factor which should not be overlooked in attempts to treat choriocarcinoma by immunotherapy. The allogeneic nature of this tumour has long made it a target for this type of treatment but, so far, the results are equivocal. Almost twenty years ago, Doniach et al. (1958) treated a patient with choriocarcinoma by repeated intradermal injections of buffy coat lymphocytes from the husband. Sensitisation was demonstrated by the subsequent accelerated rejection of husband's skin graft compared with that of a graft from an unrelated donor. The patient survived for over a year but she was also treated with methotrexate at the same time, so it is difficult to judge the contribution made by immunotherapy. A similar regime was tried by Hackett and Beech (1961) but their patient died of widespread metastases in spite of showing accelerated rejection of husband's skin graft and treatment with methotrexate. However, no lymphocytic infiltration was observed histologically around the tumour deposits which seems to reflect a lack of immunogenicity on the part of the tumour.

12.3 Foetal-maternal histocompatibility

A factor in the genesis of trophoblast neoplasms which has been much discussed is the possibility that close genetic compatibility between husband and wife can result in a foetus whose antigenic specificities are so similar to those of the mother that no immunological recognition will occur. The epidemiological observations that choriocarcinoma has a high frequency in certain countries of the Near East where endogamous marital customs frequently result in a high degree of compatibility between husband and wife, would seem to support this hypothesis (Iliya et al. 1967). Detailed analyses of the ABO and HL-A iso-antigenic systems, however, revealed that the situation is likely to be much more complicated.

12.3.1 ABO antigens

The original analyses by Schmidt et al. (1961) showed no significant difference in blood group distribution among 28 patients with choriocarcinoma compared to their husbands' blood group or the expected distribution as calculated from ABO gene frequencies. On the other hand, subsequent larger series did detect a preponderance of groups 'A' and 'AB' over 'O' among women with trophoblast neoplasms, both in America (Scott 1962) and in the Far East (Llewellyn-Jones 1965). These data were considered to be in support of the hypothesis that foetal-maternal compatibility in ABO blood groups was an important aetiological factor in trophoblast neoplasia, because a group 'O' mother would be incompatible with all foetuses except those who were also group 'O', but a group 'AB' mother would be analogous to a 'universal recipient' as in transfusion serology. However, these two series were too small to permit a statistical analysis. A further complicating factor was that while Scott's series (1962) consisted only of choriocarcinoma, Llewellyn-Jones's (1965) included both benign hydatidiform mole and choriocarcinoma. A later and much larger series from Singapore (Dawood et al. 1971) did not entirely confirm the earlier findings. In 351 cases of hydatidiform mole, no significant shift in the ABO blood group distribution was apparent in patients compared with the control population. On the other hand, in 87 cases of choriocarcinoma, there was a significant increase in the incidence of blood group 'A' and a significant decrease in blood group 'B' as compared to controls. From Japan, Tomoda et al. (1976) reported no deviation of ABO blood groups in patients with all types of trophoblast tumours compared to controls.

As regards ABO compatibility between husband and wife pairs, again there does not appear to be any significant difference between those women with trophoblast tumours and their husbands and control couples (Mittal et al. 1975; Tomoda et al. 1976).

Thus, it would appear that compatibility in the ABO antigen system is not such an important factor in the aetiology of trophoblast tumours as original reports suggested. The apparent preponderance of group 'A' patients may indicate an increased susceptibility to develop trophoblast neoplasms in these women. The association between a certain blood group and incidence of carcinoma has been observed for other neoplasms, like carcinoma of the stomach, which occurs more frequently in group 'A' individuals, although the exact mechanism of operation is unclear. The increased risk of group 'A' women in developing choriocarcinoma is confirmed by a series from Britain (Bagshawe et al. 1971), but this only holds true when the group 'A' women are married to group 'O' husbands. Group 'A' women married to group 'A' husbands have a low risk of developing choriocarcinoma. The relative risk of A ♀ × O ♂ ngs compared to A ♀ x A ♂ matings is 10.4 to 1. Since both types of matings can produce only foetuses which are ABO compatible with the mother, it is clear that other factors are involved over and above that of compatibility of the conceptus with the patient. It was suggested that perhaps a group 'O' trophoblast could react against maternal group 'A' antigens to produce a 'graft-versus-host' situation with overproliferation and increased cytolytic activity, finally resulting in choriocarcinoma. On this hypothesis, one would expect that from the A♀ × O♂ mating, the group 'O' conceptus would be the one associated with choriocarcinoma and not the group 'A' conceptus. This, however, was not observed for in 13 A♀ × O♂ couples where choriocarcinoma developed after term delivery of a child, the tumour was associated with a group 'A' child in seven instances and a group 'O' child in six instances. Mittal et al. (1975), from the United States, did not confirm that there is a higher incidence of choriocarcinoma in A♀ × O♂ matings. In their series, women of group 'A' with spouses of group 'O' occurred 18 times among 95 control couples as opposed to 13 times among an equal number of patient couples. Similarly, women of group 'A' with spouses of group 'A' occurred 16 times among control couples as opposed to 13 times among patient couples.

Thus, the position at present is that data pertaining to ABO blood groups in relation to trophoblast neoplasia are still highly conflicting. One observation which has so far not suffered from contradictory evidence is that choriocarcinoma patients who are group 'AB' have an increased mortality with rapidly progressive tumours and do not respond well to chemotherapy (Bagshawe et al. 1971; Dawood et al. 1971). This may have an immunological basis but the relationship is likely to be more complicated than is explainable by current concepts of foetal-maternal interaction.

12.3.2 HL-A antigens

Mogensen and Kissmeyer-Nielsen (1968, 1971) and Mogensen et al. (1969), on the basis of tissue-typing of the husbands and children of women with choriocarcinoma, first presented the hypothesis that 'the survival of the placental choriocarcinoma in the maternal host presupposes a high degree of histocompatibility between the foetus and the mother as regards strong transplantation antigens'. In a system as polymorphic as that of HL-A, foetal-maternal compatibility can still be achieved even when the husband possesses one or more antigens not possessed by the wife, because the child will not necessarily receive all the paternal specificities if the father is heterozygous. If choriocarcinoma develops following delivery of a viable infant, the histocompatibility between tumour and patient can be ascertained by typing the infant and the patient. In those large numbers of cases of choriocarcinoma which follow molar pregnancies or abortions, family studies of the other children can reveal the parental HL-A haplotypes. From these data, the possibility or otherwise of a couple producing a foetus histocompatible with the mother may be deduced. Lewis and Terasaki (1971) observed there was foetal-maternal compatibility or possible compatibility in seven out of 31 women with choriocarcinoma. This seems a higher frequency than in random matings, so the data fit the hypothesis formulated by Mogensen. It should be noted that there were 11 other siblings in these families in whom the HL-A patterns were identical to those of the offsprings associated with choriocarcinoma and yet there were no apparent abnormalities in these pregnancies, so that histocompatibility alone cannot be responsible for the causation of the disease.

Using a scoring system based on the maternal/paternal haplotypes, Lawler et al. (1971) studied 50 patient/husband pairs and found that they were not more compatible as a group than a control group of couples for HL-A antigens. Similar results were obtained by Mittal et al. (1975), who found no increase in the incidence of HL-A compatible couples among choriocarcinoma patients than among control couples. In a later analysis of HL-A phenotypes in 75 patient/husband pairs and comparing this with the expected frequency calculated according to each antigenic combination (Klouda et al. 1972), it was found that mating in choriocarcinoma patients was random so that the risk of a woman getting choriocarcinoma is apparently not influenced by her choice of mate as far as the HL-A system is concerned. In contrast, the choice of mate would appear to be important from the data of Ivavkova et al. (1968). They investigated 15 women with trophoblast tumours and their husbands in Prague and found a peculiar distribution of HL-A1. While 11 of the 14 husbands were HL-A1 positive, 12 of the 15 patients were HL-A1 negative, the frequency of the HL-A1 phenotype in Prague being 42%. It is tempting to postulate that perhaps the production of anti-HLA1 antibodies by the patient may have enhancing properties.

Lawler et al. (1971) reported that there was a slight suggestion from their results that treatment was more successful in those choriocarcinoma patients with no HL-A antigens in common with their husbands than in those with one or more antigens in common. There was one death in 16 in the former group compared to five deaths in 29. These figures are far from being statistically significant, so it seems that the influence of HL-A compatibility on prognosis is also unlikely to be very important.

Further evidence against the histocompatibility hypothesis can be seen in the results obtained using the mixed lymphocyte reaction. In a two-way MLR between husband and wife pairs, Halbrecht and Komlos

(1968) reported a mean percentage of transformed cells of 5.7% in a control group of normal fertile couples, while the equivalent percentage of transformed cells in a group of six women with hydatidiform moles and their husbands was 21.6%, indicating an increased husband/wife incompatibility. Rudolf and Thomas (1970), investigating two women with choriocarcinoma and one with invasive mole and their 14 children found that all 14 children's lymphocytes stimulated the mother' lymphoyctes in a one-way MLR. It is of interest to note that, if the children/mother pairs were investigated by serotyping alone, then six of the 14 children showed only those antigens also present on their mothers' lymphocytes, and would therefore be judged as histocompatible by this test. Therefore, the present conclusion seems to be that histocompatibility for HL-A antigens has very little influence on either the risk of developing trophoblast neoplasms or the prognosis.

Recent interest in the association between the HL-A system and diseases have prompted many investigations on HL-A phenotypes and the risk of trophoblast neoplasia. As is to be expected with such a polymorphic system, no definite trend has so far emerged. While Lawler et al. (1971) found a greater frequency of HL-A1 and HL-A8 among 53 patients with trophoblast neoplasms, as compared to controls tested in the same laboratory, Mittal et al. (1975) found no significant deviation in HL-A phenotype frequencies between 111 patients and controls. Tomoda et al. (1976) came to similar conclusions. However, Mittal et al. (1975) did observe an increased frequency of HL-All and W18 in patients who currently still have choriocarcinoma, and suggest that, if the results are valid for larger patient populations, then these two antigens may be associated with morbidity or progress in trophoblast neoplasia rather than predisposition.

12.4 Sex of trophoblast neoplasms

Original observations on the sex of the foetus associated with trophoblast neoplasms did not show any bias towards male or female. Schoen et al. (1954) analysed 13 cases of choriocarcinoma where the sex of the preceding child was recorded, and found the distribution to be eight females and five males. The difficulty here lies in the fact that the tumour may present a long time afterwards, and it is not always possible to exclude an intervening undiagnosed abortion as the causal pregnancy for the choriocarcinoma. Beischer (1966) reviewed the literature from 1903—1964 on cases of hydatidiform mole associated with a coexistent foetus but found only 12 cases where the sex of the foetus was recorded. Males and females occurred with an equal frequency. Tominaga and Page (1966), on the other hand, found nine female to three male foetuses associated with hydatidiform moles recorded in the literature from 1938—1960. Besides being small, these samples are not truly representative in that the presence of a coexistent foetus is unusual. The vast majority of hydatidiform moles and choriocarcinomas are not associated with a foetus, viable or otherwise, and it is these cases which should be investigated.

Varying methods have been used to directly sex these chorionic lesions. Analyses of the chromosomes revealed a preponderance of female karyotypes. Makino et al. (1963) studied the chromosomes in cultured cells from seven hydatidiform moles, two destructive moles, and two choriocarcinomas, and found female karyotypes in all specimens. Even those with tetraploid chomosomes exhibited exact duplication of the female somatic complement. Atkin (1965) analysed the chromosomes of six hydatidiform moles and found four had XX karyotypes, one had an XY karyotype and one had counts of 69 chromosomes with two sex chromatins. Wei and Chiang (1967) looked at the sex chromatin of cells cultured from 14 hydatidiform moles and found that cells from 10 (71.4%) of these exhibited the sex chromatin body and were, therefore, females while four were chromatin negative.

To obtain sufficient numbers of cultured cells from trophoblast neoplasms for chromosome and chromatin analyses is a laborious procedure. Investigators, therefore, explored the possibility of using histological sections of trophoblast neoplasms stained by the Fuelgen method to reveal the sex chromatin. The main advantage of this method is that it permits the retrospective examination of a large number of tumours. Tominaga and Page (1966) studied the sex chromatin in cytotrophoblast cells of 30 cases of hydatidiform mole and invasive mole and judged 29 cases (97%) to be chromatin positive. Of 18 cases of choriocarcinoma, 14 (78%) were found to be chromatin positive. They also collected the scattered observations from the literature spanning 1957—1966 and calculated that 86 of 98 cases (88%) were chromatin positive. Similar findings were recorded by Baggish et al. (1968) who found that 79 out of 90 cases (88%) of hydatidiform mole were chromatin positive, and by Atkin (1965) who observed that 47 out of 53 hydatidiform moles were chromatin positive. In general, chromatin sex was in agreement with chromosome analyses in those cases where this was done.

It may be argued that, since trophoblast neoplasms are frequently heteroploid or polyploid, the interpretation of genetic sex by using the chromatin body is extremely hazardous. However, male polyploid cells do not usually exhibit the sex chromatin body (Klinger and Schwarzacher 1960), and cells with double sex chromatins are rarely observed in hydatidiform moles (Marquez-Monter 1962). Furthermore, the sex chromatin is frequently absent in carcinoma cells arising from female patients which seems to indicate that abnormal karyotype is more likely to be associated with a loss of chromatin. Therefore, false negatives are more likely to complicate the picture than false positives, where there is an increase in ploidy.

Not all female cells exhibit the chromatin body nor are all male cells negative. It is generally agreed that male tissues contain no more than about 5% of cells exhibiting the chromatin body, while female tissues should have 15% or more of chromatin positive cells. When trophoblast cells of hydatidiform moles were analysed for their sex chromatin status as in the study by Baggish et al. (1968), it is clear that there was a further difficulty in interpretation because a large number of cases fell between 5% and 15% and it was, therefore, difficult to allot them into male or female categories. The data of Park (1957) showed a similar continuous distribution without separation into high and low incidence groups. Thus, Loke (1969) decided to analyse the stromal cells of the hydatidiform mole villi for sex chromatin rather than trophoblast. This revealed a distinct bimodal distribution of the incidence of cells exhibiting the sex chromatin, with one peak between 0—4% and the other around 25—29%, so there was no ambiguity in the demarcation between male and female cases (Fig. 12.3). In this study, 78 cases were chromatin positive (83%) and 14 cases were chromatin negative.

The balance of evidence from clinical observations as well as chromosome and chromatin analyses seems to suggest that there is a greater tendency for trophoblast neoplasms to be derived from a female placenta. In addition, chromatin positive hydatidiform moles tend to be more aggressive in their behaviour than chromatin negative ones, as revealed by their greater degree of trophoblastic proliferation and apparent deeper invasion of the uterine musculature (Loke and Borland 1969). It is not known why there is this unusual sex distribution in trophoblast neoplasms. The possible influence of a Y-linked antigen on human foetal-maternal interaction has already been discussed in

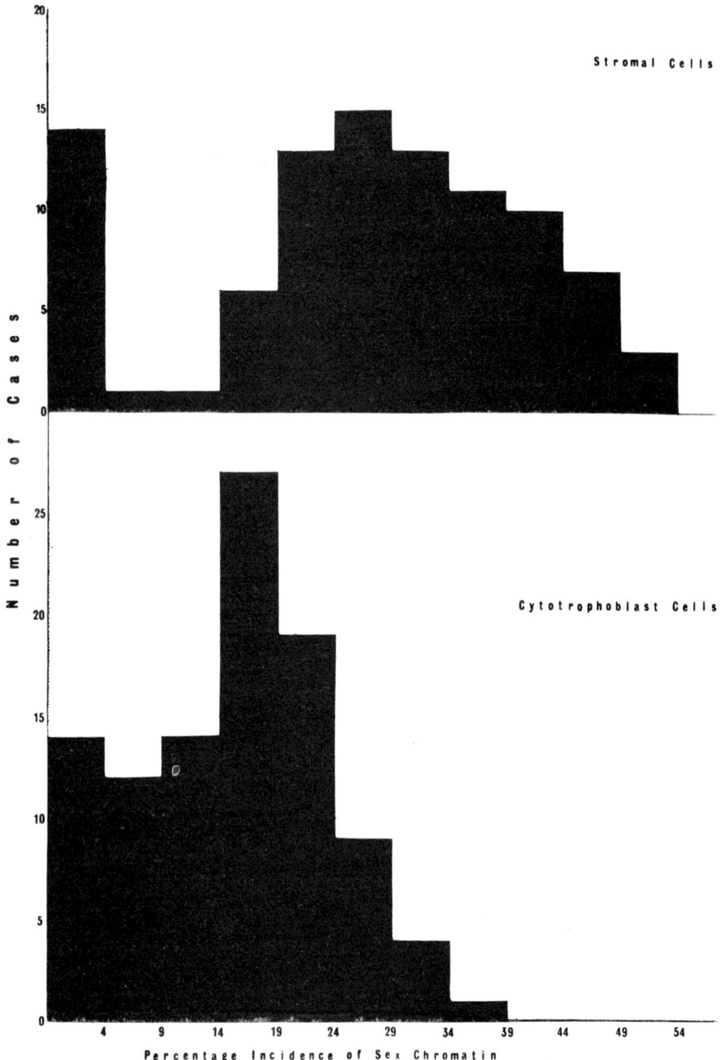

Fig. 12.3 Percentage incidence of sex chromatin in cytotrophoblast cells and in stromal cells. From Loke, Y. W. (1969) *J. med. Genet.* 6, 22—25.

Chapter 10. In the present context the reason why XX trophoblast is more susceptible than XY trophoblast to neoplastic transformation may be because this form of malignancy behaves in a recessive manner. Recent experiments with human cells have shown that fusion between malignant and normal cells resulted in the suppression of malignancy, as measured by tumour formation in immunosuppressed mice, while malignant-malignant hybrids retained their cancerous characteristics (Stanbridge 1976). These experiments used variants of malignant HeLa cells fused with normal fibroblasts. It remains to be seen if this suppression of malignancy is a general phenomenon of all human somatic cells. Japanese workers (Kajii and Ohama 1977) have recently postulated that hydatidiform moles receive all their chromosomes from a paternal source, due to fertilisation of an ovum whose nucleus is absent or inactivated. If malignancy is due to a recessive mutation, the high malignancy rate of hydatidiform moles may be explained by the homozygous nature of these tumours. Fertilisation by a haploid sperm followed by duplication of the chromosomes can give rise to the apparent diploid constitution seen in hydatidiform moles. Perhaps those with YY chromosomes are not viable, leaving only the XX ones to give rise to the high incidence of 'female' trophoblast neoplasms.

12.5 Production of HCG by trophoblast neoplasms

Trophoblast neoplasms retain the capacity to produce HCG. This can be seen clinically and also in studies of choriocarcinoma cells grown in tissue culture. Indeed, the BeWo line of choriocarcinoma cells established by Pattillo and Gey (1968) was the first hormone-synthesising cell-line to be established in vitro. These cultured cells have so far continued to produce HCG, even after many generations of sub-culture. HCG has also been demonstrated histochemically in both syncytial and cytotrophoblast cells of trophoblast neoplasms (Gärtner et al. 1975). This hormone, therefore, has become a reliable tumour marker and the development of sensitive radio-immunoassays has provided a valuable tool in the diagnosis and monitoring of progress of the disease (Bagshawe 1973).

In a previous chapter, the local and systemic immunoprotective roles of HCG in relation to normal trophoblast have already been discussed. The large amounts of HCG produced by neoplastic trophoblast may have a similar part to play in abrogating host response. The daily urinary HCG excretion in choriocarcinoma patients can reach a higher level than during the peak production period of normal pregnancy (Bagshawe 1973), but this is probably due to some tumours attaining a greater bulk. The production of HCG per choriocarcinoma cell has been calculated to be approximately 5×10^{-5} IU of HCG per day (Pattillo et al. 1971; Bagshawe 1973) compared to a figure of 1.4×10^{-2} IU of HCG per day secreted by a normal trophoblast cell (Braunstein et al. 1973), so it appears that individual choriocarcinoma cells do not have a greater capacity to synthesise the hormone compared to their normal counterparts. Qualitative differences between HCG produced by normal trophoblast and neoplastic trophoblast have also been reported. It appears that HCG produced by neoplastic trophoblast contains more sialic acid and hexose but less hexosamine than normal HCG (Reisfeld and Hertz 1960; Ashitaka et al. 1972). Whether these structural differences in HCG composition have any part to play in the behaviour of trophoblast neoplasms remains to be elucidated.

Antibody to HCG has no direct effect on the growth of choriocarcinoma cells in vitro but when given to hamsters with serially transplanted choriocarcinoma in their cheek pouches will markedly reduce the size of these tumours (Nisula and Kohler 1974). This suggests that the mode of action of HCG may be a modification of the HCG protective layer on the surface of the tumour cells, so they are now susceptible to attack by host effector lymphocytes. The importance of host cell-mediated response receives further support from the observation that treatment of hamsters with transplanted choriocarcinoma with heterologous anti-lymphocyte serum resulted in a higher incidence of tumour growth, increased tumour volume, and longer tumour survival (Lewis et al. 1969). These observations raise the hope that antiserum generated to HCG may be successful as an immunotherapeutic approach to the treatment of choriocarcinoma. It is thought that the danger of immunological enhancement of tumour growth is less likely to occur when antibody is generated against a product of cellular metabolism like HCG, rather than against structural constituents of tumour cell membrane. It is hoped that the anti-HCG may further neutralise the systemic effects of the hormone and thereby alleviate some of the patients' symptoms. Initial observations on human patients with choriocarcinoma, however, do not seem promising. Dr. Bagshawe in a discussion following Stevens' (1976) paper reported infusing up to 160 ml of a potent rabbit anti-HCG into patients with residual drug-resistant choriocarcinomas, but there were no discernible cytotoxic effects on the tumour cells, in spite of the amount of antiserum given being calculated to be in excess of that required to neutralise all the HCG/LH in the body fluids of these patients.

13

Transmission of immunity after birth

13.1 Absorption of immunoglobulins from neonatal intestine

In many animal species, the transmission of immunity occurs predominantly and sometimes even solely after birth by suckling (Brambell 1970). In man, however, this route has generally been considered to be unimportant relative to the transplacental transfer of antibodies before birth. A major argument in favour of this conclusion has been the repeated failure by investigators to demonstrate that antibodies in colostrum or milk can be absorbed through the human neonatal intestine.

As early as 1923, Kuttner and Ratner reported they could find no increase in the antitoxin titre of the infant's serum after ingestion of colostrum containing diptheria antitoxin. Diptheria antibodies in serum also did not appear to be absorbed in any significant amounts when given orally to newborns and older infants (Vahlquist and Högstedt 1949). In a study of 97 mothers with anti-A, anti-B and anti-Rh antibodies in their sera and colostra, Boorman et al. (1958) were unable to detect any rise in the serum titre of these antibodies in infants who were breast fed. Sussman (1961) examined the antibody titre to E. coli in 27 mothers and their infants. All maternal sera and colostra were found to contain antibody to E. coli 0111-B4 and in 19 cases the titre in colostrum on the first day after birth was higher than in the corresponding serum. In spite of this high colostral titre, only two infants manifested a rise in serum antibody level after suckling.

Antibodies contained in heterologous colostra have been observed to behave in a similar manner to those in human colostra. Nordbring (1957b) fed cow's colostrum containing paratyphoid 'H' agglutinins to nine premature infants but no detectable agglutinins appeared in their sera. Newborn infants and older children given cow's milk and serum containing diptheria antitoxin also showed no increase in antitoxin titre in their sera (Dixon et al. 1959).

The only observation suggestive of intestinal absorption was that by Leissring et al. (1962). They fed pooled human hyperimmune serum against S. typhi and S. paratyphi B and tetanus toxoid to seven infants ranging in ages from 12 hours to five days. In every case, a rise in circulating levels of these antibodies was detected. In several instances, the final titre attained in the infants' sera was only one dilution less than that of the serum administered, an efficiency of intestinal absorption which is rather difficult to accept.

Thus, until further evidence is available, it must be concluded that substantial amounts of immunoglobulins are probably not absorbed via the human neonatal intestine. Undoubtedly, small amounts of intact proteins do gain access to the circulation by this route as is illustrated by the occurrence of food-induced systemic anaphylactic reactions, but significant transfer of passive immunity appears unlikely. For this reason, the immunology of human colostrum and milk has, in the past, received little attention compared to that which has been directed at bovine lacteal secretions. However, the recognition of local immuno-protective qualities of IgA antibodies and the preponderance of this class of immunoglobulin in exocrine secretions including colostrum have provided fresh impetus for re-evaluation of the role of colostrum and milk in the protection of the human foetus. The recent detection of immunocompetent cells in human milk indicates that perhaps cell-mediated immunity as well as humoral immunity may be transferred.

13.2 Epidemiological evidence that breast-feeding is beneficial to the infant

Robinson (1951) observed in Great Britain that infant mortality occurred almost six times as frequently in bottle-fed babies than in breast-fed babies while the incidence of morbidity in bottle-fed babies was twice that of breast-fed babies. Those infants who were partly bottle-fed had incidence rates between the two groups (Table 13.1). In a survey

Table 13.1 Relationship between feeding and mortality and morbidity.

Feeding	No. of infants	Mortality (per/1000)	Morbidity (per/1000)
Breast-fed	971	10.2	223.4
Partly bottle-fed	1441	25.7	464.2
Bottle-fed	854	57.3	573.7
Total	3266	29.3	421.3

With kind permission from Robinson, M. (1951) *Lancet* 1, 788–794.

in Scandinavia under more controlled conditions, Mellander et al. (1959) also concluded that mortality and morbidity rates in infants favoured the breast-fed, but this favourable influence was mostly limited to the first three months of life. The advantage of breast-feeding is also manifested in lower socio-economic areas of the world like Central America where it has been reported that breast-fed village children experienced fewer infections with enteropathogenic E. coli (Mata and Urrutia 1971) as well as systemic infections (Mata and Wyatt 1971).

Further evidence that human milk may indeed interfere with intestinal colonisation by microbial pathogens are provided by the observations on infant vaccination by oral administrations of attenuated poliomyelitis virus. In a survey of over 1,000 infants vaccinated in this way during the first three months of life (Warren et al. 1964), it was found that breast-fed babies were less susceptible to infection by these viruses as monitored by the secretion of virus in their stools (Sabin et al. 1963) and the development of antibodies (Lepow et al. 1961). It was postulated that this could be due to neutralisation of the administered virus in the lumen of the infant's gut by antibodies in milk.

Taken altogether, the evidence would seem to favour the view that the contribution by breast-feeding to infant health is due to protective factors in human milk and not simply that it is a less frequent conveyor of pathogenic organisms than artificial milk products.

13.3 Immunoglobulins in human colostrum and milk

There are many factors in human milk which may provide a defense against infection for the neonate (Hanson and Winberg 1972; Goldman

Table 13.2 Different immunoglobulin classes in human colostrum.

	Mean values (mg/100 ml)		
	IgG	IgM	IgA
First day after delivery	43	159	1735
Fourth day after delivery	4	10	100

With kind permission from Ahmann, A. J. and Stiehm, E. R. (1966) *Proc. Soc. exp. Biol. Med.* 122, 1098–1100.

and Smith 1973). In an immunological analysis of human milk, Hanson (1959) detected 12 separate antigenic factors, eight of which were similar to those found in serum. Gamma-globulin was one of the substances found in both milk and serum, but unlike serum, the major immunoglobulin fraction in colostrum was IgA (Chodiker and Tomasi 1963) with a mean level of 151 mg/100 ml. Ahmann and Steihm (1966) recorded even higher levels of IgA in colostrum (Table 13.2). From the Table it can be seen that there was a rapid fall in colostral immunoglobulin levels after delivery, which is a point worth remembering in the interpretation of data relating to immunoglobulin levels of milk taken at various stages of the post-parturient period. In spite of the high levels of colostral IgA, serum levels of IgA in breast-fed and bottle-fed babies were found to be the same which is further evidence that milk antibodies are not absorbed through the intestine in any appreciable quantities.

Human colostral IgA appears to be immunologically identical to that of parotid saliva (Tomasi and Zigelbaum 1963). When extracted in a purified state, human colostral IgA has a molecular weight of 393,000 with a sedimentation coefficient of 11.7S. Further characterisation revealed it to be made up of two molecules of monomer IgA and a secretory piece which has a molecular weight of about 76,000 (Newcomb et al. 1968). It would appear, therefore, that the IgA in colostrum is very similar to the SIgA of mucous secretions.

IgE has also been detected in the colostrum and milk of two women (Bennich and Johansson 1971).

13.4 Specific antibodies in human colostrum and milk

Specific antibodies to a variety of potential pathogens have been detected in human colostrum and milk. As to bacterial diseases, colostrum has been reported to contain antibodies against pertussis (Adams et al. 1947), streptolysin and staphylolysin (Nordbring 1957a), and pneumococci which were both group and type specific against Types 3, 6, 9, 14 and 24 (Mouton et al. 1970). In general, the antibody titre is lower in colostrum than in the corresponding serum. Rather surprisingly, antibodies against enterobacteria are also frequently found in high titres in human colostrum. Arnon et al. (1959) detected antibodies to two strains of E. coli as well as to Shigella sonnei. Allardyce et al. (1974) compared the levels of antibody of S. typhi in colostrum and serum in three patients who developed clinical gastro-intestinal infection during pregnancy. Colostrum was found to contain IgA agglutinins against both salmonella flagellar and somatic antigens at a titre which exceeded that found in the patient's serum. Gindrat et al. (1972) detected antibodies against the 'O' antigens of E. coli belonging to serogroups most commonly associated with neonatal infections in 17 out of 19 milk samples tested. The titre of this antibody was very high (over 1 in 2,000) immediately after birth and then fell gradually within the next few days.

Antibodies to bacterial enterotoxins have also been demonstrated. Pooled colostrum from Guatemalan mothers obtained 2—4 days post partum was found to inhibit the induced fluid accumulation in rabbit ileal loops when incubated with V. cholerae or E. coli enterotoxin (Stoliar et al. 1976). This factor resided mainly in the IgA fraction. Similarly, Holmgren et al. (1976) demonstrated the presence of neutralising antibodies to E. coli and V. cholerae enterotoxins in milk obtained from Pakistani mothers but only rarely in Swedish mothers. This was thought to be due to a difference in antigenic exposure between the two population groups.

Human colostrum and milk also contain antibodies to enteroviruses like polio (Michaels 1965). Sabin and Fieldsteel (1962) examined colostrum and late milk of 71 mothers and detected activity against Type 2 polio virus in all of them, this activity residing in the γ-globulin fraction. The concentration in colostrum was higher than in the corresponding serum. Athreya et al. (1964) detected antibody to all three types of poliovirus in milk and serum of nursing mothers. The immunodiffusion pattern of the antibodies in serum and milk showed precipitin lines of identity. As emphasised by Hodes (1964), the presence of reaction lines of identity does not necessarily mean that the anti-polio antibody in milk and in serum are of the same immunoglobulin class, although they are probably directed against the same antigenic determinants. This was subsequently confirmed by the observation that poliovirus antibody in colostrum resided in the β-2A globulin fraction with a sedimentation of 10.5—14.8S while serum polio antibody was mainly γ-2 and β-2M globulins (Hodes et al. 1964).

Beside antibodies to pathogenic organisms, human milk has also been found to contain antibodies to foreign proteins. Hanson et al. (1977) found high titres of SIgA against purified cow's milk α-casein, β-casein and β-lactoglobulin in all 20 samples of human milk analysed.

The presence of all these antibodies in milk directed against a variety of potentially pathogenic enteric organisms as well as foreign proteins could provide the necessary protection for the neonate's gastro-intestinal tract against food allergens and infections. This hypothesis is supported by evidence that colostral antibodies seem able to survive their passage through neonatal intestine without being degraded. Kenny et al. (1967) noticed that stools of newborn breast-fed infants contained significant amounts of haemagglutinating antibody to enteropathogenic E. coli and neutralising antibody to polio viruses. Similarly Gindrat et al. (1972) observed that when infants were fed with milk with high titres of E. coli antibodies, their stool samples also showed significant amounts of the same antibody, reaching titres of 1 in 128 to 1 in 4,000. This ability to survive in the gastro-intestinal environment appears to be associated with the property of colostral IgA of being able to resist proteolytic digestion. Even when treated with trypsin and chymotrypsin, colostral IgA can maintain its 11S quaternary structure and secretory piece (Brown et al. 1970). It is not known how this resistance is brought about. Human colostrum contains a trypsin inhibitor which may neutralise some of the effects of intestinal proteolytic enzymes (Laskowski and Laskowski 1951). It has been further suggested that the secretory piece can act as a built-in protector for colostral IgA against tryptic digestion (Shim et al. 1969).

13.5 Cellular content of human colostrum and milk

As well as antibodies, recent investigations have shown that viable immunocompetent cells are also normal constituents of human colostrum and milk. Lawton and Shortridge (1977) reported a cell count ranging from 0.5×10^6 to 10×10^6/ml in colostrum, these cells being represented by polymorphs, macrophages and lymphocytes. In an examination of colostrum from 60 mothers, Smith and Goldman (1968) found a mean concentration of 2,100/mm^3 of macrophages, 205/mm^3 of lymphocytes, and 150/mm^3 of neutrophils. Both T-lymphocytes and B-lymphocytes are present (Diaz-Jouanen and Williams 1974). Parmely et al. (1977) found that 50.2% of milk lymphocytes were T-cells as judged by spontaneous sheep red cell rosette formation.

Some of the cells in milk exhibit phagocytic properties (Pitt 1976) and can be stimulated to secrete an interferon-like substance with strong antiviral activity (Emödi and Just 1974; Lawton and Shortridge 1977). The lymphocytes have been shown to respond to a variety of stimuli known to activate T-cells. Smith and Goldman (1968) found that the majority of milk cells (80—90%) underwent transformation when stimulated with non-specific stimuli like PHA, while a variable proportion (10—25%) were stimulated by tetanus toxoid, penicillin, diptheria, and PPD. Mohr et al. (1970) also noticed the manifestation of sensitivity to tuberculin by milk lymphocytes which correlated closely with the peripheral leucocyte response of the donor and with skin reactivity of the donor to the same antigen. In a detailed comparison of the reactivity of milk lymphocytes and peripheral blood lymphocytes from the corresponding donor, Parmely et al. (1976) noticed four main differences:

(1) milk lymphocytes were less responsive to non-specific stimuli like PHA and Con A compared to peripheral lymphocytes, as judged by thymidine incorporation;

(2) the response by milk lymphocytes to allogeneic stimulation was also less than by peripheral lymphocytes;

(3) milk lymphocytes from candida-sensitive donors did not respond to candida antigen, while peripheral lymphocytes from the same donors responded significantly; and

(4) milk lymphocytes responded to E. coli of K1 serotype while peripheral lymphocytes did not.

There was thus a marked disparity in the response of milk lymphocytes and peripheral blood lymphocytes from the same individual to certain antigenic stimulation. This may be a reflection of the presence of certain antigen-reactive clones in one population and not in the other. It is interesting to note that milk lymphocytes are particularly sensitised to gut-derived antigens from potentially pathogenic organisms like E. coli. The adoptive transfer of these specifically sensitised maternal lymphocytes to the neonatal intestine via milk could, therefore, aid in the defense against these enteropathogens.

Many immunoglobulin-producing cells are also present in human colostrum and milk. Using a radio-immunoelectrophoretic method, Murillo and Goldman (1970) detected synthesis of IgA and β1C by colostral cells. Macrophages, which are abundant in colostrum, are probably responsible for producing the complement component. No evidence of IgG or IgM synthesis was found which was a significant point of difference from peripheral blood lymphocytes. About 8% of human colostral lymphocytes were found to synthesise IgA antibodies (Ahlstedt et al. 1975).

13.6 Origin of colostral antibody and antigen-reactive cells

There has been much discussion on the origin of the antibodies found in colostrum and milk. Are they locally synthesised or are they derived from serum? If they have come from serum, then the fact that IgA is the major class of immunoglobulin in milk must be explained on the basis of a selective concentration mechanism in the breast. On the other hand, since IgA-synthesising cells have been demonstrated in milk, it seems that local immunoglobulin production in the breast is perhaps a more likely mechanism. Like the observations on T-cells, colostral IgA-producing lymphocytes have also been found to react against entero-bacterial antigens. In an indirect plaque assay technique used by Ahlstedt et al. (1975), IgA production was stimulated by pooled E. coli 'O' antigens. There is, therefore, a population of T-lymphocytes and B-lymphocytes in breast milk with activities towards bacterial antigens connected with the gut.

How is the gastro-intestinal immunological experience transmitted to the breast? Two mechanisms are possible. The bacterial infection may be disseminated from the gut via the systemic circulation to come into contact with antigen-sensitive cells in the breast. However, the observed disparity in antigen sensitivity between milk lymphocytes and peripheral blood lymphocytes and the lack of correlation between milk and serum specific antibody levels are against this hypothesis. The demonstration of milk neutralising antibodies against E. coli and V. cholerae enterotoxins by Holmgren et al. (1976) and Stoliar et al. (1976) favours an alternative mechanism. These enterotoxins do not usually enter deeper tissues or reach the circulation, so the presence of specific enterotoxin antibodies in breast milk suggests that immunocompetent cells may be originally primed in the intestine and then selectively migrate to the breast. This mechanism is further supported by the findings of Goldblum et al. (1975). They fed to three pregnant women just before parturition a suspension of E. coli 083, a non-pathogenic strain which is known to colonise human intestine for just a short period. Within three days of ingestion, cells producing antibody against the 'O' somatic antigen of this E. coli strain were detected in the colostrum of all three women by the indirect plaque assay technique. At the same time, an increased concentration of IgA antibodies to E. coli 083 was noted in colostrum but there was no significant increase in IgM or IgG. Serum antibody level of any immunoglobulin class was not increased.

The observations, therefore, strongly support the de novo synthesis of specific IgA antibodies by colostral cells and that these cells have probably been sensitised in the gut and then migrated to the breast. The presence in milk of reactive clones to other antigens like diptheria and tuberculin may be explained by a similar mechanism where the original sensitisation takes place in the bronchus-associated lymphoid tissue rather than in the gut-associated lymphoid tissue. The two tissues share many morphological similarities (Bienenstock et al. 1973a) and may both function as sites where lymphocytes are sensitised to specific antigens as they gain entry to the body via these natural body channels. These committed lymphocytes are then disseminated through the lymphatics or blood stream to other organs like the breast (Bienenstock et al. 1973b). This postulate of immune sensitisation seems, at least, to have the merit of cellular economy.

13.7 Mode of action of colostral antibody and cells

It is not clear by what mechanism colostral antibody combats infection. The antibodies to enterotoxins can presumably prevent the onset of clinical symptoms by neutralising the effects of the toxins in the gut but their activity on the organisms themselves is less readily apparent. Purified human colostral 11S secretory IgA does not appear to have any opsonic activity (Zipursky et al. 1973). While all nine complement components are present in human colostrum (Nakajima et al. 1977), they may not be operative, for colostral IgA has no demonstrable complement-fixing ability (Quie et al. 1968). However, it seems that IgA (Götze and Müller-Eberhard 1971), especially when aggregated (Boackle et al. 1974) can stimulate the alternate pathway of complement activation via C3 proactivator. Colostral cells have been found to produce β1C globulin and a C3 proactivator has been demonstrated immunochemically in human milk (André et al. 1964) and colostrum

(Ballow et al. 1974). Nakajima et al. (1977) found that colostral C3 activity was reduced by cobra venom factor, indicating that Factor B for the generation of C3-cleaving factor for the alternate pathway is present. Thus, all the appropriate ingredients are available in human milk to activate C3 in vivo with the resultant generation of beneficial inflammatory products like opsonins, anaphylotoxins, and chemotactic factors in the neonatal intestine.

It has been reported that colostral IgA is bacteriocidal, even in the absence of complement components (Burden 1973), but Adinolfi et al. (1966) have shown that the bacteriolytic action of colostral antibody is dependent on the presence of lysozyme. Significant amounts of lysozyme have been detected in human colostrum (Jolles and Jolles 1961; Chandan et al. 1964; Adinolfi et al. 1966), so this substance may contribute towards the protective action of colostrum.

The exact significance of the adoptive transfer of maternal sensitised T-cells to the foetus via milk is also unclear. It is possible that these cells can help B-cell clones to produce specific IgA locally in the foetal intestine. Alternatively, there may actually be a passive transfer of local cell-mediated immunity to the foetal gut. A more intriguing question is whether these sensitised maternal cells can pass through the foetal gut to be disseminated and thus lead to the adoptive transfer of systemic cell-mediated immunity. There are data in support of such an occurrence. Mohr (1972, 1973) tested breast-feeding mothers and their infants for PPD skin-sensitivity. Five mothers were found to react positively. There were 11 children born to these positive reacting mothers, nine of whom were breast-fed and two were not. Five of the nine breast-fed infants, had positive PPD skin reactions while the two non-breast-fed infants, although from the same household, did not react. None of the 78 children breast-fed by PPD negative mothers had skin reactions to PPD. Repeated attempts to isolate TB bacilli from the PPD reactive mothers failed. Similar results were obtained by Schlesinger and Covelli (1977). They analysed three groups of infants. Group A consisted of 13 infants who were breast-fed by tuberculin positive mothers. Group B consisted of 13 infants who were not breast-fed by tuberculin positive mothers. Group C consisted of nine infants breast-fed by tuberculin negative mothers. It was found that eight out of 13 infants in Group A had tuberculin reactive cells in their peripheral blood after four weeks of breast-feeding compared to one infant out of 13 in Group B and none in Group C. Earlier studies on cord blood lymphocytes of these infants showed no transformation with PPD indicating no significant transplacental transmission. All the mothers were clinically free from tuberculosis.

The results from these studies are consistent with the adoptive transfer of systemic cell-mediated immunity from mother to infant via milk. Since all the mothers were clinically normal, this is probably not mediated by the transfer of antigens. Whether this is due to the actual passage of sensitised cells or to some soluble transfer factor cannot be decided with certainty at present. Some animal studies support the concept of transfer of antigen-reactive cells from mother to infant via milk. The observations by Head et al. (1977) that the induction of tolerance in rodents by neonatal intravenous injections of allogeneic cells is influenced by suckling, that the growth of a transplantable tumour is influenced by foster nursing, and that nude mice can receive T-lymphocytes from their mothers, would indicate that maternal cells from milk can influence the development of immunocompetence in rodents. Unfortunately, these conclusions are not shared by Silvers and Poole (1975) who, in a similar series of experiments did not find any evidence that foster nursing mice or rats on mothers of a different strain could alter the infants' survival or their immunological competence. Furthermore, when stained smears of milk taken from the stomachs of 12-hour newborn animals were examined, no viable cells were detected, so it is doubtful whether maternal immunocompetent cells can survive to any extent in neonatal intestinal tract. The importance of the adoptive transfer of cellular immunity from mother to young via milk must, therefore, await more definitive evidence.

14

Immunological interruption of pregnancy

As we have seen, the mother is surprisingly tolerant to her antigenic foetus during pregnancy. It has occurred to investigators that if somehow this immunological equilibrium can be altered, it may provide a method for the artificial interruption of pregnancy. Of necessity, most of the experiments to be described are based on animal studies including sub-human primates but small controlled human trials are being initiated. It is hoped that soon the efficacy of this form of human fertility control will be known.

14.1 Immunisation against placental antigens

An obvious procedure is to sensitise the mother against placental antigens in the hope that this might provoke an immunological hostile reaction directed against the conceptus. Many experiments of this nature have been performed on a variety of animal species using both passive and active immunisation schedules as well as heterologous, homologous and isologous placental tissue as antigens.

14.1.1 Abortifacient effects

Seegal and Loeb (1940) administered intravenously to pregnant rats on the 11—12th day of gestation rabbit antiserum to whole rat placental homogenate. They found that this antiserum affected development of the foetuses resulting in death and resorption of 66% of them. A similar injection of rabbit anti-rat whole blood antiserum, even in small doses, induced a greater degree of foetal death with resorption of 79% of the foetuses. It is, therefore, not clear from these experiments what antigens are involved. The fact that absorption of the anti-placental serum with rat red blood cells did not alter its abortifacient potency suggested that there could be a factor in the antibody which was directed against placental tissue. No extra-placental lesions were observed in the aborted rats. In the same year, Cohen and Nedzel (1940) reported similar findings in guinea pigs. Rabbit antiserum to full term guinea pig placental homogenate when injected intraperitoneally into pregnant guinea pigs resulted in abortions in five out of six animals a few days later. The antibody was absorbed with guinea pig liver and kidney tissues and its administration caused no lesions in these organs.

14.1.2 Cross reaction with kidney

Initial optimism that anti-placental antiserum acted on placental tissue alone was soon dispelled when Seegal and Loeb (1946) found that if the injected animals were not sacrificed immediately after the experiments but followed up over longer periods of 3—14 months, many of them (eight out of 32) developed a chronic glomerulonephritis. These lesions were identical to those produced by actually injecting rabbit anti-rat kidney antiserum. Therefore, there appears to be a high degree of cross reactivity between anti-placental and anti-kidney antibodies. Pregnant animals were even more susceptible to the nephrotoxic action of anti-placental serum than non-pregnant animals (Loeb et al. 1949).

Renal damage following the passive administration of anti-placental antiserum was subsequently noted in a variety of experimental animals. Beveans et al. (1955) found that intravenous infusion of rabbit anti-dog placental antibodies would produce nephritis in both pregnant and non-pregnant dogs. Similar lesions were observed in mice given rabbit anti-mouse placental antiserum on the 10—14th day of gestation. Although this interrupted the pregnancy in nearly all the treated animals and immunofluorescent localisation of rabbit immunoglobulin in the necrotic placentae confirmed the placenta to be a target organ for the reaction, extra-uterine lesions in the liver and kidneys were also observed (Koren et al. 1968). In fact, the antiserum did contain a mixture of antibodies as shown by the development of several precipitin lines on immuno-electrophoresis against mouse placental homogenate.

It has been repeatedly demonstrated that antibodies produced towards human placental antigens also cross react with kidney tissue in vitro (Steblay 1962; Boss 1965; Curzen 1970). Even an antibody raised against purified glycoproteins from human chorionic villi will localise in vitro to chorionic villi as well as to Bowman's capsule, and glomerular and tubular basement membrane of the kidney (Schwartz, E. S., et al. 1974). Passive immunisation of pregnant and non-pregnant rats with this antiserum resulted in nephritis, with immunoglobulin and C3 deposited in linear diffuse pattern in the glomeruli. The rats all suffered from proteinuria (Gang et al. 1974). Surprisingly, there was no interruption of pregnancy in spite of the antibody localising to chorionic villi in vitro.

Active immunisation studies have led to similar conclusions. Menge (1968) demonstrated that immunisation of rabbits with homologous homogenised conceptus material led to interference with implantation but again cross reaction with kidney remained a problem. Injection of homologous placental tissue intraperitoneally into rats similarly resulted in nephritis (Lee et al. 1970). Even isologous placental tissue extract, when injected with complete Freund's adjuvant, induced a nephritis in rats (Okuda and Grollman 1966). These animals exhibited albuminuria and hypertension and electronmicroscopic examination of the kidneys revealed swelling of the glomerular basement membrane, dense granular deposition along the capillary basement membrane and swelling and proliferation of glomerular epithelium (Irino et al. 1967), changes which are very similar to those associated with human toxaemia of pregnancy.

14.1.3 Toxic side effects

In the experiments of Koren et al. (1968), 10% of the passively immunised pregnant mice died, indicating the presence of some toxic factors in the anti-placental serum. It seems that careful absorption of the serum will go some way towards abrogating these unwanted side-effects. In a subsequent study, Kometani and Behrman (1971) noticed a diminution in toxicity after anti-mouse placental serum was repeatedly absorbed with normal mouse serum. This absorbed serum could still produce abortions in all animals when injected on day 2 or later of gestation. Even after absorption, this antiserum was found still to be directed towards at least four different placental proteins on immunodiffusion. Beer et al. (1972) also found they could remove the toxic effects of a rabbit anti-rat trophoblast serum by absorbing it with rat red blood cells and lymphocytes. This absorbed serum which previously had killed 12% of the immunised animals was no longer toxic but still maintained its abortifacient activity when given to pregnant rats on the 7—8th day post conception.

14.1.4 Teratogenic effects

Another potential hazard of immunisation against placental tissue is the production of foetal malformations. Brent (1967) observed that rabbit anti-rat placental serum would lead to foetal death as well as malformations when injected into pregnant rats. Similar results were obtained by administering anti-rat kidney serum. Kidney and placental antiserum had precipitin lines in common and absorption with kidney tissue could protect against the teratogenic effects of both kidney and placental antiserum. These findings suggest there could be one or more identical antibodies responsible for foetal loss and teratogenesis in kidney and placental antiserum.

The mechanism involved in the teratogenic activity of anti-placental serum was studied by Slotnick and Brent (1966). Sheep antiserum to rat placental homogenate was injected into 8 days pregnant rats. The animals were sacrificed 2—5 days later in order to localise the deposition of antibody in maternal organs and embryonic sites. Antibody was found in the basement membrane of kidney glomeruli, adrenal, liver and spleen among the maternal organs and in the parietal yolk sac membrane of the foetus. No antibody was detected in the embryo proper nor in the placental trophoblast. It was, therefore, concluded that the teratogenic action of anti-placental serum was not directly on the foetus or placenta but was on the yolk sac. Alternatively, foetal malformation was an indirect consequence of maternal disease due to the antiserum causing pathological lesions in her organs.

Again, contaminating factors in anti-placental serum could be responsible for its teratogenic effects for it was found that absorption of rabbit anti-mouse placental serum with mouse red cells completely abolished its teratogenic action while preserving its abortifacient activity (Nemirovsky 1970).

14.1.5 *Defining the placental antigens involved*

The main difficulty in all these studies employing immunisation against placental tissue or homogenate is that the target antigen on the placenta to which the abortifacient activity is directed has not been clearly defined. This is not surprising since there are likely to be many antigens on trophoblast cells. Allo-antigens may be involved for there is evidence that immunisation against these antigens can affect pregnancy in mice (Breyere and Sprenger 1969). Virgin female C57 BI/Bre mice were immunised against DBA/2 and against C_3H tissues and then mated to males of either type. It was found that there was a reduction in litter size in C_3H-immunised females when mated with C_3H males but this was not observed when DBA-immunised females were mated with C_3H males. Similarly, there was again a reduction in litter size when DBA-immunised females were mated with DBA males but not when C^3H-immunised females were mated with DBA males. The data of A. G. Clarke (1971) support these findings. Allo-antigens, however, are unlikely to be of much use as 'targets' for an abortifacient immune reaction for they will be shared by other tissues beside the placenta.

Developmental antigens present at a certain stage of differentiation may be involved. These antigens normally disappear from normal adult tissues but are sometimes re-expressed on malignant cells. It is, therefore, of some interest that immunisation of mice with malignant cells has been shown to interrupt pregnancy (Parmiani and Della Porta 1973). Mice were inoculated with a methylcholanthrene-induced syngeneic tumour and then mated. The immunised animals had a significantly reduced rate of pregnancy both in the first as well as the second pregnancy. A further group of mice immunised with syngeneic embryos also showed a significant inhibition of pregnancy rate. Thus, these results indicate that immune rejection of the conceptus can result from the immunisation of mothers against embryonic differentiation antigens which are shared by syngeneic embryonic cells and sarcoma cells. Obviously, these antigens will only be of use as 'target' antigens for abortifacient reactions at one specific phase of development.

It may be that the action of abortifacient antisera are not directed at any foetal or placental antigens at all but at some essential foetal products. For instance, it has been reported that rabbits injected intravenously with sheep anti-α-foetoprotein on the 21st day of gestation showed a high incidence of foetal mortality (Slade 1973). The biological role of α-foetoprotein is not known. There is evidence that it is produced by the yolk sac, so it is possible that the effect of the antibody is directed here rather than at the foetus itself.

It is clear that the ideal antigen would be a trophoblast-specific antigen to which an effective immune reaction can be directed. An attempt was made recently to find such an antigen in monkeys which could be used to interrupt pregnancy (Behrman et al. 1974). It was found that placental antigens from rhesus and squirrel monkeys were separable into three peaks on fractionation with Sephadex G-100. Antibody to Fractions I and II when used to passively immunise pregnant squirrel monkeys had no abortifacient effects but administration of antibody to Fraction III resulted in abortions in 14 out of 19 animals. Subsequent pregnancies occurred normally so this procedure has the merit of being reversible. This Fraction III placental antigen has a molecular weight of 35,000 and appears to have none of the activities associated with placental hormones or enzymes like HPL, HCG, alkaline phosphatase or leucine aminopeptidase. Furthermore, this Fraction III cross reacts with the pregnancy-specific β_1-glycoprotein of Bohn so this may well turn out to be the elusive trophoblast-specific antigen.

14.2 Immunisation against placental hormones

In the quest for a placental-specific protein, many investigators have turned their attention to the possibility of using one of the placental hormones. The two human placental protein hormones which have been most studied are:
(1) human placental lactogen (HPL), sometimes also known as human chorionic somatomammotrophin (HCS); and
(2) human chorionic gonadotrophin (HCG).

14.2.1 Immunisation against human placental lactogen (HPL)

El Tomi et al. (1971a) immunised pregnant rats with heterologous rabbit anti-HPL. When this was done early in gestation on days 1—5, the process of implantation was affected with the number of implantation sites observed at laparotomy significantly reduced. If the rats were immunised late from days 6—10 of gestation, this resulted in some foetal resorption. The mechanism of action is not clear, for it

Table 14.1 Effects of various procedures on pregnancy in rats.

Procedure	No. of animals	Litter size (mean)
Untreated	100	10.1 ± 4.3
Injected with normal rabbit serum	40	10.2 ± 3.9
Injected with rabbit anti-human serum albumin	20	9.6 ± 3.9
Injected with rabbit anti-HPL	45	0

With kind permission from Gusdon, J. P. (1972) *Amer. J. Obstet. Gynecol.* 112, 472–475.

appears that HPL antibodies can neutralise the action of more than one biological component in the rat. Similar experiments by Gusdon (1972) were even more dramatic. Pregnant rats injected with rabbit anti-HPL delivered no infants at all (Table 14.1). Examination of the uterine horns at autopsy showed inflammatory cells and signs of foetal resorption, so the antibody probably acted after implantation. Similar abortifacient activity of anti-HPL was also observed in mice (Yamini et al. 1972) and in baboon using homologous baboon anti-HPL (Stevens 1974).

Active immunisation with HPL has also been found to affect pregnancy. El Tomi et al. (1970) immunised rats with a purified preparation of HPL. The implantation rate was slightly reduced but the main effect was in the post-implantation period where there was marked reduction in the number of surviving foetuses. Similar effects were observed in rabbits by investigators from the same laboratory (El Tomi et al. 1971b). Rabbits were injected with purified HPL and then mated when their serum anti-HPL titre reached 1 in 5,000 or more. It was found that immunisation did not significantly reduce ovulation or implantation rates as demonstrated by the number of corpora lutea and implantation sites observed at laparotomy. Again, the action seemed to be at the post-implantation period, for many of the immunised rabbits failed to maintain their pregnancies and there was evidence of partial or complete foetal resorption. Preliminary results on squirrel monkeys have been reported by Gusdon (1976) who immunised a total of 16 animals with alum-precipitated HPL bi-weekly for three weeks before the mating season. In the preceding year, each of these animals delivered their first baby, but after immunisation, only half of these animals delivered an infant. In fact, this reduction continued for the next two mating seasons when still only half the immunised animals delivered. This long-term effect of HPL immunisation was already noted by Gusdon (1974) when he followed up his sample of rats passively immunised with anti-HPL serum. None of these rats delivered any babies even two years later in spite of being repeatedly mated. Eventual necropsies showed enlargements of uteri with residual cellular infiltration, so it seems that anti-HPL can lead to some long-term derangement of uterine physiology.

At present, the reason why immunisation against HPL leads to interruption of pregnancy is far from clear. This is because the physiological role of this hormone in normal pregnancy has yet to be fully elucidated. A further complication is the lack of detailed characterisation of the antisera or HPL preparations used. In a careful reappraisal of their previous studies which used different HPL preparations, Gusdon et al. (1974) concluded that the most effective abortifacient was the anti-HPL serum which had been prepared against the least pure HPL preparation. This antiserum had antibodies reacting also against embryonic and foetal antigens when checked immunochemically. So it is possible that the abortifacient effects of immunisation against HPL are due to interaction with other antigenic determinants rather than HPL itself. Yamini et al. (1972) similarly suspected that the activity on pregnancy of their anti-HPL serum could be caused by the presence of anti-lymphocyte antibodies.

Even if the specificity of anti-HPL serum can be confirmed, it is difficult to visualise how its abortifacient action is mediated. If it acts by neutralising the circulating hormone, the feed-back mechanism should come into play to stimulate the animal to produce some more. This possibility was brought up by Stevens in a discussion following Gusdon's (1976) paper. Preliminary results were presented where baboons were immunised with a highly purified preparation of homologous baboon placental lactogen. This was highly specific and the only other protein tested with which it would cross react was HPL. Hapten-coupling of this hormone generated high titres of antibody in the immunised animals. All these animals conceived. By the 30th day of gestation, the antibody levels came down sharply, and shortly afterwards, normal placental lactogen circulating levels were again achieved. None of the animals aborted. It seemed that hormone synthesis might have outstripped the production of antibodies and abortion was averted.

A direct cytotoxic action on HPL-producing cells of the placenta would be more effective either via sensitised lymphocytes or complement-mediated antibody destruction but, so far, there is no evidence to show that any of these reactions in fact occur. Thus, immunisation studies with HPL pose more questions than they answer, and much more work is needed before a more accurate picture can emerge.

14.2.2 Immunisation against human chorionic gonadotrophin (HCG)

HCG has been shown to possess both local and systemic immunosuppressive properties and many investigators feel that it may have an important role to play in the prevention of maternal rejection of her foetus. It is, therefore, the ideal candidate for antibody neutralisation in immunological attempts to interrupt pregnancy. There are, however, several obstacles in the way of in vivo studies of this hormone. Although antibodies raised in animals to HCG are serologically active and will neutralise HCG (Rao and Shahani 1961), these antibodies appear to have very little cross reactivity with the animals' own production of endogenous hormone (Glass and Mroueh 1967). It is, therefore, not possible to study the effects of anti-HCG on pregnancy functions using lower animals. Cross reactivity between HCG and non-human primate chorionic gonadotrophin also appears to be low (Stevens 1976), in spite of the relative similarity in chemical structure between the human hormone and those from the gorilla, chimpanzee and rhesus monkey (Hodgen et al. 1973). A possible explanation for the lack of cross reactivity in vivo when passive immunisation schedules with heterologous anti-HCG sera are used, is interference by antibodies developed in the recipient animals against the heterologous serum proteins. This was shown by Schlumberger and Anderer (1969), who found that injection of rabbit anti-HCG into female mice made tolerant to rabbit γ-globulin, induced prolonged oestrus and phases of sterility. This indicates that anti-HCG can cross react with mouse endogenous gonadotrophic activity in vivo and can neutralise its biological activity. These effects, however, were markedly decreased when immunocompetent mice were used.

Studies on homologous species present their own problems. Homologous hormones similar to those already present in the host are rarely antigenic and it is usually difficult to generate a high titre of antibodies towards them without the aid of noxious adjuvants. Stevens (1973) appears to have found a way round this problem by hapten-coupling the homologous hormone to a diazonium salt. Baboons, immunised with a homologous pituitary gonadotrophin altered in this matter and injected in an oil vehicle, were found to produce antibodies which cross reacted and neutralised the biological effects of endogenous unaltered hormone.

Perhaps the most serious problem is that antibody to HCG can cross react with other hormones. Structural studies of HCG have shown that it is made up of an α- and a β-subunit. The α-subunit resembles that of three other hormones, TSH, FSH and LH, so there is the obvious danger of cross reactions if the whole HCG molecule is used. The β-subunit of HCG, on the other hand, shows homology only to the β-subunit of LH but can be distinguished from the latter by the presence of 28 additional residues at the carboxyl terminus of the peptide chain (Carlsen et al. 1973). These findings offer the hope that immunisation against HCG β-subunit, particularly to the extra amino-acid residues, will lead to the production of an antibody which is highly specific to HCG alone.

From this background, we can now evaluate some of the experimental studies which have recently been performed on non-human primates and on a few women. Stevens and Crystle (1973) and Stevens (1976) studied a series of pre- and post-menopausal women and confirmed that antibodies could be elicited when these women were immunised with a highly purified intact HCG preparation hapten-coupled to para-amino sulphonic acid (PASA) and administered in mannide manoleate. Unfortunately, these antibodies generated to whole HCG would also cross react with endogenous LH as predicted, leading to a marked reduction in circulating LH levels.

Heterologous immunisation studies on baboons, rabbits and sheep using β-subunit of HCG (Stevens 1976) have shown that in 16 baboons immunised in this manner, no pregnancy resulted from 30 matings. Conception rates of non-immunised animals in the colony were usually in excess of 90%. Interruption of pregnancy could also be achieved by passive immunisation with anti-HCGβ-subunit serum. When 50 ml of a sheep anti-HCG β were administered intravenously to a pregnant baboon at about the 20th day of gestation, menstrual bleeding began 36 hours after the antibody infusion. Unfortunately, these studies have further confirmed the conclusion from structural analyses that the antibody so raised in all three species would cross react with human

LH. Thus, the cross reactivity even of an antibody raised against the β-subunit of HCG is unacceptably high to permit its use in full scale clinical trials.

Attempts, therefore, have been made to raise antibodies against the terminal amino-acid residues in HCG β-subunits which have no analogues in LH β-subunits. Since it is difficult to obtain sufficient quantities of this peptide from native HCG, immunisation with a synthetic 35 amino-acid peptide have been tried (Stevens 1976). Preliminary results are encouraging and have shown that antibodies to this synthetic peptide reacted on radioimmunoassay with intact HCG, β-subunit of HCG, a natural 39 amino-acid peptide obtained from chymotryptic digestion of HCG-β, and the synthetic peptide itself. Human LH did not cross react at doses of up to 2.5 IU. Dr. Talwar from India, in a discussion following Stevens' paper (1974), presented a slightly different method of ridding the LH cross reacting portion from the β-subunit of HCG. Repeated absorption with an immunoabsorbent against heterologous LH preparation finally produced an HCG preparation with negligible cross reactive sites with human LH. To induce antibody production, this purified HCG-β preparation was conjugated to a proteinic carrier rather than modified by haptenic groups like Stevens' procedure. Tetanus toxoid was used as this protein carrier which has the merit of being a substance which is approved for human use and also has highly desirable immunising properties. It was found that this HCG-β and tetanus toxoid complex was highly immunogenic in a variety of species ranging from mouse, rabbit, goat, monkey to man. The antibody produced reacted immunologically with total HCG molecule but not with HGH, HPL, FSH, TSH or LH at physiological concentrations. Some controlled clinical trials using this purified HCG-β preparation have begun in India and, so far, careful monitoring of the immunised patients' kidney, liver, thyroid, adrenal and pituitary functions have revealed no detectable abnormalities.

These studies have indicated that it may soon be feasible to immunise against a specific portion of HCG with no cross reactivity with other hormones. If it can be shown subsequently that this immunisation can disrupt pregnancy, then the goal towards an immunological control of human fertility is one step nearer. In addition, there is the hope that a similar regime could be used to combat the neoplastic equivalent of trophoblast, choriocarcinoma.

There are several possible mechanisms through which anti-HCG serum can act to achieve its anti-pregnancy effects. It may neutralise the hormone's endocrinological functions which are responsible for extending the life of the corpus luteum during pregnancy, so that the appropriate uterine environment cannot be maintained. The antiserum may abrogate the hormone's known immunosuppressive activity and thereby bring about the rejection of the placenta. A direct action on HCG-producing trophoblast cells of the placenta is a further possibility. The hormone is found on the surface of trophoblast cells and may even be incorporated as an integral component of the cell membrane so an antibody reacting against these HCG determinants may be expected to lead to damage of the membrane. Currie (1967) has reported that rabbit antibody to HCG, even at high dilutions, was cytotoxic to cultured human trophoblast cells in vitro in the presence of complement. Morisada et al. (1976) have, similarly, shown that organ culture of human trophoblast in the presence of rabbit anti-HCG resulted in severe degeneration, particularly of the syncytial layer. This effect was also seen in human trophoblast cultured in diffusion chambers in the peritoneal cavity of rabbits immunised against HCG (Morisada et al. 1972). These results, however, are somewhat difficult to interpret, for the antigenic source of HCG was from commercial preparations of no more than about 5,900 IU/mg. It has been shown that these crude preparations are frequently contaminated with impurities like human serum proteins so that an antiserum prepared against these HCG preparations is likely to contain antibodies directed at human species antigens rather than HCG alone, especially if used unabsorbed as would appear to be the case in Morisada's studies. The fact that non-immunised rabbits permitted the growth of human trophoblast for a relatively longer period does not clarify the situation. Perhaps a more important control would be to see if other human embryonic tissues behave in a similar way in the presence of rabbit antiserum to HCG.

That anti-HCG may not have a direct cytotoxic action on HCG-secreting trophoblast cells is suggested by the data of Nisula and Kohler (1974). These investigators observed that anti-HCG had no demonstrable effects on the growth of choriocarcinoma cells in vitro but when given to hamsters with transplanted choriocarcinoma, would markedly reduce the size of these tumours. This was interpreted as due to the antiserum modifying the protective layer of HCG on the surface of the tumour cells so that they became susceptible to attack by host lymphocytes in vivo. The action of the antiserum, therefore, is an indirect one.

There is evidence that HCG is produced very early during human pregnancy at around the 8th day post-ovulation (Wide 1969; Mishell et al. 1974; Saxena et al. 1974). This may be indicative of HCG production by the pre-implantation human blastocyst. Gonadotrophin secretion has been reported for the rabbit blastocyst (Haour and Saxena 1974). This raises the hope that anti-HCG serum may act on the blastocyst before implantation. For medical as well as non-medical (e.g. religious) reasons, this mechanism of fertility control by preventing implantation is obviously far preferable to repeated abortions induced by post-implantation effects of antiserum on the placenta.

14.3 Application to human fertility control

It is clear that many of the experimental procedures described in this chapter are unlikely to be clinically applicable. Immunisation with placental antigens, no matter how purified, are too crude, with their attendant dangers of cross reactivity, nephrotoxicity and teratogenicity. What is needed is an antigen whose specificity can be clearly defined. The main hope of isolating such a placental-specific protein to which immunisation can be directed probably lies in one of the placental hormones. Of these, HCG would seem to be the prime candidate for many reasons. It is a hormone with known immunosuppressive properties so its neutralisation would be expected to have the prospect of boosting maternal immunological reactivity against her conceptus. HCG is presumably only produced by the trophoblast during pregnancy so its ablation by antiserum would not lead to any derangement of the body's self-regulatory feed-back mechanism, as would be the case for immunological intervention against pituitary gonadotrophins. Detailed studies of the structure of HCG have revealed a portion of the molecule which is unique to it and investigators are optimistic that immunisation against this peptide will be directed specifically at HCG with negligible cross reactions with other hormones. It remains to be seen whether this immunisation procedure will achieve its objective of interrupting human pregnancy.

Although the fundamental problems associated with the isolation of a specific placental protein as 'target' for immunological attack is nearing a solution, there are still some misgivings about whether this form of fertility control is advisable in man. These doubts have recently been aired in a symposium in the Karolinska Institute in Stockholm

(Celada 1974; Mitchison 1974). A decision has to be made whether active or passive immunisation is the method of choice. Initially, during clinical trials when the potential dangers are still unknown, it may be argued that passive immunisation is to be preferred for the effects will not be too long lasting. Passive immunisation has a further merit in that it is quick acting and can, therefore, be used only when needed like after the discovery of a missed period. The main disadvantage, of course, is the danger of hypersensitivity resulting from repeated administration of heterologous antiserum. The use of homologous antiserum will circumvent this problem but it is probably impracticable to find enough human volunteers for this task. Hence, active immunisation as envisaged by Stevens and Talwar remains the more feasible procedure.

A related question is that of reversibility. Passive immunisation is obviously transient but the disadvantage will be the need for repeated re-immunisation. Active immunisation tends to be more long lasting. From experience with other types of immunisation, this kind of immunity will also wane in time unless there is some form of persistence of antigen. In the case of immunisation against HCG, it is not known whether the cross reacting endogenous LH can provide the stimulus. This may lead to a permanent state of sterility which will be difficult to reverse.

The possible occurrence of immunopathological phenomena should also be carefully explored. Immune neutralisation of hormone or destruction of trophoblast tissue could lead to immune-complex disease. Stimulation by environmental antigens is very different from stimulation by antigens related to self components and auto-immunity is another danger which should be kept in mind. Although immunisation against a specific part of the HCG molecule will prevent the induction of autoimmunity via shared antigenic determinants with other self components, other mechanisms of T-B cell cooperation may come into play. When T-cells are sensitised to this sub-component of HCG, they may then serve as helper-cells to present other parts of the host's own -subunits to B-cells. These B-cells will then produce antibodies which will cross react with other host's components bearing the appropriate β-subunit antigenic configuration (Mitchison 1974). In other words, cross reactivity with LH can still result.

It must also be pointed out that immune reaction can work both ways, that is, rejection as well as facilitation. This will be particularly relevant if immunisation results in a response directed at embryonic or developmental antigens which are sometimes re-expressed on neoplastic cells. The immunopotentiation of tumour growth may upset the normal immune-surveillance mechanism, leading to a higher incidence of cancer.

The possible effects on the population, as opposed to the individual, must also be considered. Immunological control of human fertility could impose a selective pressure in favour of those who cannot mount an adequate immune response. The genetical consequence of immunoselection against the immune response genes has yet to be determined.

From what has been said, it is evident that many problems are still to be surmounted before an immunological method of human fertility control can be considered as an alternative to those which are already available. We have, of course, only dealt with the possible immune attack on the conceptus for this is related to our discussion on the foetal-maternal interaction. There are, however, other stages in the human reproductive process which are susceptible to immunological interference (Diczfalusy 1974; Edwards 1976). Indeed, pre-fertilisation periods may be even more amenable to immunological manipulations like, for example, local immunisation of the female genital tract against spermatozoa. It may well be that human fertility regulation of the future will be directed at one of these early stages of the reproductive cycle rather than against the already implanted conceptus.

15

Conclusion

The evolution of placentation and viviparity has undoubted survival advantage for the newborn but, at the same time, this form of reproduction creates many problems. The placenta is especially developed in those species, like man, which also have the most efficient immune system so there must be some means by which the mother is prevented from rejecting her antigenically alien conceptus during the period of gestation. At present, it is not clear how this immunological equilibrium is maintained but multiple factors are likely to be involved.

Prime consideration must be given to the placenta for it is this extra-embryonic organ, and not the embryo itself, which lies in intimate contact with maternal tissue over a wide surface area. Evidence would seem to indicate that trophoblast cells of the human placenta do possess special surface characteristics which could, at least in theory, confer on the organ special immunologically neutral properties. For instance, surface antigens are more difficult to demonstrate on trophoblast cells in vitro than on equivalent cells from other foetal tissues and trophoblast cells are also less immunogenic in in vivo transplantation studies. This relative deficiency of antigenic expression may be due to structural surface characteristics, for it has been observed that trophoblast cells have a peri-cellular layer of sialic acid-rich mucoprotein material which could mask antigens. Although an attractive hypothesis, direct confirmatory evidence is lacking. Attempts to dissolve away this layer by enzymatic treatment have generally failed to uncover any underlying antigenic determinants. The alternative concept that this mucoprotein coat could affect the efferent arc of the maternal immune response by increasing the surface negative charge or by its surface hydration properties, thereby preventing close contact with maternal effector lymphocytes, again has not been vindicated by direct experimentation. Nevertheless, many investigators would like to believe that this special surface characteristic on trophoblast cells is not entirely fortuitous but may play some useful immunological role in the survival of the placenta. The observation that all neoplastic cells studied have an alteration in cell surface glycoprotein profile with an increased neuraminidase-sensitive glycosylation of certain glycopeptides may be relevant. It is, therefore, tempting to entertain the idea that both neoplastic and trophoblast cells may evade host immune attack by a similar mechanism of an increased sialylation of cell surface glycoprotein. It may be more than coincidence that the immunosuppressive action of α-foetoprotein appears to be related to its degree of sialylation and that the migration inhibition factor (MIF) produced by sensitised lymphocytes is also dependent on the presence of terminal sialic acid residues for its migration inhibition activity.

What may have led to this change in cell surface glycoprotein on trophoblast cells? It so happens that the placental hormone HCG is a sialoglycoprotein and it can be demonstrated on the surface of syncytial trophoblast cells. There is evidence that the hormone may even be incorporated as an integral component of the plasma membrane of these cells. This finding is somewhat surprising in terms of purely hormonal functions, for other hormones do not appear to be similarly integrated into the cell membranes of their secretory cells. This has led to the suggestion that the intrinsic nature of HCG on trophoblast plasma membranes may contribute to these cells' special surface characteristics. The hormone thus subserves an immunoprotective as well as an endocrine function during pregnancy. It is curious that many (perhaps even all?) neoplasms, even of non-trophoblast origin, have been observed to secrete HCG. This may be merely another manifestation of a regression towards a foetal phenotype by tumour cells but it is intriguing that there should be this re-expression of a trophoblast property in particular. Can it be that an ability to produce HCG and the membrane integration of this hormone is a primary change responsible for the invasive nature of neoplastic cells? There are other similarities in cell surface characteristics between tumour cells and trophoblast, like the presence of receptors for wheat germ agglutinin and Fc receptors for IgG. That the study of the foetal-maternal interaction may also throw light on the tumour-host relationship is exciting.

Besides being locally protective, HCG also appears to have systemic immunosuppressive properties and could contribute to the immunosuppressive action of pregnancy sera. This conclusion is supported by much experimental evidence which, however, may be faulted on the grounds that the possibility has not been entirely excluded that the immunosuppression observed may be due to contaminants in the HCG preparations used rather than to the hormone itself. To some extent, the same reservations extend to the reported immunosuppressive activities of other pregnancy-associated proteins like α-macroglobulin, β_1-glycoprotein and α-foetoprotein, so the true importance of these substances in vivo remains to be determined.

From what has been said, it is clear that the human placenta possesses many characteristics and produces various substances which may aid its survival. Does the pregnant mother make any concessions on her part? There is no doubt that she is immunologically aware of her conceptus, for she develops both humoral antibodies and cell-mediated immunity towards foetal antigenic specificities. Maternal peripheral lymphocyte populations are not strikingly altered nor is there any detectable inherent defect in in vitro lymphocyte reactivity so there is probably no marked alteration of maternal immunocompetence. Any hyporeactivity which has been observed seems to be mediated by serum factors. Some of these are likely to be the trophoblast-derived proteins already mentioned. In addition, other substances in pregnancy serum like 'blocking' antibodies, soluble foetal antigens alone or complexed with antibody, and products liberated by foetal suppressor cells have all been thought to play a part in helping the placenta to evade maternal immune rejection.

The placenta plays a central role in the foetal-maternal interaction, for it effectively separates the two circulations. Of necessity, this barrier cannot be an absolute one because the whole purpose of placentation is the transmission of beneficial substances from mother to foetus. There is, however, a remarkable selectivity in this transplacental transport which seems to be based on a more sophisticated mechanism than the simple exclusion of large molecular weight proteins by ultrafiltration of maternal plasma. The transmission of maternal IgG is especially favoured which seems to be due to the presence of appropriate IgG Fc receptors on the plasma membrane of trophoblast cells. This surface binding and subsequent invagination of the membrane to form micropinocytotic vesicles is thought to protect the IgG molecule from intracellular enzymes, enabling the immunoglobulin to be transported intact without degradation across trophoblast layer to the foetal circulation. The main function of this process is, of course, the transfer of passive immunity so that maternal immunological experience may benefit the foetus. But how is the placenta to distinguish between beneficial IgG and potentially harmful IgG? That it cannot always do so is clearly demonstrated by the occurrence of erythroblastosis foetalis due to the materno-foetal transmission of anti-D. Nevertheless, apart from this, other iso-immune reactions are uncommon. This has generally been attributed to the presence of the relevant antigens on the majority of other foetal tissues or to the presence of soluble antigenic substances, so that the deleterious effect of maternal antibody is diluted and not concentrated against just one cell type like the Rh antigen on red cells. However, studies on the specificities of antibodies eluted from placental cells have suggested the alternate explanation that this organ may act by selectively absorbing out all those potentially harmful maternal iso-antibodies directed at foetal specificities, thereby preventing them from reaching the foetal circulation. The failure of this method of selective transmission according to antibody specificity in the case of anti-D may be because placental cells do not possess the relevant Rh antigens. Another group of antibodies which can escape this placental selection are some tissue-specific maternal auto-antibodies. When transmitted, these antibodies may lead to transient manifestations of auto-allergic diseases in the neonate. The trans-placental transmission of maternal auto-antibodies, therefore, affords a natural experimental opportunity to distinguish those auto-antibodies with a pathogenic significance like LATS in thyrotoxicosis from those which are merely secondary products of an underlying immunological derangement like the L-E factor. The observation that foetal pathological conditions can result from the transmission of maternal iso-antibodies and auto-antibodies indicates that the selective transplacental transport of immunoglobulins in man is, as yet, far from perfect.

Blood cellular constituents can also be exchanged between the foetus and mother across the placenta. Among mammals, the haemo-monochorial human placenta has the fewest intervening layers between foetal and maternal circulations and this may explain the relative ease for cellular exchange. However, it seems that most of the cells cross during delivery, presumably following separation of the placenta-decidua interphase while the few cells which have succeeded in being transmitted during pregnancy have probably done so through breaks in the placenta. The transplacental exchange of cells, therefore, may be an accidental rather than a physiological phenomenon. Certainly, the effects of this cellular exchange is, in the main, detrimental rather than beneficial to either mother or foetus. Thus, the foeto-maternal transfer of blood cells merely serves to act as antigenic stimuli for inducing maternal production of potentially harmful iso-antibodies like anti-D. The effects of maternal cells on the foetus is less clear. Confrontation with maternal antigens during a period when the foetus is not yet immunocompetent might be expected to lead to tolerance. This, of course, is of great interest to transplantation biologists, for the possibility of in utero induction of tolerance to histocompatibility antigens could be manipulated to benefit future allograft survival. However, this prospect appears unlikely since the balance of evidence shows that contact with antigens, even early in gestation, usually leads to sensitisation and not tolerance. This observation attests to the early maturation of the immune system in the human foetus. Many supporting data are now available indicating that the ontogeny of humoral immunity, cellular immunocompetence, and the complement system occurs very early in human foetal development. Foetal sensitisation from intra-uterine infections has also been documented. This raises the hope that pre-natal active immunisation of the foetus by administering the vaccine to the mother may be feasible.

The transfer of immunocompetent maternal leucocytes to the allogeneic foetus will be expected to have harmful consequences. Creation of similar conditions in animals has led to the development of graft-versus-host disease. Fortunately in man, apart from a few reported cases of lymphoid chimerism and immunodeficiency syndromes, there is no definite evidence that maternally-induced 'runt disease' actually occurs. There may be, however, other less overt manifestations, for it has been suggested that some cases of lymphoid tumours and also auto-allergic conditions may be caused by maternal lymphocyte clones which have colonised the foetus during gestation. This means that some diseases in man may be initiated before birth. That these pathological conditions do not occur more often is perhaps testimony for the impermeability of the placenta to cellular traffic and for the early maturation of foetal immunocompetence which will destroy any predator maternal lymphocytes that have been accidentally transmitted. The rarity of metastases of malignant neoplasms between mother and foetus further supports this conclusion. Maternal tumour cells in placental blood spaces have been observed to lie in close proximity to chorionic villi and yet to be unable to penetrate the trophoblast layer. There is a belief that trophoblast cells may themselves be immunocompetent and are capable of destroying foreign maternal cells. The concept of the placenta as an active immune barrier is an aspect which has been somewhat neglected in the past.

It will be appreciated from the foregoing discussion that, in spite of numerous immunological hurdles, human gestation is remarkably successful. Some investigators have actually come to the conclusion from animal studies that antigenic disparity may even be beneficial to foetal survival, although this may be an over-interpretation of the data. In human pregnancy, antigenic incompatibility does not appear to have any easily discernible effects on reproductive performance as a whole. There is some suggestion that sex-linked antigens, especially when acting in concert with other major histocompatibility systems, may influence the sex ratio at birth, and that blood group or HL-A incompatibility could be associated with increased early foetal wastage. However, the reverse has also been observed where increased homozygosity is related to abortions. The available evidence, therefore, may be regarded as inconclusive. This is really not surprising, for in an outbred population like man with a polymorphic antigen system, foetal-maternal incompatibility is the rule rather than the exception. Any correlation between the degree of incompatibility and foetal well-being would be extremely difficult to measure.

While the effect of foetal-maternal antigenic disparity on the foetus is not obvious, can it influence the development of maternal diseases during pregnancy? An example may be provided by pre-eclampsia and eclampsia. The aetiology of these conditions is not known but it has long been suspected that immunological factors may have an important part to play in the pathogenesis. In Chapter 11, a mechanism has been proposed whereby an increased degree of foetal-maternal antigenic disparity is thought to increase the intensity of maternal immunological reaction against foetal antigens in decidual blood vessels which leads to placental ischaemia and infarction. It is also possible that this incompatibility may increase placental mass and thus place an additional burden on the blood supply of this organ.

Another pregnancy disease which may have a similar immunological basis is trophoblast neoplasia. Since this is essentially an allogeneic tumour, it is logical to suppose that its successful colonisation of the maternal host could be aided by an unduly close antigenic compatibility between tumour and patient. However, detailed analyses of ABO and HL-A antigens between patients and their husbands or children have failed to provide any definitive supporting evidence for this hypothesis. One observation emerges which may be relevant and that is that almost all these tumours seem to have originated from an apparently female placenta. In the context of foetal-maternal interaction, this could either be a sex-linked phenomenon with an XX placenta being more compatible to the mother than an XY placenta and therefore having a survival advantage, or it may be sex-associated in that there is a differential production of essential immunoprotective substances like HCG between a male and female placenta. On the other hand, there is the alternative interpretation of the inheritance of some recessive malignant characteristics in trophoblast neoplasia.

There is increasing evidence that maternal immunological influence on her foetus does not end at birth but may continue afterwards via colostrum and milk. This mainly takes the form of the transfer of specific IgA antibodies which protect the foetal intestine against enteropathogens. These colostral IgA antibodies against enteric organisms appear to be produced in situ in the breast which is somewhat surprising, but it seems that maternal gut-associated lymphocytes, after being sensitised in the intestine, can then selectively migrate to the breast to secrete the appropriate specific antibodies. This is really a rather wonderful example of cellular economy and adaptation. Human colostrum also contains immunocompetent T-cells and some investigators believe that sensitised maternal cells may actually gain access to the foetal circulation via absorption through the intestine. At the moment, opinion still differs as to whether this actually occurs in man, but if it does, then the protective value of colostrum extends from a passive local intestinal immunity to a transfer of systemic cell-mediated immunity. The modern trend towards artificial feeding may well be depriving the neonate of a very important means of defence.

The elucidation of the pathogenesis of erythroblastosis foetalis and the eventual prevention of Rh sensitisation by the administration of anti-D are well known success stories where observations made from a study of the foetal-maternal interaction have been applied to clinical practice. A potential application for the not too distant future could be in the development of an immunological method for human fertility control. The main obstacle has been the lack of a specific 'target' antigen to which immunisation could be directed but this problem appears to be nearing a solution with the discovery that one portion of the HCG molecule has sufficient specificity to serve as the immunogen. It remains to be seen whether this form of immunological fertility control possesses sufficient advantages to replace those methods which are already available.

References

Aase, J. M., Noren, G. R., Reddy, D. V. and Geme, J. W. St. (1972) Mumps-virus infection in pregnant women and the immunologic response of their offspring. *New Engl. J. Med.* 286, 1379—1382.

Abbas, T. M. and Tovey, J. E. (1960) Proteins of the liquor amnii. *Brit. med. J.* 1, 476—479.

Abelev, G. I. (1971) Alpha-foetoprotein in ontogenesis and its association with malignant tumours. *Adv. Cancer Res.* 14, 295—358.

Abelev, G. I. (1974) α-fetoprotein as a marker of embryo-specific differentiation in normal and tumour tissues. *Transplant. Rev.* 20, 1—37.

Abilgaard, H. and Jensen, K. G. (1964) The influence of maternal leucocyte antibodies on infants. *Scand. J. Haemat.* 1, 47—62.

Ablin, R. U., Bruns, G. R., Guinan, P. and Bush, I. M. (1974) The effect of estrogen on the incorporation of ^{3}H-thymidine by PHA stimulated human peripheral blood lymphocytes. *J. Immunol.* 113, 705—707.

Ackerman, D. R. (1967) Antibodies of the ABO system and the metabolism of human spermatozoa. *Nature (London)* 213, 253—256.

Adams, D. D. and Kennedy, T. H. (1967) Occurrence in thyrotoxicosis of a gamma globulin which protects LATS from neutralisation by an extract of thyroid gland. *J. clin. Endocrinol.* 27, 173—177.

Adams, D. D. and Kennedy, T. H. (1971) Evidence to suggest that LATS protector stimulates the human thyroid gland. *J. clin. Endocrinol.* 33, 47—51.

Adams, J. M., Kimball, A. C. and Adams, F. H. (1947) Early immunization against pertussis. *Amer. J. Dis. Child.* 74, 10—18.

Adcock, E. W., Teasdale, F., August, C. S., Cox, S., Meschia G., Battaglia, F. C. and Naughton, M. A. (1973) Human chorionic gonadotropin: its possible role in maternal lymphocyte suppression. *Science* 181, 845—847.

Adinolfi, M. (1965) Anti-I antibody in normal human newborn infants. *Immunology* 9, 43—52.

Adinolfi, M. (1972) Ontogeny of components of complement and lysozyme. In: *Ontogeny of Acquired Immunity*. CIBA Foundation Symposium. Eds.: Porter and Knight. Associated Scientific Publishers, Amsterdam, pp. 65—85.

Adinolfi, M. (1975) The human placenta as a filter for cells and plasma proteins. In: *Immunobiology of Trophoblast.* Eds.: Edwards, Howe and Johnson. Cambridge University Press, Cambridge, pp. 193—210.

Adinolfi, M., Glynn, A. A., Lindsay, M. and Milne, C. M. (1966) Serological properties of γA antibodies to Escherichia coli present in human colostrum. *Immunology* 10, 517—526.

Adinolfi, M., Gardner, B. and Wood, C. B. S. (1968) Ontogenesis of two components of human complement: β1E and β1C—1A globulins. *Nature (London)* 219, 189—191.

Ahlstedt, S., Carlsson, B., Hanson, L. Å. and Goldblum, R. M. (1975) Antibody production by human colostral cells. I. Immunoglobulin class, specificity and quantity. *Scand. J. Immunol.* 4, 535—539.

Ahmann, A. J. and Stiehm, E. R. (1966) Immune globulin levels in colostrum and breast milk, and from formula- and breast-fed newborns. *Proc. Soc. exp. Biol. Med.* 122, 1098—1100.

Ahrons, S. (1971a) HL-A antibodies. Influence on the human foetus. *Tissue Antigens* 1, 129—136.

Ahrons, S. (1971b) Leucocyte antibodies: occurrence in primigravidae. *Tissue Antigens* 1, 178—183.

Alexander, P. (1974) Escape from immune destruction by the host through shedding of surface antigens: is this a characteristic shared by malignant and embryonic cells? *Cancer Res.* 34, 2077—2082.

Alford, C. A, Schaefer, J., Blankenship, W. J., Straumfjord, J. V. and Cassady, G. (1967) A correlative immunologic, microbiologic and clinical approach to the diagnosis of acute and chronic infections in newborn infants. *New Engl. J. Med.* 277, 437—449.

Allan, T. M. (1959) ABO blood groups and sex ratio at birth. *Brit. med. J.* 1, 553—554.

Allardyce, R. A., Shearman, D. J. C., McClelland, D. B. L., Marwick, K., Simpson, A. J. and Laidlaw, R. B. (1974) Appearance of specific colostrum antibodies after clinical infection with Salmonella typhimurium. *Brit. med. J.* 3, 307—309.

Allen, C. M. (1964) Blood groups and abortions. *J. chronic Dis.* 17, 619—626.

Allen, J. C. (1967) Evidence for anti-Gm(a) antibody in γA immunoglobulins. *Proc. Soc. exp. Biol. Med.* 124, 138—144.

Alper, C. A. Boenisch, T. and Watson, L. (1972) Genetic polymorphism in human glycine-rich beta-glycoprotein. *J. exp. Med.* 135, 68—80.

Anderson, J. M. (1972) *Nature's Transplant. The Transplantation Immunology of Viviparity.* Butterworths, London.

Anderson, J. M. and Ferguson-Smith, M. A. (1971). Nature's transplant. *Brit. med. J.* 2, 166—167.

André, A., Peetoom, F. and Rondman, K. W. (1964) Mise en évidence, dans le lait de mère, d'un facteur influençant le complexe intermédiaire de C' dans la réaction d'immunohémolyse. *Vox San.* 8, 99—102.

Andresen, R. H. and Monroe, C. W. (1962) Experimental study of the behaviour of adult human skin homografts during pregnancy. *Amer. J. Obstet. Gynecol.* 84, 1096—1101.

Andrews, G. S. (1959) Blood groups and toxaemia of pregnancy. *Brit. med. J.* 2, 806—807.

Arala-Chawes M. and Meirinho, M. (1972) Immunological responses in pregnancy. *Brit. med. J.* 4, 49.

Armstrong, M. Y. K., Schwartz, R. S. and Beldotti, L. (1967) Neoplastic sequelae of allogeneic disease. III. Histological events following transplantation of allogeneic spleen cells. *Transplantation* 6, 1380—1391.

Armstrong, M. Y. K., Ruddle, N. H., Lipman, M. B. and Richards, F. F. (1973) Tumour induction by immunologically activated murine leukaemia virus. *J. exp. Med.*'137, 1163-1179.

Arnaiz-Villena, A. and Festenstein, H. (1976) HLA genotyping by using spermatozoa: evidence for haploid gene expression. *Lancet* 2, 707—709.

Arnon, H., Salzberger, M. and Olitzki, A. L. (1959) The appearance of anti-bacterial and antitoxic antibodies in maternal sera, umbilical-cord blood and milk: observations on the specificity of antibacterial antibodies in human sera. *Pediatrics* 23, 86—91.

Aronsson, S. (1963) A case of transplacental tumour metastasis. *Acta paediat.* 52, 123—124.

Ashitaka, Y., Mochizuki, M. and Tojo, S. (1972) Purification and properties of chorionic gonadotropin from the trophoblastic tissue of hydatidiform mole. *Endocrinology* 90, 609—617.

Asma, G. E. M., Pichler, W., Schnit, H. R. E., Knapp, W. and Humans, W. (1977) The development of lymphocytes with T- or B-membrane determinants in the human foetus. *Clin. exp. Immunol.* 29, 278—285.

Aster, R. H., Miskovich, B. H. and Rodey, G. E. (1973) Histocompatibility antigens of human plasma. Localisation to the HLD-3 lipoprotein fraction. *Transplantation* 16, 205—210.

Astor, S. H., and Frick, O. S. (1973) Cellular immunity in the newborn infant: Is cellular immunity passed from mother to fetus? *J. Allergy clin. Immunol.* 51, 104.

Athreya, B. H., Coriell, L. L. and Charney, J. (1964) Poliomyelitis antibodies in human colostrum and milk. *J. Pediat.* 64, 79—82.

Atkin, H. B. (1965) Sex chromosome studies in trophoblast. In: *The Early Conceptus, Normal and Abnormal.* Ed.: Park. Univ. of St. Andrew's. pp. 130—134.

Attwood, H. D. and Park, W. W. (1961) Embolism to the lungs by trophoblast. *J. Obstet. Gynaecol. Brit. Commonw.* 68, 611—617.

Auer, I. O. and Kress, H. G. (1977) Suppression of the primary cell-mediated immune response by human α_1-fetoproteins in vitro. *Cell. Immunol.* 30, 173—179.

August, C. S., Berkel, I., Driscoll, S. and Merler, E. (1971) Onset of lymphocyte function in the developing human fetus. *Pediat. Res.* 5, 539—547.

Aycock, W. L. and Kramer, S. D. (1930) Immunity to poliomyelitis in mother and the newborn as shown by neutralisation tests. *J. exp. Med.* 52, 457—464.

Ayoub, J. and Kasakura, S. (1971) In vitro response of foetal lymphocytes to PHA, and a plasma factor which suppresses the PHA response of adult lymphocytes. *Clin. exp. Immunol.* 8, 427—434.

Bach, S., Ruddy, S., MacLaren, A. J. and Austen, K. F. (1971) Electrophoretic polymorphism of the fourth component of human complement (C4) in paired maternal and foetal plasmas. *Immunology* 21, 869—878.

Baehner, R. L. (1974) Molecular basis for functional disorders of phagocytes. *J. Pediat.* 84, 317—327.

Baggish, M. S., Woodruff, J. D., Tow, S. H. and Jones, H. W. (1968) Sex chromatin pattern in hydatidiform mole. *Amer. J. Obstet. Gynecol.* 102, 362—370.

Bagshawe, K. D. (1973) Recent observations related to the chemotherapy and immunology of gestational choriocarcinoma. *Adv. Cancer Res.* 18, 231—263.

Bagshawe, K. D., Rawlings, G., Pike, M. C. and Lawler, S. D. (1971) ABO blood-groups in trophoblastic neoplasia. *Lancet* 1, 553—557.

Bahl, O. P. (1969) Human chorionic gonadotropin. I. Purification and physico-chemical properties. *J. biol. Chem.* 244, 567—574.

Baines, M. G., Millar, K. G. and Mills, P. (1974) Studies of complement levels in normal human pregnancy. *Obstet. Gynecol.* 43, 806—810.

Baines, M. G., Pross, H. F. and Millar, K. G. (1977) Lymphocyte populations in peripheral blood during normal human pregnancy. *Clin. exp. Immunol.* 28, 453—457.

Balfour, A. and Jones, E. A. (1976) The binding of IgG to human placental membranes. In: *Maternofoetal Transmission of Immunoglobulins.* Ed.: Hemmings. Cambridge University Press, Cambridge, pp. 61—72.

Ballow, M., Fang, F., Good, R. A. and Day, N. K. (1974) Developmental aspects of complement components in the newborn. The presence of complement components and C3 proactivator (properdin factor B) in human colostrum. *Clin. exp. Immunol.* 18, 257—266.

Bangham, D. R., Hobbs, K. R. and Terry, R. J. (1958) Selective placental transfer of serum proteins in the Rhesus. *Lancet* 2, 351—354.

Bardawil, W. A., Mitchell, G. W., McKeogh, R. P. and Marchant, D. J. (1962) Behaviour of skin homografts in human pregnancy. I. Habitual abortion. *Amer. J. Obstet. Gynecol.* 84, 1283—1295.

Barnes, E. W., MacCuish, A. C., Landon, N. B., Jordan, J. and Irvine, W. J. (1974) Phytohaemagglutinin-induced lymphocyte transformation and circulating autoantibodies in women taking oral contraceptives. *Lancet* 1, 898—900.

Barr, M., Glenny, A. T. and Randall, K. J. (1949) Concentration of diptheria antitoxin in cord blood, and rate of loss in babies. *Lancet* 2, 324—326.

Baumgarten, A. (1976) E-rosette-formation in the presence of α-fetoprotein and ferritin. *Clin. Immunol. Immunopathol.* 6, 42—46.

Bayliss, R. I. S., McC. Brown, J. C., Round, B. P. and Steinbeck, A. W. (1955) Plasma-17-hydroxycorticosteroids in pregnancy. *Lancet* 1, 62—64.

Beasley, R. A. (1953) Haemolytic disease in first-born infants. *Brit. med. J.* 2, 1389.

Beck, D., Ginsburg, H. and Naot, Y. (1977) Modulating effect of human chorionic gonadotropin on lymphocyte blastogenesis. *Amer. J. Obstet. Gynecol.* 129, 14—20.

Beck, J. S. and Rowell, N. R. (1963) Transplacental passage of antinuclear antibody. *Lancet* 1, 134—135.

Becker, J. C. (1948) Aetiology of eclampsia. *J. Obstet. Gynaecol. Brit. Emp.* 55, 756—765.

Beer, A. E. (1969) Fetal erythrocytes in maternal circulation of 155 Rh-negative women. *Obstet. Gynecol.* 34, 143—150.

Beer, A. E. and Billingham, R. E. (1973) Maternally acquired runt disease. Immune lymphocytes from the maternal blood can traverse the placenta and cause runt disease in the progeny. *Science* 179, 240—243.

Beer, A. E. and Billingham, R. E. (1976) The Immunobiology of Mammalian Reproduction. Eds.: Osler and Weiss. Prentice-Hall Foundations of Immunology Series, New Jersey, U.S.A.

Beer, A. E. and Billingham. R. E. (1977) Histocompatibility gene polymorphisms and maternal-fetal interaction. *Transplant. Proc.* 9, 1393—1401.

Beer, A. E., Billingham, R. E. and Yang, S. L. (1972) Further evidence concerning the autoantigenic status of the trophoblast. *J. exp. Med.* 135, 1177—1184.

Behrman, S. J., Buettner-Janusch, J., Heglar, R., Gershowitz, H. and Tew, W. L. (1960) ABO(H) blood incompatibility as a cause of infertility: a new concept. *Amer. J. Obstet. Gynecol.* 79, 847—855.

Behrman, S. J., Yoshida, T., Amano, Y. and Paine, P. (1974) Rhesus and squirrel monkey placental specific antigen(s). *Amer. J. Obstet. Gynecol.* 118, 616—625.

Beierwaltes, W. H., Dodson, V. N. and Wheeler, A. H. (1959) Thyroid autoantibodies in families of cretins. *J. clin. Endocrinol.* 19, 179—182.

Beischer, N. A. (1966) Hydatidiform mole with coexistent foetus. *Aust. N.Z. J. Obstet. Gynaecol.* 6, 127—141.

Beleil, D. M., Mickey, M. R. and Terasaki, P. I. (1972) Comparison of male and female kidney transplant survival rates. *Transplantation* 13, 493—500.

Beling, C. G. and Weksler, M. E. (1974) Suppression of mixed lymphocyte reactivity by human chorionic gonadotrophin. *Clin. exp. Immunol.* 18, 537—541.

Bell, S. D. and Erickkson, Z. (1931) Studies in the transmission of sensitization from mother to child in human beings. I. Transfer of skin sensitizing antibodies. *J. Immunol.* 20, 447—458.

Bellanti, J. A. and Jackson, A. L. (1967) Characterization of the serum immunoglobulins to the somatic antigen of S. typhosa in an infant following intrauterine immunization. *J. Pediat.* 71, 783—789.

Bender, S. (1950) Placental metastases in malignant disease complicated by pregnancy. *Brit. med. J.* 1, 980—981.

Bennett, J. H. and Brandt, J. (1954) Some more exact tests of significance for O-A maternal-foetal incompatibility. *Ann. Eugen.* 18, 302—310.

Bennich, H. and Johansson, S. G. O. (1971) Structure and function of human immunoglobulin E. *Adv. Immunol.* 13, 1—55.

Bergström, H., Nilsson, L-A., Nilsson, L. and Ryttinger, L. (1967) Demonstration of Rh antigens in a 38-day fetus. *Amer. J. Obstet. Gynecol.* 99, 130—133.

Berlyne, G. M., Short, S. A. and Vickers, C. F. H. (1957) Placental transmission of the L.E. factor. Report of two cases. *Lancet* 2, 15—16.

Beveans, M., Seegal, B. C. and Kaplan, R. (1955) Glomerulonephritis produced in dogs by specific antiserum. II. Pathologic sequences following the injection of rabbit antidog-placenta serum or rabbit antidog-kidney serum. *J. exp. Med.* 102, 807—821.

Bienenstock, J., Johnston, N. and Perey, D. Y. E. (1973a) Bronchial lymphoid tissue. I. Morphologic characterisation. *Lab. Invest.* 28, 686—692.

Bienenstock, J., Johnston, N. and Perey, D. Y. E. (1973b) Bronchial lymphoid tissue. II. Functional characteristics. *Lab. Invest.* 28, 693—698.

Bierman, H. R., Aggeler, P. M., Thelander, H., Kelly, K. H. and Cordes, F. L. (1956) Leukaemia and pregnancy. A problem in transmission, *J. Amer. med. Assoc.* 161, 220—223.

Billingham, R. E. (1967) Transplantation immunity and the trophoblast. In: *Choriocarcinoma.* Eds.: Holland and Hreshchyshyn. Springer, New York, N.Y. pp. 9—17.

Billington, W. D. (1964) Influence of immunological dissimilarity of mother and foetus on size of placenta in mice. *Nature (London)* 202, 317—318.

Billington, W. D. (1975) Organisation, ultrastructure and histochemistry of the placenta: immunological consideration. In: *Immunobiology of Trophoblast.* Eds.: Edwards, Howe and Johnson. Cambridge University Press, Cambridge. pp. 67—78.

Birner, W. F. (1961) Neuroblastoma as a cause of antenatal death. *Amer. J. Obstet. Gynecol.* 82, 1388—1391.

Blizzard, R. M., Chandler, R. W., Landing, B. H., Pettit, M. D. and West, C. D. (1960) Maternal auto-immunization to thyroid as a probable cause of athyrotic cretinism. *New Engl. J. Med.* 263, 327—336.

Boackle, R. J., Pruitt, K. M. and Mestecky, J. (1974) The interaction of human complement with interfacially aggregated preparations of human secretory IgA. *Immunochemistry* 11, 543—548.

Boettcher, B. (1977) Haploid expression of HLA genes on spermatozoa. *Lancet* 1, 363—364.

Bohn, H. (1976) Isolation and characterisation of placental specific proteins SP1 and PP5. In: *Protides of Biological Fluids.* 24th Colloquium. Ed.: Peeters. Pergamon Press, Oxford. pp. 117—124.

Bonnar, J., McNicol, G. P. and Douglas, A. S. (1969) Fibrinolytic enzyme system and pregnancy. *Brit. med. J.* 3, 387—389.

Bonnar, J., McNicol, G. P. and Douglas, A. S. (1971) Coagulation and fibrinolytic system in pre-eclampsia and eclampsia. *Brit. med. J.* 2, 12—16.

Bonnard, G. D. and Lemos, L. (1972) The cellular immunity of mother versus child at delivery: sensitisation in unidirectional mixed lymphocyte culture and subsequent ^{51}Cr-release cytotoxicity test. *Transplant. Proc.* 4, 177—180.

Bonneau, M., Latour, M., Revillard, J. P., Robert, M. and Traeger, J. (1973) Blocking antibodies eluted from human placenta. *Transplant. Proc.* 5, 589—592.

Boorman, K. E., Dodd, B. E. and Mollison, P. L. (1945) Isoimmunization to the blood group factors A,B and Rh. *J. Pathol. Bacteriol.* 57, 157—169.

Boorman, K. E., Dodd, B. E. and Gunther, M. (1958) A consideration of colostrum and milk as source of antibodies which may be transferred to the newborn baby. *Arch. Dis. Childh.* 33, 24—29.

Booth, P. B., Dunsford, J., Grant, J. and Murray, S. (1953) Haemolytic disease in first born infants. *Brit. med. J.* 2, 41—42.

Borland, R. (1975) Placenta as an allograft. In: *Comparative Placentation. Essays in Structure and Function.* Ed.: Steven. Academic Press, London. pp. 268—280.

Borland, R., Loke, Y. W. and Oldershaw, P. J. (1970) Sex difference in trophoblast behaviour on transplantation. *Nature* (Lond.) 228, 572.

Borland, R., Loke, Y. W. and Wilson, D. (1975) Immunological privilege resulting from endocrine activity of trophoblast in vivo. In: *Immunobiology of Trophoblast.* Ed.: Edwards, Howe and Johnson. Cambridge University Press, Cambridge. pp. 158—169.

Boroditsky, R. S., Reyes, F. I., Winter, J. S. D. and Faiman, C. (1975) Serum human chorionic gonadotropin and progesterone patterns in last trimester of pregnancy — relationship to fetal sex. *Amer. J. Obstet. Gynecol.* 212, 238—241.

Boss, J. H. (1965) Antigenic relationships between placenta and kidney in humans. *Amer. J. Obstet. Gynecol.* 93, 574—582.

Bowley, C. C. and Dunsford, I. (1957) Blood group chimeras. *Brit. med. J.* 2, 408.

Boyde, J. D., Hamilton, W. J. and Boyde, C. A. R. (1968) The surface of the syncytium of the human chorionic villus. *J. Anat.* 102, 553—563.

Boyse, E. A. and Abbott, J. (1975) Surface reorganization as an initial inductive event in the differentiation of prothymocytes to thymocytes. *Fed. Proc. Fed. Amer. Soc. exp. Biol.* 34, 24—27.

Boyse, E. A., Old, L. J. and Luell, S. (1963) Antigenic properties of experimental leukaemias. II. Immunological studies in vivo with C57BL/6 radiation-induced leukaemias. *J. nat. Cancer Inst.* 31, 987—995.

Bradbury, S., Billington, W. D., Kirby, D. R. S. and Williams, E. A. (1969) Surface mucin of human trophoblast. *Amer. J. Obstet. Gynecol.* 104, 416—417.

Bradbury, S., Billington, W. D., Kirby, D. R. S. and Williams, E. A. (1970) Histochemical characterisations of the surface mucoprotein of normal and abnormal human trophoblast. *Histochem. J.* 2, 263—274.

Brain, P. (1968) Leucocyte agglutinins and birth weight. *Med. J. Aust.* 1, 1046—1047.

Brain, P., Marston, R. H. and Gordon, J. (1972) Immunological responses in pregnancy. *Brit. med. J.* 4, 488.

Brambell, F. W. R. (1966) The transmission of immunity from mother to young and the catabolism of immunoglobulins. *Lancet* 2, 1087—1093.

Brambell, F. W. R. (1970) *The Transmission of Passive Immunity from Mother to Young.* North-Holland Publ. Co., Amsterdam.

Brambell, F. W. R., Brierley, J., Halliday, R. and Hemmings, W. A. (1954) Transference of passive immunity from mother to young. *Lancet* 1, 964—965.

Brambell, F. W. R., Hemmings, W. A., Oakley, C. L. and Porter, R. R. (1960) The relative transmission of the fractions of papain hydrolysed homologous γ-globulin from the uterine cavity to the foetal circulation in the rabbit. *Proc. roy. Soc., B.* 151, 478—482.

Brasher, G. W. and Hartley, T. F. (1969) Quantitation of IgA and IgM in umbilical cord serum of normal infants. *J. Pediat.* 74, 784—788.

Braun, E. H., Buckwold, A. E., Emson, H. E. and Russel, A. V. (1960) Familial neonatal neutropenia with maternal leucocyte antibodies. *Blood 16,* 1745—1752.

Braunstein, G. D., Grodin, J. M., Vaitukaitis, J. and Ross, G. T. (1973) Secretory rates of human chorionic gonadotropin by normal trophoblast. *Amer. J. Obstet. Gynecol.* 115, 447—450.

Brent, R. L. (1967) Production of congenital malformations using tissue antisera. III. Placental antiserum. *Proc. Soc. exp. Biol. Med.* 125, 1024—1029.

Brewer, J. I. and Gerbie, A. B. (1966) Early development of choriocarcinoma. *Amer. J. Obstet. Gynecol.* 94, 692—710.

Breyere, E. J. and Sprenger, W. W. (1969) Evidence of allograft rejection of the conceptus. *Transplant. Proc.* 1, 71—75.

Bridge, R. G. and Foley, F. E. (1954) Placental transmission of the lupus erythematodes factor. *Amer. J. med. Sci.* 227, 1—8.

Bridges, R. A., Condie, R. M., Zak, S. J. and Good, R. A. (1959) The morphologic basis of antibody formation. Development during the neonatal period. *J. Lab. clin. Med.* 53, 331—357.

British medical Journal (1954) Fitness, fertility, and blood group. *Brit. med. J.* 1, 1197—1198.

British medical Journal (1966) Placental transmission of autoimmune diseases. *Brit. med. J.* 1, 1554—1555.

British medical Journal (1974) Pre-eclampsia and the kidney. *Brit. med. J.* 1, 468—469.

British medical Journal (1976) Immunological factors in pre-eclampsia. *Brit. med. J* 3, 604—605.

Brochier, J. P., Roitt, I. and Festenstein, H. (1974) Inhibition of lymphocyte proliferative responses by anti-HL-A alloantisera. *Eur. J. Immunol.* 4, 709—715.

Broder, L. E., Weintraub, B. D., Rosen, S. W., Cohen, M. H. and Tejada, F. (1977) Placental proteins and their subunits as tumor markers in prostatic carcinoma. *Cancer* 40, 211—216.

Brodsky, I., Baren, M., Kahn, S. B., Lewis, G. and Tellem, M. (1965) Metastatic malignant melanoma from mother to fetus. *Cancer* 18, 1048—1054.

Brody, J. I., Oski, F. A. and Wallach, E. E. (1968) Neonatal lymphocyte reactivity as an indicator of intrauterine bacterial contact. *Lancet* 1, 1396—1398.

Brown, E. S. (1963) Foetal erythrocytes in the maternal circulation. *Brit. med. J.* 1, 1000—1001.

Brown, W. R., Newcomb, R. W. and Ishizaka, K. (1970) Proteolytic degradation of exocrine and serum immunoglobulins. *J. clin. Invest.* 49, 1374—1380.

Browne, J. C. M. and Veall, N. (1953) The maternal placental blood flow in normotensive and hypertensive women. *J. Obstet. Gynaecol. Brit. Commonw.* 60, 141—147.

Bryce, L. M., Jakobcwicz, R., McArthur, N. and Penrose, L. S. (1950) Blood group frequencies in a mother and infant sample of the Australian population. *Ann. Eugen.* 15, 271—275.

Buchanan, D. I., Bell, R. E., Beck, R. P. and Taylor, W. C. (1969) Use of different doses of anti-Rh IgG in the prevention of Rh isoimmunisation. *Lancet* 2, 288—290.

Buckell, E. W. C. and Owen, T. K. (1954) Chorioepithelioma in mother and infant. *J. Obstet. Gynaecol. Brit. Emp.* 61, 329—330.

Buckley, R. H., Schiff, R. I. and Amos, D. B. (1972) Blocking of autologous and homologous leucocyte responses by human alloimmune plasmas: a possible in vitro correlate of enhancement. *J. Immunol.* 108, 34—44.

Bulmer, R. and Hancock, K. W. (1977) Depletion of circulating T lymphocytes in pregnancy. *Clin. exp. Immunol.* 28, 302—305.

Burden, D. W. (1973) The bactericidal action of immunoglobulin A. *J. med. Microbiol.* 6, 131—139.

Burke, J. and Johansen, K. (1974) The formation of HL-A antibodies in pregnancy. The antigenicity of aborted and term fetuses. *J. Obstet. Gynaecol. Brit. Commonw.* 81, 227—228.

Burman, D. and Oliver, R. A. M. (1958) Placental transfer of the lupus erythematosus factor. *J. clin. Path.* 11, 43—44.

Burstein, R. H. and Blumenthal, H. T. (1969) Immune reactions of normal pregnancy. *Amer. J. Obstet. Gynecol.* 104, 671—677.

Caffrey, M. and James, D. C. O. (1973) Human lymphocyte antigen association in ankylosing spondylitis. *Nature (London)* 242, 121.

Caldwell, J. L., Stites, D. P. and Fudenberg, H. H. (1975) Human chorionic gonadotropin: effects of crude and purified preparations on lymphocyte responses to phytohaemagglutinin and allogeneic stimulation. *J. Immunol.* 115, 1249—1253.

Cambiasco. C. L. Ricconi, H. and Masson, P. L. (1977) Automated determination of immune complexes by their inhibitory effect on the agglutination of IgG-coated particles by rheumatoid factor or Clq. *Ann. rheum. Dis.* 36, suppl. I, 40—44.

Campbell, A. C., Waller, C., Wood., J., Aynsley-Green, A. and Yu, V. (1974) Lymphocyte populations in the blood of newborn infants. *Clin. exp. Immunol.* 18, 469—482.

Campbell, D. H., Sturgeon, P. and Vinograd, J. R. (1955) Separation of complete and incomplete Rh antibodies by centrifugation. *Science* 122, 1091—1092.

Campbell, D. M., MacGillivray, I. and Thompson, B. (1977) Twin zygosity and pre-eclampsia. *Lancet* 2, 97.

Campion, P. D. and Currey, H. L. F. (1972) Cell-mediated immunity in pregnancy. *Lancet* 2, 830.

Camus, D., Carlier, Y., Bina, J. C., Borojevic, R., Prata, A. and Capron, A. (1976) Sensitization to Schistosoma mansoni antigen in uninfected children born to infected mothers. *J. infect. Dis.* 134, 405—408.

Carbonara, A., Trinchieri, G., Massobrio, M. and Pilone, N. (1974) Antibodies in parous women detected by antibody dependent cell mediated cytotoxicity. *Tissue Antigens* 4, 558—563.

Carlsen, R. B., Bahl, Om. P. and Swaminathan, N. (1973) Human chorionic gonadotropin. Linear amino acid sequence of the β subunit. *J. biol. Chem.* 248, 6810—6827.

Carr, M. C. and Stites, D. P. (1972) Reactivity of maternal lymphocytes to phytohaemagglutinin. *Lancet* 1, 1073—1074.

Carr, M. C., Lieber, E. and Fudenberg, H. H. (1970) In vitro cytolysis by human fetal lymphocytes. *Cell Immunol.* 1, 455—458.

Carr, M. C., Stites, D. P. and Fudenberg, H. H. (1972) Cellular immune aspects of the human fetal-maternal relationship. I. In vitro response of cord blood lymphocytes to phytohaemagglutinin. *Cell. Immunol.* 5, 21—29.

Carr, M. C., Stites, D. P. and Fudenberg, H. H. (1973a) Cellular immune aspects of the human fetal maternal relationship. II. In vitro response of gravida lymphocytes to phytohaemagglutinin. *Cell. Immunol.* 8, 448—454.

Carr, M. C., Stites, D. P. and Fudenberg, H. H. (1973b) Dissociation of response to phytohaemagglutinin and adult allogeneic lymphocytes in human foetal lymphoid tissues. *Nature (London) New Biol.* 241, 279—281.

Carr, M. C., Stites, D. P. and Fudenberg, H. H. (1974) Cellular immune aspects of the human fetal-maternal relationship. III. Mixed lymphocyte reactivity between related maternal and cord blood lymphocytes. *Cell. Immunol.* 11, 332—341.

Carr, M. C., Stites, D. P. and Fudenberg, H. H. (1975) The numerical development of lymphoid cells during human embryogenesis. *Transplantation* 20, 410—413.

Catty, D. and Lowe, J. A. (1976) Effect of maternal anti-immunoglobulin (anti-allotypic) antibody on the synthesis of immunoglobulin in the neonatal rabbit. In: *Maternofoetal Transmission of Immunoglobulins.* Ed.: Hemmings. Cambridge University Press, Cambridge. pp. 261—271.

Cavell, B. (1963) Transplacental metastasis of malignant melanoma. Report of a case. *Acta paediat.* Suppl. 146, 37—40.

Cederqvist, L. L. and Litwin, S. D. (1974) Production of alpha$_1$ and alpha$_2$ immunoglobulin heavy chains during fetal life. *J. Immunol.* 112, 1605—1608.

Cederqvist, L. L., Francis, L. C., Zervoudakis, I. A., Becker, C. G. and Litwin, S. D. (1976) Fetal immune response following prematurely ruptured membranes. *Amer. J. Obstet. Gynecol.* 126, 321—327.

Cederqvist, L. L., Ewool, L. C. and Litwin, S. D. (1977a) IgD and the fetal immune response. *Scand. J. Immunol.* 6, 821—825.

Cederqvist, L. L., Kimball, A. C., Ewool, L. C. and Litwin, S. D. (1977b) Fetal immune response following congenital toxoplasmosis. *Obstet. Gynecol.* 50, 200—204.

Celada, F. (1974) Concepts and methods in immunology applicable to the control of human fertility. In: *Immunological Approaches to Fertility Control.* Karolinska Symposia on Research Methods in Reproductive Endocrinology. Ed.: Diczfalusy. Karolinska Institute, Stockholm. pp. 419—435.

Ceppellini, R. (1971) Old and new facts and speculations about transplantation antigens in man. In: *Progress in Immunology.* Ed.: Amos, Acad. Press, London. pp. 973—1019.

Ceppellini, R., Bonnard, G. D., Coppo, F., Miggiano, V. C., Pospisil, M., Curtoni, E. S. and Pellegrino, M. (1971) Mixed leucocyte cultures and HL-A antigens. I. Reactivity of young fetuses, newborns and mothers at delivery. *Transpl. Proc.* 3, 58—63.

Cerni, C., Tatra, G., Bohn, H. (1977) Immunosuppression by human placenta lactogen (HPL) and the pregnancy-specific β_1-glycoprotein (SP-1). Inhibition of mitogen-induced lymphocyte transformation. *Arch. Gynäk.* 223, 1—7.

Chan. D. P. C. (1967) The natural history of choriocarcinoma. In: *Choriocarcinoma.* Eds. Holland and Hreshcyshyn. Springer-Verlag, New York. pp. 37—44.

Chandan, R. C., Shahani, K. M. and Holly, R. C. (1964) Lysozyme content of human milk. *Nature* (Lond.) 204, 76—77.

Chandra, R. K. (1976) Levels of IgG subclasses, IgA, IgM, and tetanus antitoxin in paired maternal and foetal sera: Findings in healthy pregnancy and placental insufficiency. In: *Maternofoetal Transmission of Immunoglobulins.* Ed.: Hemmings. Camb. Univ. Press, Cambridge, pp. 77—87.

Chaplin, H. Jr., Cohen, R., Bloomberg, G., Kaplan, H. J., Moore, J. A. and Dorner, I. (1973) Pregnancy and idiopathic haemolytic anaemia: a prospective study during 6 months gestation and 3 months post-partum. *Brit. J. Haematol.* 24, 219—229.

Chargaff, E. (1945) The isolation of preparations of thromboplastic protein from human organs. *J. biol. Chem.* 161, 389—394.

Charlton, R. K. and Zmijewski, C. M. (1970) Soluble HL-A7 antigen: localisation in β-lipoprotein fraction of human serum. *Science* 170, 636—637.

Charpentier, B., Guttman, R. D., Shuster, J. and Gold, P. (1977) Augmentation of proliferation of human mixed lymphocyte culture by human α-fetoprotein. *J. Immunol.* 119, 897—900.

Chase, P. S. (1972) The effects of human serum fractions on phytohaemagglutinin- and concanavalin A- stimulated human lymphocyte cultures. *Cell. Immunol.* 5, 544—554.

Chattoraj, A., Gilbert, R. and Josephson, A. M. (1968) Serological demonstration of fetal production of blood group iso-antibodies. *Vox Sang.* 14, 289—291.

Chesley, L. C., Annitto, J. E. and Cosgrove, R. A. (1968) The familial factor in toxaemia of pregnancy. *Obstet. Gynec.* 32, 303—311.

Chipperfield, E. J. and Evans, B. A. (1972) The influence of local infection on immunoglobulin formation in the human endocervix. *Clin. exp. Immunol.* 11, 219—223.

Chodirker, W. B. and Tomasi, T. B. (1963) Gamma-globulins: quantitative relationships in human serum and non-vascular fluids. *Science* 142, 1080—1081.

Chown, B. (1954) Anaemia from bleeding of the foetus into the mother's circulation. *Lancet* 1, 1213—1215.

Chung, H. K., McLimans, W. F., Horoszewicz, J. and Hreshchyshyn, M. M. (1969) In vitro studies of human trophoblast. *Amer. J. Obstet. Gynecol.* 104, 945—952.

Clarke, A. G. (1971) The effects of maternal pre-immunization on pregnancy in the mouse. *J. Reprod. Fertil.* 24, 369—375.

Clarke, B. C. and Kirby, D. R. S. (1966) Maintenance of histocompatibility polymorphisms. *Nature (London)* 211, 999—1000.

Clarke, C. A. (1968) Immunology of pregnancy: significance of blood group incompatibility between mother and foetus. *Proc. roy. Soc. Med.* 61, 1213.

Clarke, C. A. (1971) The mechanism of action of Rh immune globulin. *Clin. Obstet. Gynecol.* 14, 611—624.

Cochron, T. E. and Good, W. (1974) The distribution of immunoglobulins and albumin between maternal and cord serum at delivery. *J. Obstet. Gynaecol. Brit. Commonw.* 81, 980—987.

Coen, R., Grush, O. and Kauder, E. (1969) Studies on bactericidal activity and metabolism of the leucocyte in full term neonates. *J. Pediat.* 75, 400—406.

Cohen, B. H. (1970) ABO and Rh incompatibility. I. Fetal and neonatal mortality with ABO and Rh incompatibility. *Amer. J. hum. Genet.* 22, 412—440.

Cohen, F. and Zuelzer, W. W. (1964) Identification of blood group antigens by immunofluorescence and its application to the detection of the transplacental passage of erythrocytes in mother and child. *Vox Sang.* 9, 75—78.

Cohen, F., Zuelzer, W. W., Gustafson, D. C. and Evans, M. M. (1964) Mechanisms of iso-immunization. I. The transplacental passage of fetal erythrocytes in homospecific pregnancies. *Blood* 23, 621—646.

Cohen, F., Zuelzer, W. W., Kadowaki, J., Thompson, R. and Kennedy, D. (1965) Temporary persistence of replicating donor cells after intrauterine transfusions. *J. Pediat.* 67, 937—938.

Cohen, H. R. and Nedzel, A. J. (1940) Specific action of an antiserum for placental proteins on placenta and normal progress of pregnancy. *Proc. Soc. exp. Biol. Med.* 43, 249—250.

Colten, H. R. (1972) Ontogeny of the human complement system: in vitro biosynthesis of individual complement components by fetal tissues. *J. clin. Invest.* 51, 725—730.

Colten, H. R., Gordon, J. M., Borsos, T. and Rapp, H. J. (1968) Synthesis of the first component of human complement in vitro. *J. exp. Med.* 128, 595—603.

Combined Study (1966) Prevention of Rh haemolytic disease. Results of the Clinical Trial. A combined study from Centres in England and Baltimore. *Brit. med. J.* 2, 907—914.

Comings, D. E. (1967) Lymphocyte transformation in response to phytohaemagglutinin during and following a pregnancy. *Amer. J. Obstet. Gynecol.* 97, 213—217.

Constandoulkis, M. and Kay, H. E. M. (1962) A and B antigens of the human foetal erythrocyte. *Brit. J. Haematol.* 8, 57—63.

Contractor, S. F. and Davies, H. (1973) Effect of human chorionic somatomammotrophin and human chorionic gonadotrophin on phytohaemagglutinin-induced lymphocyte transformation. *Nature (London)* New Biol. 243, 284—285.

Contractor, S. F. and Krakauer, K. (1976a) Immunofluorescent localisation of cathepsin D in trophoblastic cells in tissue culture. *Beitr. Pathol.* 158, 445—449.

Contractor, S. F. and Krakauer, K. (1976b) Pinocytosis and intracellular digestion of ^{125}I-labelled haemoglobin by trophoblastic cells in tissue culture in the presence and absence of serum. *J. Cell Sci.* 21, 595—607.

Cooper, M. D., Lawton, A. A. and Bockman, D. E. (1971) Agammaglobulinaemia with B lymphocytes. Specific defect of plasma-cell differentiation. *Lancet* 2, 791—794.

Cooperband, S. R., Davis, R. C., Schmid, K. and Mannick, J. A. (1969) Competitive blockade of lymphocyte stimulation by a serum immunoregulatory alpha globulin (IRA). *Transplant. Proc.* 1, 516—523.

Cooperband, S. R., Badger, A. M., Davies, R. C., Schmid, K. and Mannick, J. A. (1972) The effect of immunoregulatory αglobulin (IRA) upon lymphocytes in vitro. *J. Immunol.* 109, 154—163.

Cornelius, E. A. (1972a) Induction of both host- and donor-type tumours as a result of the graft-versus-host reaction. *Transplantation* 13, 589—591.

Cornelius, E. A. (1972b) Rapid viral induction of murine lymphomas in the graft-versus-host reaction. *J. exp. Med.* 136, 1533—1544.

Cramer, D. V., Kunz, H. W. and Gill, T. J. (1974) Immunologic sensitization prior to birth. *Amer. J. Obstet. Gynecol.* 120, 431—439.

Crawford, H., Cutbush, M. and Mollison, P. L. (1953) Haemolytic disease of the newborn due to anti-A. *Blood* 8, 620—639.

Creger, W. P. and Steele, M. R. (1957) Human fetomaternal passage of erythrocytes. *New Engl. J. Med.* 256, 158—161.

Currie, G. A. (1967) Immunological studies of trophoblast in vitro. *J. Obstet. Gynaecol. Brit. Commonw.* 74, 841—848.

Currie, G. A. and Bagshawe, K. D. (1967a) The antigenicity of normal and malignant trophoblast: Some implications. In: *Advance in Transplantation.* Eds.: Dausset, Hamburger and Mathé. Munksgaard, Copenhagen. pp. 523—530.

Currie, G. A. and Bagshawe, K. D. (1967b) The masking of antigens on trophoblast and cancer cells. *Lancet* 1, 708—710.

Currie, G. A. and Basham, C. (1972) Serum mediated inhibition of the immunological reactions of the patient to his own tumour: a possible role for circulating antigen. *Brit. J. Cancer* 26, 427—438.

Currie, G. A., Van Doorninck, W. and Bagshawe, K. D. (1968) Effect of neuraminidase on the immunogenicity of early mouse trophoblast. *Nature (London)* 219, 191—192.

Curzen, P. (1968) The antigenicity of human placenta. *J. Obstet. Gynaecol. Brit. Commonw.* 75, 1128—1133.

Curzen, P. (1970) The antigenicity of the human placenta. *Proc. roy. Soc. Med.* 63, 65—66.

Curzen, P., Jones, E. and Gaugas, J. (1972) Immunological responses in pregnancy. *Brit. med. J.* 4, 49.

Daamen, C. B. F., Bloem, G. W. D. and Westerbeck, A. J. (1968) Chorio-epithelioma in mother and child. *J. Obstet. Gynaecol. Brit. Emp.* 68, 144—149.

Dancis, J., Lind, J., Oratz, M., Smolens, J. and Vara, P. (1961) Placental transfer of proteins in human gestation. *Amer. J. Obstet. Gynecol.* 82, 167—171.

Dancis, J., Douglas, G. W. and Fierer, J. (1966) Immunologic competence of mouse placental cells in irradiated hosts. *Amer. J. Obstet. Gynecol.* 94, 50—56.

Dattwyler, R. J., Murgita, R. A. and Tomasi, T. B. (1975) Binding of α-foeto-protein to murine T cells. *Nature (London)* 256, 656—657.

Davis, J. C. and Hipkin, L. J. (1974) Depression of lymphocyte transformation in women taking oral contraceptives. *Lancet* 2, 217.

Davis, R. H. and Galant, S. P. (1975) Non-immune rosette formation: a measure of the newborn infant's cellular immune response. *J. Pediat.* 87, 449—452.

Dawood, M. Y., Teoh, E. S. and Ratnam, S. S. (1971) ABO blood group in trophoblastic disease. *J. Obstet. Gynaec. Brit. Commonw.* 78, 918—923.

De Ikonikoff, L. K. and Cedard, L. (1973) Localisation of human chorionic gonadotropic and somatomammotropic hormones by the peroxidase immunohisto-enzymologic method in villi and amniotic epithelium of human placentas (from six weeks to term). *Amer. J. Obstet. Gynecol.* 116, 1124—1132.

Den Oudsten, S. A., Van Loghem-Langereis, P. D. and Dorfmeijer, H. (1958) Difference in the behaviour of the 'Rose' factor and the L. E. factor in regard to placental transmission. *Vox Sang.* 3, 193—196.

Derrington, M. M. and Soothill, J. F. (1961) An immunochemical study of the proteins of amniotic fluid and of maternal and foetal serum. *J. Obstet. Gynaecol. Brit. Commonw.* 68, 755—761.

Desai, R. G. and Creger, W. P. (1963) Maternal-fetal passage of leucocytes and platelets in man. *Blood* 21, 665—673.

Desai, R. G., McCutcheon, E., Little, B. and Driscoll, S. G. (1966) Fetomaternal passage of leucocytes and platelets in erythroblastosis fetalis. *Blood* 27, 858—862.

Diamondopoulos, G. T. and Hertig, A. T. (1963) Transmission of leukaemia and allied diseases from mother to fetus. *Obstet. Gynecol.* 21, 150—154.

Diaz-Jouanen, E. P. and Williams, R. C. (1974) T and B lymphocytes in human colostrum. *Clin. Immunol. Immunopathol.* 3, 248—255.

Diaz-Jouanen, E., Williams, R. C. and Strickland, R. G. (1975) Age-related changes in T and B cells. *Lancet* 1, 688—689.

Dickens, A. M., Richardson, J. R. E. and Pike, L. A. (1956) Further observations on ABO blood group frequencies and toxaemia of pregnancy. *Brit. med. J.* 1, 776—777.

Diczfalusy, E. (1974) Steps in the human reproductive process susceptible to immunological interference. In: *Immunological Approaches to Fertility Control. Karolinska Symposia on Research Methods in Reproductive Endocrinology.* Ed.: Diczfalusy. Karolinska Institute, Stockholm. pp. 13—36.

Dirmikis, S. M., Munro, D. S., Hiller, E. J., Crawford, M. J., Wynne, J. and Purcell, M. (1974) Placental transmission of LATS-protector. *Lancet* 2, 1579—1580.

Dixon, F. J., Vazquez, J. J., Weigle, W. O. and Cochrane, C. G. (1958) Pathogenesis of serum sickness. *Arch. Pathol.* 65, 18—28.

Dixon, F. J., Kuhns, W., Weigle, W. O. and Taylor, P. (1959) The lack of absorption of ingested bovine antibody in humans. *J. Immunol.* 83, 437—441.

Dodson, M. G., Kerman, R. H., Lange, C. F., Stefani, S. S. and O'Leary, J. A. (1977) T and B cells in pregnancy. *Obstet. Gynecol.* 49, 299—302.

Doniach, D. and Roitt, I. M. (1968) Thyroid auto-allergic disease. In: *Clinical Aspects of Immunology.* 2nd Ed. Eds.: Gell and Coombs. Blackwell, Oxford. pp. 933—958.

Doniach, I., Crookston, J. H. and Cope, T. I. (1958) Attempted treatment of a patient with choriocarcinoma by immunisation with her husband's cells. *J. Obstet. Gynaecol. Brit. Emp.* 65, 553—556.

Dossett, J. H., Williams, R. C. Jr. and Quie, P. G. (1969) Studies on interaction of bacteria, serum factors and polymorphonuclear leucocytes in mothers and newborns. *Pediatrics* 44, 49—57.

Doughty, R. W. and Gelsthorpe, K. (1974) An initial investigation of lymphocyte antibody activity through pregnancy and in eluates prepared from placental material. *Tissue Antigens* 4, 291—298.

Doughty, R. W. and Gelsthorpe, K. (1976) Some parameters of lymphocyte antibody activity through pregnancy and further eluates of placental material. *Tissue Antigens* 8, 43—48.

Douglas, G. W., Thomas, L., Carr, M., Cullen, N. M. and Morris, R. (1959) Trophoblasts in the circulating blood during pregnancy. *Amer. J. Obstet. Gynecol.* 78, 960—969.

Douthwaite, R. M. and Urbach, G. I. (1971) In vitro antigenicity of trophoblast. *Amer. J. Obstet. Gynecol.* 109, 1023—1029.

Dray, S. (1972) Allotype suppression. In: *Ontogeny of Acquired Immunity*. CIBA Foundation Symposium. pp. 87—112.

Dreskin, R. B., Spicer, S. S. and Greene, W. B. (1970) Ultrastructural localization of chorionic gonadotropin in human term placenta. *J. Histochem. Cytochem.* 18, 862—874.

Dunsford, I. (1957) Proof of foetal antigens entering the maternal circulation. *Vox Sang.* 2, 125—127.

Dwyer, J. M. and Mackay, I. M. (1970) Antigen-binding lymphocytes in human foetal thymus. *Lancet* 1, 1199—1202.

Dwyer, J. M., Warner, N. L. and Mackay, I. R. (1972) Specificity and nature of the antigen combining sites on fetal and mature thymus lymphocytes. *J. Immunol.* 108, 1439—1446.

Edgecombe, K. (1930) Isohemagglutinins: the influence of the fetus upon the titer of the mother's blood during pregnancy. *J. Pathol. Bacteriol.* 33, 963—979.

Edidin, M. (1966) The release of soluble H-2 alloantigens during disaggregation of mouse embryo tissue by a chelating agent. *J. Embryol. exp. Morphol.* 16, 519—530.

Edwards, J. H. (1957) A critical examination of the reputed primary influence of ABO phenotype on fertility and sex ratio. *Brit. J. prev. soc. Med.* 11, 79—89.

Edwards, R. G. (1976) Immunity and the control of human fertility. In: *Immunology of Human Reproduction*. Eds.: Scott and Jones. Academic Press, London. pp. 415—470.

Edwards, R. G. and Coombs, R. R. A. (1975) Immunological interactions between mother and fetus. In: *Clinical Aspects of Immunology*. 3rd Ed. Eds.: Gell, Coombs, Lachman. Blackwell, Oxford. pp. 561—598.

Eichenwald, H. F. and Shinefield, H. R. (1963) Antibody production by the human fetus. *J. Pediat.* 63, 870.

Eichwald, E. J. and Silmser, C. R. (1955) Communication. *Transplant. Bull.* 2, 148—149.

Eife, R., Eife, G., Kuhre, W. and August, C. (1974) Lymphotoxin production and blast cell transformation by newborn lymphocytes. *Clin. Res.* 22, 227A.

El-alfi, O. S. and Hathout, H. (1969) Maternofetal transfusion: immunologic and cytogenetic evidence. Amer. J. Obstet. Gynecol. 103, 599—600.

Elston, C. W. (1969) Cellular reaction to choriocarcinoma. J. Pathol. 97, 261—268.

El Tomi, A. E. F., Boots, L. and Stevens, V. C. (1970) Effects of immunization with human placental lactogen on reproduction in female rats. *Endocrinology* 87, 1181—1185.

El Tomi, A. E. F., Boots, L. and Stevens, V.C. (1971a) Effects of antibodies to human placental lactogen on reproduction in pregnant rats. *Endocrinology* 88, 805—809.

El Tomi, A. E. F., Crystle, C. D. and Stevens, V. C. (1971b) Effects of immunization with human placental lactogen on reproduction in female rabbits. *Amer. J. Obstet. Gynecol.* 109, 74—77.

Emödi, G. and Just, M. (1974) Interferon production by lymphocytes in human milk. *Scand. J. Immunol.* 3, 157—160.

Epstein, R. D., Lozner, E. L. and Cobbey, T. S. (1950) Congenital thrombocytopenic purpura. Purpura haemorrhagica in pregnancy and in the newborn. *Amer. J. Med.* 9, 44—56.

Fahey, J. L. (1960) Separation of serum antibody activities by anion-exchange cellulose chromatography. *Science* 131, 500—501.

Fahey, J. L. and Morrison, E. G. (1960) Separation of 6.6S and 18S gamma globulins with isohemagglutinin activity. *J. Lab. clin. Med.* 55, 912—916.

Faulk, W. P. and Johnson, P. M. (1977) Immunological studies of human placentae: identification and distribution of proteins in mature chorionic villi. *Clin. exp. Immunol.* 27, 365—375.

Faulk, W. P. and Temple, A. (1976) Distribution of β_2 microglobulin and HL-A in chorionic villi of human placentae. *Nature (London)* 262, 799—802.

Faulk, W. P., Goodman, J. R., Maloney, M. A., Fudenberg, H. H. and Yoffey, J. M. (1973) Morphology and nucleoside incorporation of human neonatal lymphocytes. *Cell. Immunol.* 8, 166—172.

Faulk, W. P., Jeannet, M., Creighton, W. D. and Carbonara, A. (1974a) Immunological studies of the human placenta. Characterisation of immunoglobulins on trophoblastic basement membranes. *J. clin. Invest.* 54, 1011—1019.

Faulk, W. P., Van Loghem, E. and Stickler, G. B. (1974b) Maternal antibody to foetal light-chain (Inv) antigens. *Amer. J. Med.* 56, 393—397.

Faulk, W. P., Sanderson, A. and Temple, A. (1977) Distribution of MHC antigens in human placental chorionic villi. *Transplant. Proc.* 9, 1379—1384.

Faulkner, W. and Borella, L. (1970) Measurement of IgA levels in human cord serum by a new radioimmunoassay. *J. Immunol.* 105, 786—790.

Fellous, M. and Dausset, J. (1970) Probable haploid expression of HL-A antigens on human spermatozoa. *Nature (London)* 225, 191—193.

Ferrone, S., Mickey, M. R., Terasaki, P. I., Reisfeld, R. A. and Pellegrino, M. A. (1976) Humoral sensitisation in parous women: cytotoxic antibodies to non HL-A antigens. *Transplantation* 22, 61—68.

Field, E. J. and Caspary, E. A. (1971) Is maternal lymphocyte sensitisation passed to the child? *Lancet* 2, 337—341.

Fikrig, S. M., Valenti, C. and Kehaty, T. (1967) Masking of antigens on trophoblast. *Lancet* 1, 1055.

Fingleton, A. M. (1971) Leucocytotoxic antibodies and pre-eclampsia of pregnancy. *Transplantation* 12, 319—321.

Finn, R., Clarke, C. A., Donohoe, W. T. A., McConnell, R. B., Sheppard, P. M. and Lehane, D. (1961a) Transplacental passage of red cells in man. *Nature (London)* 190, 922—923.

Finn, R., Clarke, C. A., Donohoe, W. T. A., McConnell, R. B., Sheppard, P. M., Lehane, D. and Kulke, W. (1961b) Experimental studies on the prevention of Rh haemolytic disease. *Brit. med. J.* 1, 1486—1490.

Finn, R., St. Hill, C. A., Govan, A. J., Ralfs, I. G., Gurney, F. J. and Denye, V. (1972) Immunological responses in pregnancy and survival of fetal homograft. *Brit. med. J.* 3, 150—152.

Fireman, P., Zuchowski, D. A. and Taylor, P. M. (1969) Development of human complement system. *J. Immunol.* 103, 25—31.

Fishel, C. W. and Pearlman, D. S. (1961) Complement components of paired mother-cord sera. *Proc. Soc. exp. Biol. Med.* 107, 695—699.

Fisher, J. M. and Taylor, K. B. (1967) Placental transfer of gastric antibodies. *Lancet* 1, 695—698.

Ford, W. H., Caspary, E. A. and Shenton, B. (1973) Purification and properties of a lymphocyte inhibition factor from human serum. *Clin. exp. Immunol.* 15, 169—179.

Forman, M. L. and Stiehm, E. R. (1969) Impaired opsonic activity but normal phagocytosis in low birthweight infants. *New Engl. J. Med.* 281, 926—931.

Fowler, R. Jr., Schubert, W. K. and West, C. D. (1960) Acquired partial tolerance to homologous skin grafts in the human infant at birth. *Ann. N.Y. Acad. Sci.* 87, 403—428.

Franklin, E. C. and Kunkel, H. G. (1958) Comparative levels of high molecular weight (19S) gamma globulin in maternal and umbilical cord sera. *J. Lab. clin. Med.* 52, 724—727.

Fraser, I. D. and Raper, A. B. (1962) Observation of compatible and incompatible foetal red cells in the maternal circulation. *Brit. med. J.* 2, 303—304.

Freda, V. J. (1958) A-B-O (H) blood group substances in the human maternal-fetal barrier and amniotic fluid. *Amer. J. Obstet. Gynecol.* 76, 407—416.

Freda, V. J. (1962) Placental transfer of antibodies in man. *Amer. J. Obstet. Gynecol.* 84, 1756—1777.

Freda, V. J. and Carter, B. (1962) Placental permeability in the human for anti-A and anti-B isoantibodies. *Amer. J. Obstet. Gynecol.* 84, 1351—1367.

Freda, V. J., Gorman, J. G., Galen, R. S. and Treacy, N. (1970) The threat of Rh immunisation from abortion. *Lancet* 2, 147—148.

Freda, V. J., Gorman, J. G. and Pollack, W. (1977) Prevention of Rh-hemolytic disease with Rh-immune globulin. *Amer. J. Obstet. Gynecol.* 128, 456—460.

Freedman, W. L. and McMahon, F. J. (1960) Placental metastasis. Review of literature and report of case of malignant melanoma. *Obstet. Gynecol.* 16, 550—560.

Fudenberg, H. H. and Fudenberg, B. R. (1964) Antibody to hereditary human gamma-globulin (Gm) factor resulting from maternal-foetal incompatibility. *Science* 145, 170—171.

Fujikura, T. and Klionsky, B. (1975) Transplacental passage of maternal erythrocytes with sickling. *J. Pediat.* 87, 781—783.

Gailami, S., Chu, T. M., Nussbaum, A., Ostrander, M. and Christoff, N. (1976) Human chorionic gonadotrophins (hCG) in non-trophoblastic neoplasms. *Cancer* 38, 1684—1686.

Gang, N. F., Schwartz, E. S., Majerovics, A., De Champlain, M-L. and Trachtenberg, E. (1974) Studies on the placenta. II. Nephrotoxicity of antibodies produced against a chorionic glycoprotein. *Amer. J. Obstet. Gynecol.* 120, 73—82.

Garrett, J. V., McC. Giles, H., Coombs, R. R. A. and Gurner, B. W. (1960) Neonatal purpura with platelet iso-antibody in maternal serum. *Lancet* 1, 521.

Gärtner, A., Larsson, L-I. and Sjöberg, N-O (1975) Immunohistochemical demonstration of chorionic gonadotrophin in trophoblastic tumours. *Acta obstet. gynaecol. scand.* 54, 161—163.

Gatti, R. A., Yunis, E. J. and Good, R. A. (1973) Characterisation of a serum inhibitor of MLC reactions. *Clin. exp. Immunol.* 13, 427—437.

Gau, G. and Chard, T. (1976) Location of the protein hormones of the placenta by the immunoperoxidase technique. *Brit. J. Obstet. Gynaecol.* 83, 876—878.

Gaugas, J. M., Jones, E. and Curzen, P. (1975) Spontaneous lymphocyte transformation in pregnancies complicated by pre-eclampsia. *Amer. J. Obstet. Gynecol.* 121, 542—544.

Gelfand, H. M., Strean, G. J., Pavilanis, V. and Sternberg, J. (1960a) Studies in placental permeability. Transmission of poliomyelitis antibodies, lipoproteins and cholesterol in single and twin newborn infants. *Amer. J. Obstet. Gynecol.* 79. 117—133.

Gelfand, H. M., Fox, J. P., LeBlanc, D. R. and Elveback, L. (1960b) Studies on the development of maternal immunity to poliomyelitis in Louisiana. V. Passive transfer of polioantibody from mother to fetus, and natural decline and disappearance of antibody in the infant. *J. Immunol.* 85, 46—55.

George, K. P. (1970) Cytochemical differentiation along human chromosomes. *Nature (London)* 226, 80—81.

George, P. A., Fortner, J. P. and Pack, G. T. (1960) Melanoma with pregnancy. A report of 115 cases. *Cancer* 13, 854—859.

Gerhard, O. and Terasaki, P. I. (1977) Influence of sex on histocompatibility matching in renal transplantation. *Lancet* 2, 419—421.

Germuth, F. G. (1953) A comparative histologic and immunologic study in rabbits of induced hypersensitivity of the serum sickness type. *J. exp. Med.* 97, 257—282.

Gershowitz, H., Behrman, S. J. and Neel, J. V. (1958) Hemagglutinins in uterine secretions. *Science* 128, 719—720.

Ghosh, N. K. and Cox, R. P. (1976) Production of human chorionic gonadotropin in HeLa cell cultures. *Nature (London)* 259, 416—417.

Gill, T. J. (1973) Maternal-fetal interactions and the immune response. *Lancet* 1, 133—135.

Gindrat, J-J., Gothefors, L., Hanson, L. Å. and Winberg, J. (1972) Antibodies in human milk against E. coli of the serogroups most commonly found in neonatal infections. *Acta paediat. scand.* 61, 587—590.

Githens, J. A., Muschenheim, S., Sulginiti, V. A., Robinson, A. and Kay, H. E. M. (1969) Thymic alymphoplasia with XX/XY lymphoid chimerism secondary to probable maternal-fetal transfusion. *J. Pediat.* 75, 87—94.

Gitlin, D. and Biasucci, A. (1969) Development of γG, γA, γM, β_1c, β_1a, C'_1 esterase inhibitor, ceruloplasmin, transferrin, hemopexin, haptoglobin, fibrinogen, plasminogen, α_1 anti-trypsin, orosomucoid, β lipoprotein, α_2 macroglobulin, and prealbumin in the human conceptus. *J. clin. Invest.* 48, 1433—1446.

Gitlin, D. and Boesman, M. (1966) Serum α-fetoprotein, albumin, and γG-globulin in the human conceptus. *J. clin. Invest.* 45, 1826—1838.

Gitlin, D., Kumate, J., Urrusti, J. and Morales, C. (1964a) The selectivity of the human placenta in the transfer of plasma proteins from mother to fetus. *J. clin. Invest.* 43, 1938—1951.

Gitlin, D., Kumate, J., Urrusti, J. and Morales, C. (1964b) Selective and directional transfer of 7S γ_2-globulin across the human placenta. *Nature (London)* 203, 86—87.

Gitlin, D., Kumate, J. and Morales, C. (1965) On the transport of insulin across the human placenta. *Pediatrics* 35, 65—69.

Gitlin, J. D. and Gitlin, D. (1976) Protein binding by cell membranes and the selective transfer of proteins from mother to young across tissue barriers. In: *Maternofoetal Transmission of Immunoglobulins.* Ed.: Hemmings. Cambridge University Press, Cambridge. pp. 113—119.

Glass, R. H. and Mroueh, A. (1967) Pregnancy in the rabbit following immunization with human chorionic gonadotropin. *Amer. J. Obstet. Gynecol.*, 97, 1082—1084.

Gleichmann, E., Gleichmann, H. and Schwartz, R. S. (1972) Immunologic induction of malignant lymphoma: genetic factors in the graft-versus-host model. *J. nat. Cancer Inst.* 49, 793—804.

Gluck, L. and Silverman, W. A. (1957) Phagocytosis in premature infants. *Pediatrics* 20, 951—957.

Gokel, J. M., Rjosk, H. K., Meister, P., Stelter, W-J. and Witte, J. (1977) Metastatic choriocarcinoma transplanted with cadaver kidney. *Cancer* 39, 1317—1321.

Gold, P. and Freedman, S. O. (1965) Specific carcinoembryonic antigens of the human digestive system. *J. exp. Med.* 122, 467—481.

Goldblum, R. M., Ahlstedt, S., Carlsson, B., Hanson, L. Å., Jodal, U., Lidin-Janson, G. and Sohl-Åkerlund, A. (1975) Antibody-forming cells in human colostrum after oral immunisation. *Nature (London)* 257, 797—799.

Goldman, A. S. and Smith, C. W. (1973) Host resistance factors in human milk. *J. Pediat.* 82, 1082—1090.

Goldstein, M. and Baxter, H. (1958) Fetal tissue homografts. *Ann. N.Y. Acad. Sci.* 73, 564—569.

Good, R. A. and Zak, S. J. (1956) Disturbances in gamma-globulin synthesis as 'experiments of nature'. *Pediatrics* 18, 109—149.

Good, W. (1967) Masking of antigens on trophoblast. *Lancet* 1, 1156.

Goodhall, H. B., Frances, S., Graham, F. S., Miller, M. D. and Cameron, C. (1958) Transplacental bleeding from the fetus. *J. clin. Pathol.* 11, 251—260.

Goodfellow, P. N., Barnstable, C. J., Bodmer, W. F., Snary, D. and Crumpton, M. J. (1976) Expression of HLA system antigens on placenta. *Transplantation* 22, 595—603.

Gordon, J. E. and Janney, J. H. (1941) Antistreptolysin content of the sera of normal infants and children. *J. Pediat.* 18, 587—591.

Goto, S., Hoshino, M., Tomoda, Y. and Ishizuka, N. (1977) Immunoelectron microscopy of the human chorionic villus in search of blood group A and B antigens. *Lab. Invest.* 35, 530—536.

Götze, O. and Müller-Eberhard, H. J. (1971) The C3-activator system: An alternate pathway of complement activation. *J. exp. Med.* 134, 905—1085.

Goulmy, E., Termijtelen, A., Bradley, B. A. and Van Rood, J. J. (1977) Y-antigen killing by T cells of women is restricted by HL-A. *Nature (London)* 266, 544—545.

Green, I., Inkelas, M. and Allen, L. B. (1960) Hodgkin's disease: a maternal-to-foetal lymphocyte chimaera? *Lancet* 1, 30—32.

Grogan, T. M., Broughton, D. D. and Doyle, W. F. (1975) Graft-versus-host reaction (GVHR). A case report suggesting GVHR occurred as a result of maternofetal cell transfer. *Arch. Pathol.* 99, 330—334.

Gross, S. J. (1966) Human blood group A substance in human endometrium and trophoblast localised by chromatographed rabbit antiserum. *Amer. J. Obstet. Gynecol.* 95, 1149—1159.

Grosset, L., Barrelet, V. and Odartchenko, N. (1974) Antenatal fetal sex determination from maternal blood during early pregnancy. *Amer. J. Obstet. Gynecol.* 120, 60—63.

Grubb, R. and Laurell, A. B. (1956) Hereditary serological human serum groups. *Acta pathol. microbiol. scand.* 39, 390—398.

Grubb, R. and Sjöstedt, S. (1955) Blood groups in abortion and sterility. *Ann. hum. Genet.* 19, 183—195.

Grundbacher, F. J. (1964) Changes in the human A antigen of erythrocytes with the individual's age. *Nature (London)* 204, 192—194.

Gullbring, B. (1957) Investigation on the occurrence of blood group antigens in spermatozoa from man, and serological demonstration of the segregation of characters. *Acta med. scand.* 159, 169—172.

Gupta, S. and Good, R. A. (1977) α-fetoprotein and human lymphocyte subpopulations. *J. Immunol.* 118, 405—408.

Gurchot, C. (1975) The trophoblast theory of cancer revisited. *Oncology* 31 310—333.

Gusdon, J. P. (1972) An immunologic method of pregnancy destruction and contraception. *Amer. J. Obstet. Gynecol.*, 112, 472—475.

Gusdon, J. P. (1974) A long-term follow-up of passively immunologically sterilised rats. *Amer. J. Obstet. Gynecol.* 118, 1145—1146.

Gusdon, J. P (1976) The effects of active and passive immunity to human placental lactogen. In: *Physiological Effects of Immunity against Reproductive Hormones.* Eds.: Edwards and Johnson. Cambridge University Press, Cambridge. pp. 205—228.

Gusdon, J. P., Witherow, C. C., and Iannuzzi, N. P (1974) The role of embryonic antigens in immunologic sterilization. *Amer. J. Obstet. Gynecol.* 120, 242—248.

Hackett, E. and Beech, M. (1961) Immunological treatment of a case of choriocarcinoma. *Brit. med. J.* 2, 1123—1126.

Hagen, C. and Frøland, A. (1972) Depressed lymphocyte response to PHA in women taking oral contraceptives. *Lancet* 1, 1185.

Halbrecht, I. (1944) Role of hemagglutinins anti-A and anti-B in pathogenesis of jaundice of the newborn (icterus neonatorum precox). *Amer. J. Dis. Childh.* 68, 248—249.

Halbrecht, I. (1951) Icterus precox: Further studies on its frequency, etiology prognosis and the blood chemistry of the cord blood. *J. Pediat.* 39, 185—190.

Halbrecht, I. and Komlos, L. (1968) Lymphocyte transformation in mixed wife-husband leucocyte cultures in abortions and in hydatidiform moles. *Obstet. Gynecol.* 31, 173—177.

Halbrecht, I and Komlos, L. (1976) E-rosette-forming lymphocytes in mother and new-born. *Lancet* 1, 544.

Hamilton, W. J. and Boyde, J. D. (1966) Trophoblast in human utero-placental arteries. *Nature (London)* 212, 906—908.

Han, T. (1974) Inhibitory effect of human chorionic gonadotrophin on lymphocyte blastogenic response to mitogen, antigen and allogeneic cells. *Clin. exp. Immunol.* 18, 529—535.

Hanson, L. Å. (1959) Immunological analysis of human milk. *Int. Arch. Allergy appl. Immunol.* 15, 245—256.

Hanson, L. Å. and Winberg, J. (1972) Breast milk and defense against infection in the newborn. *Arch. Dis. Childh.* 47, 845—848.

Hanson, L. Å., Ahlstedt, S., Carlsson, B. and Fällström, S. P. (1977) Secretory IgA antibodies against cow's milk proteins in human milk and their possible effect in mixed feeding. *Int. Arch. Allergy appl. Immunol.* 54, 457—462.

Haour, F. and Saxena, B. B. (1974) Detection of a gonadotropin in rabbit blastocysts before implantation. *Science* 185, 444—445.

Harlap, S. and Davies, A. M. (1974) Maternal blood group A and pre-eclampsia. *Brit. med. J.* 3, 171—172.

Harrington, W. J., Sprague, C. C., Minnich, V., Moore, C. V., Aulvin, R. C. and Dubach, R. (1953) Immunologic mechanisms in idiopathic and neonatal thrombocytopenic purpura. *Ann. intern. Med.* 38, 433—469.

Harris, R. E. and Lordon, R. E. (1976) The association of maternal lymphocytotoxic antibodies with obstetric complications. *Obstet. Gynecol.* 48, 302—304.

Harrison, M. R. (1976) Maternal immunocompetence. II. Proliferative responses of maternal lymphocytes in vitro and inhibition by serum from pregnant rats. *Scand. J. Immunol.* 5, 881—889.

Hashem, N. (1972) Is maternal lymphocyte sensitisation passed to the child? *Lancet* 1, 40—41.

Hay, F. C., Hull, M. G. R. and Torrigiani, G. (1971) The transfer of human IgG subclasses from mother to foetus. *Clin. exp. Immunol.* 9, 355—358.

Hayward, A. R. and Ezer, G. (1974) Development of lymphocyte populations in the human foetal thymus and spleen. *Clin. exp. Immunol.* 17, 169—178.

Hayward, A. R. and Soothill, J. F. (1972) Reaction to antigen by human foetal thymus lymphocytes. In: *Ontogeny of Acquired Immunity*. CIBA Foundation Symposium. Eds.: Porter and Knight. Associated Scientific Press, Amsterdam. pp. 261—273.

Head, J. R., Beer, A. E. and Billingham, R. E. (1977) Significance of the cellular component of the maternal immunologic endowment in milk. *Transplant. Proc.* 9, 1465—1471.

Hedenstedt, S. and Naeslund, J. (1946) Investigations of the permeability of the placenta with the help of elliptocytes. *Acta. med. scand.* Suppl. 170, 126—134.

Hellström, I. and Hellström, K. E. (1969) Studies on cellular immunity and its serum-mediated inhibition in Maloney virus-induced mouse sarcomas. *Int. J. Cancer* 4, 587—600.

Hellström, K. E. and Hellström, I. (1972) The role of serum factors ('blocking antibodies') as mediators of immunological non-reactivity to cellular antigens. In: *Ontogeny of Acquired Immunity*. CIBA Foundation Symposium. Eds.: Porter and Knight. Associated Scientific Press, Amsterdam. pp. 133—143.

Hellström, K. E., Hellström, I. and Brawn, J. (1969) Abrogation of cellular immunity to antigenically foreign mouse embryonic cells by a serum factor. *Nature (London)* 224, 914—915.

Hemmings, W. A. (1973) Transport of IgM antibody to the rabbit foetus. *Immunology* 25, 165—166.

Hemmings, W. A. and Williams, E. W. (1976) The attachment of IgG to cell components of transporting membranes. In: *Maternofoetal Transmission of Immunoglobulins.* Ed.: Hemmings. Cambridge University Press, Cambridge. pp. 91—111.

Henderson, A. H., Pugsley, D. J. and Thomas, D. P. (1970) Fibrin degradation products in pre-eclamptic toxaemia and eclampsia. *Brit. med. J.* 3, 545—547.

Hertz, R., Lewis, J. and Lipsett, M. B. (1961) Five years' experience with the chemotherapy of metastatic choriocarcinoma and related trophoblastic tumours in women. *Amer. J. Obstet. Gynecol.* 82, 631—640.

Hindemann, P. (1973) Maternofetal transfusion during delivery and Rh sensitisation of the newborn. *Lancet* 1, 46.

Hirsch, M. S., Black, P. H., Tracey, G. S., Leibowitz, S. and Schwartz, R. S. (1970) Leukaemia virus activation in chronic allogeneic disease. *Proc. nat. Acad. Sci.* 67, 1914—1917.

Hirsch, M. S., Phillips, S. M. and Solnik, C. (1972) Activation of leukaemia viruses by graft versus host and mixed lymphocyte reactions in vitro. *Proc. nat. Acad. Sci.* 69, 1069—1072.

Hitzig, W. H. and Gitzelmann, R. (1959) Transplacental transfer of leucocyte agglutinins. *Vox Sang.* 4, 445—456.

Hodari, A. A. (1967) Chronic uterine ischaemia and reversible experimental 'toxaemia of pregnancy'. *Amer. J. Obstet. Gynecol.* 97, 597—607.

Hodes, H. L. (1964) Poliomyelitis antibodies in human colostrum and milk. *J. Pediat.* 65, 319—320.

Hodes, H. L., Berger, L., Ainbender, E., Hevizy, M. M., Zepp, H. D. and Kockwa, S. (1964) Proof that colostrum polio antibody is different from serum antibody. *J. Pediat.* 65, 1017—1018.

Hodgen, G. D., Nixon, W. E., Vaitukaitis, J. L., Tullner, W. W. and Ross, G. T. (1973) Neutralization of primate chorionic gonadotropin activities by antisera against the subunits of human chorionic gonadotropin in radioimmunoassay and bioassay. *Endocrinology* 92, 705—709.

Hoffenberg, R. (1974) Aetiology of hyperthyroidism — II. *Brit. med. J.* 3, 508—510.

Högman, C. F. (1959) Blood group antigens A and B determined by means of mixed agglutination on cultured cells of human fetal kidney, liver, spleen, lung, heart and skin. *Vox Sang.* 4, 319—332.

Hohler, C. W., Bardawil, W. A. and Mitchell, G. W. (1972) Placental weight and water content relative to blood types of human mothers and their offspring. *Obstet. Gynecol.* 40, 799—806.

Holborow, E. J., Brown, P. C., Glynn, L. E., Hawes, M. D., Gresham, G. A., O'Brien, T. F. and Coombs, R. R. A. (1960) The distribution of the blood group A antigen in human tissues. *Brit. J. exp. Pathol.* 41, 430—437.

Hollingsworth, D. R., Mabry, C. C. and Eckerd, J. M. (1972) Hereditary aspects of Graves' disease in infancy and childhood. *J. Pediat.* 81, 446—459.

Holm, G. and Perlman, P. (1967) Cytotoxic potential of stimulated human lymphocytes. *J. exp. Med.* 125, 721—736.

Holmgren, J., Hanson, L. Å., Carlsson, B., Lindblad, B. S. and Rahimtoola, J. (1976) Neutralizing antibodies against E. coli and V. cholerae enterotoxins in human milk from a developing country. *Scand. J. Immunol.* 5, 867—871.

Horne, C. H. W., McLay, A. L. C., Tavadia, H. B., Carmichael, I., Mollinson, A. C., Laiwah, A. A. C. Y., Thomas, M. A. and MacSween, R. N. M. (1973) Studies on pregnancy-associated globulin. *Clin. exp. Immunol.* 13, 603—611.

Horne, C. H. W., Reid, I. N. and Milne, G. D. (1976a) Prognostic significance in inappropriate production of pregnancy protein by breast cancers. *Lancet* 2, 279—282.

Horne, C. H. W., Towler, C. M., Pugh-Humphreys, R. G. P., Thomson, A. W. and Bohn, H. (1976b) Pregnancy specific β_1-glycoprotein — a product of the syncytiotrophoblast. *Experientia* 32(9), 1197—1199.

Horne, C. H. W., Towler, C. M. and Milne, G. D. (1977) Detection of pregnancy specific β_1-glycoprotein in formalin-fixed tissues. *J. clin. Pathol.* 30, 19—23.

Horner, E. N. (1960) Placental metastases. *Obstet. Gynecol.* 15, 566—572.

Hostrup, H. (1963) A and B blood group substances in the serum of the newborn infant and the foetus. *Vox Sang.* 8, 557-566.

Howie, P. W., Prentice, C. R. M. and McNicol, G. P. (1971) Coagulation, fibrinolysis and platelet function in pre-eclampsia, essential hypertension and placental insufficiency. *J. Obstet. Gynaecol. Brit. Commonw.* 78, 992—1003.

Hsia, D. Y-Y. and Gellis, S. S. (1954) Studies on erythroblastosis due to ABO incompatibility. *Pediatrics* 13, 503—510.

Hsu, C. C. S. (1974) Peripheral blood lymphocytes responses to phytohaemagglutinin and pokeweed mitogen during pregnancy. *Proc. Soc. exp. Biol. Med.* 146, 771—775.

Hulka, J. F. and Brinton, V. (1963) Antibody to trophoblast during early postpartum period in toxemic pregnancies. *Amer. J. Obstet. Gynecol.* 86, 130—134.

Hulka, J. F. and Mohr, K. (1969) Placental hormones and graft rejection. *Amer. J. Obstet. Gynecol.* 104, 889—892.

Hulka, J. F. and Omran, K. F. (1969) The uterine cervix as a potential local antibody secretor. *Amer. J. Obstet. Gynecol.* 104, 440—442.

Hulka, J. F., Hsu, K. C. and Beiser, S. M. (1961) Antibodies to trophoblasts during the post-partum period. *Nature (London)* 191, 510—511.

Hulka, J. F., Brinton, V., Schaaf, J. and Baney, C. (1963) Appearance of antibodies to trophoblast during the post-partum period in normal human pregnancies. *Nature (London)* 198, 501—502.

Hummel, K. (1972) Failure of anti-D prevention in monozygotic twins. *Nature (London) New Biol.* 240, 60.

Humphries, J. O. (1960) Occurrence of hypertensive toxemia of pregnancy in mother-daughter pairs. *Bull. Johns Hopkins Hosp.* 107, 271—277.

Hurst, J. G., Taylor, H. C. and Wiener, A. S. (1946) Individual blood differences in relation to pregnancy, with special reference to the pathogenesis of pre-eclamptic toxemia. *Blood* 1, 234—246.

Hutchinson, D. L., Turner, J. H. and Schlesinger, E. R. (1971) Persistence of donor cells in neonates after fetal and exchange transfusion. *Amer. J. Obstet. Gynecol.* 109, 281—284.

Iliya, F. A., Williamson, S. and Azar, H. A. (1967) Choriocarcinoma in the Near East. Consanguinity as a possible etiologic factor. *Cancer* 20, 144—149.

Irino, T., Okuda, T. and Grollman, A. (1967) Changes induced in the glomeruli of the kidney of rats by placental extracts as observed with the electron microscope. *Amer. J. Pathol.* 50, 421—433.

Isojima, S. and Tsuzuku, O. (1968) Problem of ABO blood group incompatibility and sterility: the effect of blood group antibody on spermatozoa. *Amer. J. Obstet. Gynecol.* 102, 304—306.

Ivavkova, E., Jakoubkova, J., Zavadil, M. and Schneid, V. (1968) HL-A antigens and the choriocarcinoma. *Folia biol. (Prague)* 2, 398—401.

Jäämeri, K. E. U., Koivuniemi, A. P. and Carpen, E. O. (1965) Occurrence of trophoblasts in the blood of toxaemic patients. *Gynaecologia* 160, 315—320.

Jackson, C. E., Mann, J. D. and Schull, W. J. (1969) Xg^a blood group system and the sex ratio in man. *Nature (London)* 222, 445—446.

Jacobs, P. A. and Smith, P. G. (1969) Practical and theoretical implications of fetal/maternal lymphocyte transfer. *Lancet* 2, 745.

Jacobs, P. A., Tough, I. M. and Wright, D. H. (1963) Cytogenetic studies in Burkitt's lymphoma. *Lancet* 1, 1144—1146.

Jacobson, E. B., Herzenberg, L. A., Riblet, R. and Herzenberg, L. A. (1972) Active suppression of immunoglobulin allotype synthesis. *J. exp. Med.* 135, 1163—1176.

Jakobowicz, R., Williams, L. and Silberman, F. (1972) Immunization of Rh-negative volunteers by repeated injections of very small amounts of Rh-positive blood. *Vox Sang.* 23, 376—381.

James, D. A. (1965) Effects of antigenic dissimilarity between mother and foetus on placental size in mice. *Nature (London)* 205, 613—614.

James, D. A. (1967) Some effects of immunological factors on gestation in mice. *J. Reprod. Fertil.* 14, 265—275.

Jandl, J. H., Jones, R. A. and Castle, W. B. (1957) The destruction of red cells by antibodies in man. I. Observations on the sequestration and lysis of red cells altered by immune mechanisms. *J. clin. Invest.* 36, 1428—1459.

Javett, S. N., Senior, B., Brando, J. L. and Heymann, S. (1959) Neonatal thyrotoxicosis. *Pediatrics* 24, 65—73.

Jeannet, M., Werner, Ch., Ramirez, E., Vassalli, P. and Faulk, W. P. (1977) Anti-HLA, anti-human 'Ia-like' and MLC blocking activity of human placental IgG. *Transplant. Proc.* 9, 1417—1422.

Jeffcoate, T. N. A. (1966) Pre-eclampsia and eclampsia: the disease of theories. *Proc. roy. Soc. Med.* 59, 397—404.

Jenkins, D. M. (1976) Pre-eclampsia/eclampsia (gestosis) and other pregnancy complications with a possible immunologic basis. In: *Immunology of Human Reproduction.* Eds.: Scott and Jones. Academic Press, London. pp. 297—327.

Jenkins, D. M. and Good, S. (1972) Mixed lymphocyte reaction and placentation. *Nature (London) New Biol.* 240, 211—212.

Jenkins, D. M. and Hancock, K. W. (1972) Maternal unresponsiveness to paternal histocompatibility antigens in human pregnancy. *Transplantation* 13, 618—619.

Jenkins, D. M., Acres, M. G., Peters, J. and Riley, J. (1972) Human chorionic gonadotropin and the fetal allograft. *Amer. J. Obstet. Gynecol.* 114, 13—15.

Jenkins, D. M., Need, J. and Rajah, S. M. (1977) Deficiency of specific HL-A antibodies in severe pregnancy pre-eclampsia/eclampsia. *Clin. exp. Immunol.* 27, 485—486.

Jenkinson, E. J. and Billington, W. D. (1974) Differential susceptibility of mouse trophoblast and embryonic tissue to immune cell lysis. *Transplantation* 18, 286—289.

Jenkinson, E. J., Billington, W. D. and Elson, J. (1976) Detection of receptors for immunoglobulin on human placenta by EA rosette formation. *Clin. exp. Immunol.* 23, 456—461.

Jensen, K. G. (1960) Transplacental passage of leucocyte agglutinins occurring on account of pregnancy. *Danish med. Bull.* 7, 55—58.

Jensen, K. G. (1962) Leucocyte antibodies in serum of pregnant women serology and clinic. *Vox Sang.* 7, 454—469.

Jha, P., Talwar, G. P. and Hingorani, V. (1975) Depression of blast transformation of peripheral leukocytes by plasma from pregnant women. *Amer. J. Obstet. Gynecol.* 122, 965—968.

Johansen, K., Festenstein, H. and Burke, J. (1974) Possible relationships between maternal HL-A antibody formation and fetal sex. Evidence for a sex-linked histocompatibility system in man. *J. Obstet. Gynaecol. Brit. Commonw.* 81, 781—785.

Johansson, S. G. O. (1968) Serum IgND levels in healthy children and adults. *Int. Arch. Allergy appl. Immunol.* 34, 1—8.

Johnson, M. H. (1975) Antigens of the peri-implantation trophoblast. In: *Immunobiology of Trophoblast.* Eds.: Edwards, Howe and Johnson. Cambridge University Press, Cambridge. pp. 87—112.

Johnson, P. M., Trenchev, P. and Faulk, W. P. (1975) Immunological studies of human placentae. Binding of complexed immunoglobulin by stromal endothelial cells. *Clin. exp. Immunol.* 22, 133—138.

Johnson, P. M., Faulk, W. P. and Wang, A-C. (1976) Immunological studies of human placentae: subclass and fragment specificity of binding of aggregated IgG by placental endothelial cells. *Immunology* 31, 659—664.

Jolles, P. and Jolles, J. (1961) Lysozyme from human milk. *Nature (London)* 192, 1187—1188.

Jones, E. and Curzen, P. (1973) The immunological reactivity of maternal lymphocytes in pregnancy. *J. Obstet. Gynaecol. Brit. Commonw.* 80, 608—610.

Jones, E. A. and Waldmann, T. A. (1972) The mechanism of intestinal uptake and transcellular transport of IgG in the neonatal rat. *J. clin. Invest.* 51, 2916—2927.

Jones, T. G., Goldsmith, K. L. G. and Anderson, I. Am. (1961) Maternal and neonatal platelet antibodies in a case of congenital thrombocytopenia. *Lancet* 2, 1008—1009.

Jones, W. R. (1968a) Immunological factors in human placentation. *Nature (London)* 218, 480.

Jones, W. R. (1968b) Immunological aspects of intrauterine transfusion. *Brit. med. J.* 3, 280—282.

Jones, W. R. (1969) In vitro transformation of fetal lymphocytes. *Amer. J. Obstet. Gynecol.* 104, 586—592.

Jones, W. R., Ing, R. M. Y. and Kay, M. D. (1972) Experimental immunization against human placental antigens. *Aust. N.Z. J. Obstet. Gynaecol.* 12, 237—245.

Jonker, M., Van Leeuwen, A. and Van Rood, J. J. (1977) Inhibition of the mixed leukocyte reaction by alloantisera in man. II. Incidence and characteristics of MLC-inhibiting antisera from multiparous women. *Tissue Antigens* 9, 246—258.

Jonsson, B. (1936) Zur Frage der heterospezifischen Schwangerschaft. *Acta pathol. microbiol. scand.* 13, 424—433.

Kadowaki, J. I., Zuelzer, W. W., Brough, A. J., Thompson, R. I., Wooley, P. V. and Gruber, D. (1965) XX/XY lymphoid chimaerism in congenital immunological deficiency syndrome with thymic alymphoplasia. *Lancet* 2, 1152—1156.

Kahn, C. R., Rosen, S. W., Weintraub, B. D., Fajans, S. S. and Gorden, P. (1977) Ectopic production of chorionic gonadotropin and its subunits by Islet-cell tumours. *New Engl. J. Med.* 297, 565—569.

Kajii, T. and Ohama, K. (1977) Androgenetic origin of hydatidiform mole. *Nature (London)* 268, 633—634.

Kaku, M. (1953) Placental polysaccharide and the aetiology of the toxaemia of pregnancy. *J. Obstet. Gynaecol. Brit. Emp.* 60, 148—156.

Kalmus, H. (1946) Genetic antigenic incompatibility as a possible cause of the toxaemia occurring late in pregnancy. *Ann. Eugen.* 13, 146—149.

Kasakura, S. (1971) A factor in maternal plasma during pregnancy that suppresses the reactivity of mixed leucocyte cultures. *J. Immunol.* 107, 1296—1301.

Kasakura, S. (1973) Is cortisol responsible for inhibition of MLC reactions by pregnancy plasma? *Nature (London)* 246, 496—497.

Katz, J. (1969) Transplacental passage of fetal red cells in abortion: increased incidence after curettage and effect of oxytocic drugs. *Brit. med. J.* 4, 84—86.

Kaufman, H. S. (1971) Allergy in the newborn: skin test reactions confirmed by the Prausnitz-Küstner test at birth. *Clin. Allergy* 1, 363—367.

Kay, H. E. M. and Margoles, C. (1971) Chromosomes of human fetal lymphocytes: frequency of abnormalities and absence of maternal cells. *Lancet* 2, 733—735.

Kay, H. E. M., Playfair, J. H., Wolfendale, M. and Hopper, P. K. (1962) Development of thymus in human foetus and its relation to immunological potential. *Nature (London)* 196, 238—240.

Kay, H. E. M., Wolfendale, M. R. and Playfair, J. H. L. (1966) Thymocytes and phytohaemagglutinin. *Lancet* 2, 804.

Kay, H. E. M., Doe, J. and Hockley, A. (1970) Response of human foetal thymocytes to phytohaemagglutinin (PHA). *Immunology* 18, 393—396.

Kaye, M. D. and Jones, W. R. (1971) Effect of human chorionic gonadotropin on in vitro lymphocyte transformation. *Amer. J. Obstet. Gynecol.* 109, 1029—1031.

Kempe, C. H. and Benenson, A. S. (1953) Vaccinia. Passive immunity in newborn infants. I. Placental transmission of antibodies. II. Response to vaccinations. *J. Pediat.* 42, 525—531.

Kenny, J. F., Boesman, M. I. and Michaels, R. H. (1967) Bacterial and viral coproantibodies in breast-fed infants. *Pediatrics* 39, 202—212.

Kirby, D. R. S. (1970) The egg and immunology. *Proc. roy. Soc. Med.* 63, 59—61.

Kirby, D. R. S., Billington, W. D., Bradbury, S. and Goldstein, D. J. (1964) Antigen barrier of the mouse placenta. *Nature (London)* 204, 548—549.

Kirby, D. R. S., McWhirter, K. C., Teitelbaum, M. S. and Darlington, C. D. (1967) A possible immunological influence on sex ratio. *Lancet* 2, 139—140.

Kirk, R. L., Shield, J. W., Stenhouse, N. S., Bryce, L. M. and Jacobowicz, R. (1955) A further study of ABO blood groups and differential fertility among women in two Australian maternity hospitals. *Brit. J. prev. soc. Med.* 9, 104—111.

Kissmeyer-Nielsen, F. and Thorsby, E. (1970) Human transplantation antigens. In: *Transplantation Review*. No. 4, Munksgaard, Copenhagen.

Kitzmiller, J. L. and Benirschke, K. (1973) Immunofluorescent study of placental bed vessels in pre-eclampsia of pregnancy. *Amer. J. Obstet. Gynecol.* 115, 248—251.

Kitzmiller, J. L., Stoneburner, L., Yelenosky, P. F. and Lucas, W. E. (1973) Serum complement in normal pregnancy and pre-eclampsia. *Amer. J. Obstet. Gynecol.* 117, 312—315.

Klapper, D. G. and Mendenhall, H. W. (1971) Immunoglobulin D concentration in pregnant women. *J. Immunol.* 107, 912—915.

Klein, R. B., Rech, K. C., Biberstein, M. and Stiehm, E. R. (1976) Defective mononuclear and neutrophil phagocyte chemotaxis in the newborn. *Clin. Res.* 24, 180A.

Klinger, H. P. and Schwarzacher, H. G. (1960) The sex chromatin and heterochromatic bodies in human diploid and polyploid nuclei. *J. biophys. biochem. Cytol.* 8, 345—364.

Klouda, P. T., Lawler, S. D. and Bagshawe, K. D. (1972) HL-A matings in trophoblastic neoplasia. *Tissue Antigens* 2, 280—284.

Kochwa, S., Rosenfield, R. E., Tallal, L. and Wasserman, L. R. (1961) Isoagglutinins associated with ABO erythroblastosis. *J. clin. Invest.* 40, 874—883.

Koerner, K. A. (1954) Congenital goitre with exophthalmos and hyperthyroidism. *J. Pediat.* 45, 464—470.

Kohler, P. (1973) Maturation of the human complement system. 1. Onset time and sites of fetal Clq, C4, C3, and C5 synthesis. *J. clin. Invest.* 52, 671—677.

Kohler, P. F. and Farr, R. S. (1966) Elevation of cord over maternal IgG immunoglobulin: evidence for an active placental IgG transport. *Nature (London)* 210, 1070—1071.

Kometani, K. and Behrman, S. J. (1971) The time of onset of placental susceptibility in mice to heterologous anti-mouse placental serum. *Int. J. Fertil.* 16, 139—143.

Komlos, L., Zamir, R., Joshua, H. and Halbrecht, I. (1977) Common HL-A antigens in couples with repeated abortions. *Clin. Immunol. Immunopathol.* 7, 330—335.

Koren, Z., Abrams, G. and Behrman, S. J. (1968) Antigenicity of mouse placental tissue. *Amer. J. Obstet. Gynecol.* 102, 340—346.

Kretschmer, R. R., Stewardson, P., Papierniak, C. and Gotoff, S. P. (1976) Chemotaxis of human cord blood monocytes. *Pediat. Res.* 10, 389.

Kuhns, W. J. (1965) Studies of immediate wheal reactions and of reaginic antibodies from pregnancy and the new born infant. *Proc. Soc. exp. Biol. Med.* 118, 377—380.

Kuttner, A. and Ratner, B. (1923) The importance of colostrum to the new-born infant. *Amer. J. Dis. Child.* 25, 413—434.

Lafferty, K. J., Walker, K. Z., Scollay, R. G. and Kilby, V. A. A. (1972) Allogeneic interactions provide evidence for a novel class of immunological reactivity. *Transplant. Rev.* 12, 198—228.

Lajos, L., Gorcs, J., Székely, J., Csaba, I. and Domány, S. (1964) The immunologic and endocrinologic basis of successful transplantation of human trophoblast. *Amer. J. Obstet. Gynecol.* 89, 595—605.

Lajos, L., Csaba, I., Domány, S., Székely, J. and Saáry, Z. (1967) Effect of placentotrophin on trophoblast homografts. *Acta morphol. Acad. Sci. hung.* 15, 185—193.

Lalezari, P., Nussbaum, T., Gelman, S. and Spaet, T. K. (1960) Neonatal neutropenia due to maternal iso-immunisation. *Blood* 15, 236—243.

Lampkin, B. C., Shore, N. A. and Chadwick, D. (1966) Megaloblastic anemia of infancy secondary to maternal pernicious anemia. *New Engl. J. Med.* 274, 1168—1171.

Lancet (1975) Hypertension in pregnancy. *Lancet* 2, 487—489.

Landon, J., Ratcliffe, J. G., Rees, L. H. and Scott, A. P. (1974) Tumour associated hormonal products. *J. clin. Pathol.* 27, Suppl. 7, 127—134.

Landsteiner, K. and Levine, P. (1926) On group specific substances in human spermatoza. *J. Immunol.* 12, 415—418.

Laskowski, M. Jr. and Laskowski, M. (1951) Crystalline trypsin inhibitor from colostrum. *J. biol. Chem.* 190, 563—573.

Lau, H. L. and Linkins, S. E. (1976) Alpha-fetoprotein. *Amer. J. Obstet. Gynecol.* 124, 533—554.

Lauritsen, J. G., Grunnet, N. and Jensen, O. M. (1975) Materno-fetal ABO incompatibility as a cause of spontaneous abortion. *Clin. Genet.* 7, 308—316.

Lauritsen, J. G., Jøgensen, J. and Kissmeyer-Nielsen, F. (1976a) Significance of HL-A and blood group incompatibility in spontaneous abortion. *Clin. Genet.* 9, 575—582.

Lauritsen, J. G., Kristensen, T. and Grunnet, N. (1976b) Depressed mixed lymphocyte culture reactivity in mothers with recurrent spontaneous abortion. *Amer. J. Obstet. Gynecol.* 125, 35—39.

Lawler, S. D. (1960) A genetical study of the Gm groups in human serum. *Immunology* 3, 90—94.

Lawler, S. D., Klouda, P. T. and Bagshawe, K. D. (1971) The HL-A system in trophoblastic neoplasia. *Lancet* 2, 834—837.

Lawler, S. D., Klouda, P. T. and Bagshawe, K. D. (1974) Immunogenicity of molar pregnancies in the HL-A system. *Amer. J. Obstet. Gynecol.* 120, 857—861.

Lawler, S. D., Ukaejiofo, E. O. and Reeves, B. R. (1975) Interaction of maternal and neonatal cells in mixed lymphocyte cultures. *Lancet* 2, 1185—1187.

Lawton, A. R., Self, K. S., Royal, S. A. and Cooper, M. D. (1972) Ontogeny of B-lymphocytes in the human fetus. *Clin. Immunol. Immunopathol.* 1, 84—93.

Lawton, J. W. M. and Shortridge, K. F. (1977) Protective factors in human breast milk and colostrum. *Lancet* 1, 253.

Lee, Y. W., Lee, Y. B. and Kim, D. S. (1970) Experimental nephritis induced by homologous placental tissue as observed with the light, fluorescent and electron microscope. *Yonsei med. J.* 11, 119—125.

Leikin, S. (1972) Depressed maternal lymphocyte response to phytohaemagglutinin in pregnancy. *Lancet* 2, 43.

Leikin, S. and Oppenheim, J. J. (1971) Prenatal sensitisation. *Lancet* 2, 876—877.

Leikin, S., Mochir-Fatemi, F. and Park, K. (1968) Blast transformation of lymphocytes from newborn human infants. *J. Pediat.* 72, 510—517.

Leissring, J. C., Anderson, J. W. and Smith, D. W. (1962) Uptake of antibodies by the intestine of the newborn infant. *Amer. J. Dis. Child.* 103, 160—165.

Lepow, M. L., Warren, R. J., Gray, N., Ingram, V. G. and Robbins, F. C. (1961) Effect of Sabin type 1 poliomyelitis vaccine administered by mouth to newborn infants. *New Engl. J. Med.* 264, 1071—1078.

Leslie, G. A. and Swate, T. E. (1972) Structure and biologic functions of human IgD. I. The presence of immunoglobulin D in human cord sera. *J. Immunol.* 109, 47—50.

Lester, E. P., Miller, J. B. and Yachnin, S. (1976) Human alpha-fetoprotein as a modulator of human lymphocyte transformation — correlation of biological potency with electrophoretic variants. *Proc. nat. Acad. Sci.* 73, 4645—4648.

Levine, P. (1943) Serological factors as possible causes in spontaneous abortions. *J. Hered.* 34, 71—80.

Levine, P. (1946) Genetic and constitutional causes of fetal and neonatal morbidity. *Ann. N.Y. Acad. Sci.* 46, 939—967.

Levine, P. and Celano, M. J. (1961) The question of D (Rh_0) antigenic sites on human spermatozoa. *Vox Sang.* 6, 720—723.

Lewis, J., Whang, J., Nagel, B., Oppenheim, J. and Perry, S. (1966) Lymphocyte transformation in mixed leucocyte cultures in women with normal pregnancy or tumours of placental origin. *Amer. J. Obstet. Gynecol.* 96, 287—290.

Lewis, J. L. and Terasaki, P. I. (1971) HL-A leucocyte antigen studies in women with gestational trophoblastic neoplasms. *Amer. J. Obstet. Gynecol.* 111, 547—552.

Lewis, J. L., Davis, R. C. and Parker, J. J. (1969) Modification of the immunological response to human choriocarcinoma in the hamster cheek pouch by heterologous antilymphocyte serum. *Cancer Res.* 29, 1988—1993.

Lieberman, R. and Dray, S. (1964) Maternal-fetal mortality in mice with isoantibodies to paternal γ-globulin allotypes. *Proc. Soc. exp. Biol. Med.* 116, 1069—1074.

Lin, T. M. and Halbert, S. P. (1975) Immunological comparison of various human pregnancy-associated plasma proteins. *Int. Arch. Allergy appl. Immunol.* 48, 101—115.

Lin, T. M., Halbert, S. P., Kiefer, D., and Spellacy, W. N. (1974) Three pregnancy-associated human plasma proteins: purification, monospecific antisera and immunological identification. *Int. Arch. Allergy appl. Immunol.* 47, 35—53.

Lindahl-Kiessling, K. and Böök, J. A., (1964) Effects of phytohaemagglutinin on leucocytes. *Lancet 2*, 591.

Lindblom, J. B., Friberg, J., Hogman, C. F. and Gemzell, C. (1972) HL-A haplotypes and unexplained infertility. *Tissue Antigens* 2, 352—358.

Ling, N. R. and Kay, J. E. (1975) *Lymphocyte Stimulation.* North-Holland Publ. Co., Amsterdam.

Linnet-Jepsen, P., Gelatins-Jensen, F. and Hauge, M. (1958) On the inheritance of the Gm serum group. *Acta genet.* (*Basel*) 8, 164—196.

Linscott, W. D. (1970) Effect of cell surface antigen density on immunological enhancement. *Nature (London)* 228, 824—827.

Lipton, M. M. and Steigman, A. J. (1957) Neonatal immunity. I. Disparity in maternal-infant poliovirus antibody. *Proc. Soc. exp. Biol. Med.* 96, 348—352.

Little, C. C. (1924) The genetics of tissue transplantation in mammals. *J. Cancer Res.* 8, 75—80.

Littman, B. H., Alpert, E. and Rocklin, R. E. (1977) The effect of purified α-fetoprotein on in vitro assays of cell-mediated immunity. *Cell. Immunol.* 30, 35—42.

Litwak, O., Taswell, H. F. and Banner, E. A. (1969) Transplacental fetal bleeding in spontaneous abortion. *Lancet* 2, 1161—1162.

Litwak, O., Taswell, H. F., Banner, E. A. and Keith, L. (1970) Fetal erythrocytes in maternal circulation after spontaneous abortion. *J. Amer. med. Assoc.* 214, 531—534.

Llewellyn-Jones, D. (1965) Trophoblast tumours. Geographical variations in incidence and possible aetiological factors. *J. Obstet. Gynaecol. Brit. Commonw.* 72, 242—248.

Loeb, E. N., Knowlton, A. I., Stoerk, M. G. and Seegal, B. C. (1949) Observations on the pregnant rat injected with nephrotoxic rabbit anti-rat placenta serum and desoxycorticosterone acetate. *J. exp. Med.* 89, 287—293.

Loke, Y. W. (1969) Sex chromatin of hydatidiform moles. *J. med. Genet.* 6, 22—25.

Loke, Y. W. (1975) Tumours of the placenta: a breakdown in foetal-maternal relationships. In: *Comparative Placentation. Essays in Structure and Function.* Ed.: Steven. Academic Press, London. pp. 282—293.

Loke, Y. W. and Ballard, A-C. (1973) Blood group A antigens on human trophoblast cells. *Nature (London)* 245, 329—330.

Loke, Y. W. and Borland, R. (1969) A histological study of chromatin positive and negative hydatidiform moles. *Brit. J. Cancer* 23, 554—558.

Loke, Y. W. and Borland, R. (1970) Immunofluorescent localisation of chorionic gonadotrophin in monolayer cultures of human trophoblast cells. *Nature (London)* 228, 561—562.

Loke, Y. W. and Pepys, M. B. (1975) Effects of human chorionic gonadotropin preparations on complement in vitro. *Amer. J. Obstet. Gynecol.* 121, 37—40.

Loke, Y. W., Joysey, V. C. and Borland, R. (1971) HL-A antigens on human trophoblast cells. *Nature (London)* 232, 403—405.

Loke, Y. W., Wilson, D. V. and Borland, R. (1972) Localization of human chorionic gonadotropin in monolayer cultures of trophoblast cells by mixed agglutination. *Amer. J. Obstet. Gynecol.* 113, 875—879.

Loke, Y. W., Brook, S. S. and Allen, G. E. (1975) Increase in IgM-bearing lymphocytes in peripheral blood of pregnant women. *Amer. J. Obstet. Gynecol.* 122, 561—564.

Loke, Y. W., Brook, S. S. and Allen, G. E. (1976) In vitro lymphocyte reactivity during pregnancy. *Brit. med. J.* 4, 1134.

Loke, Y. W., Brook, S. S. and Allen, G. E. (1977) Surface IgM on lymphocytes from pregnant women. *Amer. J. Obstet. Gynecol.* 127, 846—849.

Longsworth, L. G., Curtis, R. M. and Pembroke, R. H. (1945) The electrophoretic analysis of maternal and fetal plasmas and sera. *J. clin. Invest.* 24, 46—53.

Macris, N. T., Hellman, L. M. and Watson, R. J., (1958) Transmission of transfused sickle-trait cells from mother to fetus. *Amer. J. Obstet. Gynecol.* 76, 1214—1218.

Maes, R. F. and Claverie, N. (1977) The effect of preparations of human chorionic gonadotropin on lymphocyte stimulation and immune response. *Immunology* 33, 351—360.

Maisey, M. H. and Stimmler, L. (1972) The role of long acting thyroid stimulator in neonatal thyrotoxicosis. *Clin. Endocrinol.* 1, 81—90.

Makino, S., Sasaki, M. S. and Fukushima, T. (1963) Preliminary notes on the chromosomes of human chorionic lesions. *Proc. Jap. Acas.* 39, 54—58.

Mannick, J. A. and Schmid, K. (1967) Prolongation of allograft survival by an alpha globulin isolated from normal blood. *Transplantation* 5, 1231—1238.

Manolov, G., Levan, A. and Nadkarni, J. S. (1970) Burkitt's lymphoma with female karyotype in an African male child. *Hereditas* 66, 79—100.

Mantyjarvi, R., Hirvonen, T. and Toivanen, P. (1970) Maternal antibodies in human neonatal sera. *Immunology* 18, 449—451.

Maraz, A. and Petri, I. B. (1974) Intrinsic alteration of lymphocyte reactivity in women with normal pregnancy or tumour of placental origin. *Cell. Immunol.* 10, 496—499.

Marquez-Monter, H. (1962) The superfemale mole. *Lancet* 2, 202.

Martensson, L. and Fudenberg, H. H. (1965) Gm genes and γ_G-globulin synthesis in the human fetus. *J. Immunol.* 94, 514—520.

Mason, E. O., South, M. A. and Montgomery, J. R. (1976) Cord serum IgA in congenital cytomegalovirus infection. *J. Pediat.* 89, 945—946.

Masson, P. L., Delire, M. and Cambiaso, C. L. (1977) Circulating immune complexes in normal human pregnancy. *Nature (London)* 266, 542—543.

Mata, L. J. and Urrutia, J. J. (1971) Intestinal colonization of breast-fed children in a rural area of low socioeconomic level. *Ann. N.Y. Acad. Sci.* 176, 93—109.

Mata, L. J. and Wyatt, R. G. (1971) The uniqueness of human milk. Host resistance to infection. *Amer. J. clin. Nutr.* 24, 976—986.

Mathé, G., Dausset, J., Hervet, E., Amiel, J. L. and Colombani, J. (1964) Immunological studies in patients with placental choriocarcinoma. *J. nat. Cancer Inst.* 33, 193—208.

Matoth, Y. (1952) Phagocytic and amoeboid activities of the leukocytes in the newborn infant. *Pediatrics* 9, 748—754.

Matre, R. (1977) Similarities of Fc γ receptors on trophoblasts and placental endothelial cells. *Scand. J. Immunol.* 6, 953—958.

Matre, R., Tønder, O. and Endresen, C. (1975) Fc receptors in human placenta. *Scand. J. Immunol.* 4, 741—745.

Matsunaga, E. and Itoh, S. (1958) Blood groups and fertility in a Japanese population, with special reference to intra-uterine selection due to maternal-foetal incompatibility. *Ann. hum. Genet.* 22, 111—131.

Matthews, C. D. and Matthews, A. E. B. (1969) Transplacental haemorrhage in spontaneous and induced abortion. *Lancet* 1, 694—695.

May, D. (1973) Maternal blood group A and pre-eclampsia. *Brit. med. J.* 4, 738.

McCormick, J. N., Faulk, W. P., Fox, H. and Fudenberg, M. D. (1971) Immunohistological and elution studies of the human placenta. *J. exp. Med.* 133, 1—18.

McCracken, G. H. Jr and Eichenwald, H. F. (1971) Leucocyte function and the development of opsonic and complement activity in the neonate. *Amer. J. Dis. Child.* 121, 120—126.

McDevitt, H. O. and Benacerraf, B. (1969) Genetic control of specific immune responses. *Adv. Immunol.* 11, 31—74.

McFarlane, A. and Scott, J. S. (1976) Pre-eclampsia/eclampsia in twin pregnancies. *J. med. Genet.* 13, 208—211.

McKay, D. G. (1962) The placenta in experimental toxaemia of pregnancy. *Obstet. Gynecol.* 20, 1—22.

McKay, D. G., Merrill, S. J., Weiner, A. E., Hertig, A. T. and Reid, D. E. (1953) The pathologic anatomy of eclampsia, bilateral renal cortical necrosis, pituitary necrosis and other fatal complications of pregnancy and its possible relationship to the generalised Swartzman phenomenon. *Amer. J. Obstet. Gynecol.* 66, 507—539.

McKay, E. and Thom, H. (1971) Antibodies to gamma globulin in pregnant women: incidence, aetiology and size. *J. Obstet. Gynaecol. Brit. Commonw.* 78, 345—354.

McKenzie, J. M. (1964) Neonatal Graves' disease. *J. clin. Endocrinol.* 24, 660—668.

McLaren, A. (1962) Does immunity to male antigen affect female reproductive performance? *Nature (London)* 195, 1323—1324.

McLaren, A. (1975) Antigenic disparity: does it affect placental size, implantation or population genetics? In: *Immunobiology of Trophoblast.* Eds.: Edwards, Howe and Johnson. Cambridge University Press, Cambridge. pp. 255—273.

McLarey, D. C. and Fish, S. A. (1966) Fetal erythrocytes in the maternal circulation. *Amer. J. Obstet. Gynecol.* 95, 824—830.

McManus, L. M., Naughton, M. A. and Martinez-Hernandez, A. (1976) Human chorionic gonadotropin in human neoplastic cells. *Cancer Res.* 36, 3476—3481.

McNabb, T., Koh, T. Y., Dorrington, K. J. and Painter, R. H. (1976) Structure and function of immunoglobulin domains. V. Binding of immunoglobulin G. and fragments to placental membrane preparations. *J. Immunol.* 117, 882—887.

McNeil, C., Warenski, L. C, Fullmer, C. D. and Trentelman, E. F. (1954) A study of blood groups in habitual abortions. *Amer. J. clin. Pathol.* 24, 767—773.

Medical Research Council, Working Party Report (1974) Controlled trial of various anti-D dosages in suppression of Rh sensitisation following pregnancy. *Brit. med. J.* 2, 75—80.

Mellander, O., Vahlquist, B. and Mellbin, T. (1959) Breast feeding and artificial feeding. A clinical, serological, and biochemical study in 402 infants with a survey of the literature. *Acta paediat. scand.* 48, Suppl. 116, 1—108.

Menge, A. C. (1968) Fertilization, embryo and foetal survival rates in rabbits isoimmunised with semen, testis and conceptus. *Proc. Soc. exp. Biol. Med.* 127, 1271—1275.

Mengert, W. F., Rights, C. S., Bates, C. R., Reid, A. F., Wolf, G. R. and Nabors, G. C. (1955) Placental transmission of erythrocytes. *Amer. J. Obstet. Gynecol.* 69, 678—685.

Mercer, R. D., Lammert, A. C., Anderson, R. and Hazard, J. B. (1958) Choriocarcinoma in mother and infant. *J. Amer. med. Assoc.* 166, 482—483.

Meuwissen, H. J., Bach, F. H., Hong, R. and Good, R. A. (1968) Lymphocyte studies in congenital thymic dysplasia: the one-way stimulation test. *J. Pediat.* 72, 177—185.

Michaels, R. H. (1965) Studies of antiviral factors in human milk and serum. *J. Immunol.* 94, 262—270.

Midgley, A. R. and Pierce, G. B. (1962) Immunohistochemical localisation of human chorionic gonadotropin. *J. exp. Med.* 115, 289—294.

Mijer, F. and Olsen, R. N. (1958) Transplacental passage of the L.E. factor. *J. Pediat.* 52, 690—693.

Milgrom, H. and Shore, S. L. (1977) Assessment of monocyte function in normal newborn infant by antibody-dependent cellular cytotoxicity. *J. Pediat.* 91, 612—614.

Millar, K. G. and Mills, P. (1972) C′3 and IgG levels in mothers and babies at delivery. *Obstet. Gynecol.* 39, 527—532.

Miller, F. (1976) Serum-derived immunosuppressive substances. I. Partial purification and range of action. *Transplantation* 21, 179—187.

Miller, M. E. (1969) Phagocytosis in the newborn infant: humoral and cellular factors. *J. Pediat.* 74, 255—259.

Miller, M. E. (1971) Chemotactic function in the human neonate: humoral and cellular factors. *Pediat. Res.* 5, 487—492.

Miller, M. J., Sunshine, P. J. and Remington, J. S. (1969) Quantitation of cord serum IgM and IgA as a screening procedure to detect congenital infection: results in 5,006 infants. *J. Pediat.* 75, 1287—1291.

Milton, J. D. and Mowbray, J. F. (1972) Reversible loss of surface receptors on lymphocytes. *Immunology* 23, 599—608.

Mishell, D. R., Nakamura, R. M., Barberia, J. M. and Thoneycroft, I. A. (1974) Initial detection of human chorionic gonadotropin in serum in normal human gestation. *Amer. J. Obstet. Gynecol.* 118, 990—991.

Mitchison, N. A. (1974) Long term hazards in immunological methods of fertility control. In: *Immunological Approaches to Fertility Control.* Karolinska Symposia on Research Methods in Reproductive Endocrinology. Ed.: Diczfalusy. Karolinska Institute, Stockholm. pp. 405—418.

Mittal, K. K., Kachru, R. B. and Brewer, J. I. (1975) The HL-A and ABO antigens in trophoblastic disease. *Tissue Antigens* 6, 57—69.

Miyajima, T., Hirate, A. A. and Terasaki, P. I. (1972) Escape from sensitization to, HLA antibodies. *Tissue Antigens* 2, 64—73.

Møe, N. (1969) Deposits of fibrin and plasma proteins in the normal human placenta: an immunofluorescence study. *Acta pathol. microbiol. scand.* 76, 74—88.

Mogensen, B. and Kissmeyer-Nielsen, F. (1968) Histocompatibility antigens on the HL-A locus in generalised gestational choriocarcinoma. *Lancet* 1, 721—724.

Mogensen, B. and Kissmeyer-Nielsen, F. (1971) Current data on HL-A and ABO typing in gestational choriocarcinoma and invasive mole. *Transplant Proc.* 3, 1267—1271.

Mogensen, B. and Olsen, S. (1973) Cellular reaction to gestational choriocarcinoma and invasive mole. *Acta pathol. microbiol. scand. Sect. A,* 81, 453—456.

Mogensen, B., Kissmeyer-Nielsen, F. and Hauge, M. (1969) Histocompatibility antigens on the HL-A locus in gestational choriocarcinoma. *Transplant. Proc.* 1, 76—79.

Mohr, J. A. (1972) Lymphocyte sensitisation passed to the child from the mother. *Lancet* 1, 688.

Mohr, J. A. (1973) The possible induction and/or acquisition of cellular hypersensitivity associated with ingestion of colostrum. *J. Pediat.* 82, 1062—1064.

Mohr, J. A., Leu, R. and Mabry, W. (1970) Colostral leucocytes. *J. surg. Oncol.* 2, 163—167.

Mollison, P. L. (1967) *Blood Transfusion in Clinical Medicine.* Blackwell, Oxford. 4th Ed.

Mollison, P. L. (1973) Clinical aspects of Rh immunisation. *Amer. J. clin. Pathol.* 60, 287—301.

Mollison, P. L. and Hughes-Jones, N. C. (1967) Clearance of Rh positive red cells by low concentrations of Rh antibody. *Immunology* 12, 63—73.

Moore, D. H., Du Pan, R. M. and Buxton. C. L. (1949) An electrophoretic study of maternal, fetal and infant sera. *Amer. J. Obstet. Gynecol.* 57, 312—322.

Morell, A., Terry, W. D. and Waldmann, T. A. (1970) Metabolic properties of IgG subclasses in man. *J. clin. Invest.* 49, 673—680.

Morell, A., Skvaril, F. Van Loghem, E. and Kleemola, M. (1971) Human IgG subclasses in maternal and fetal serum. *Vox Sang.* 21, 481—492.

Morisada, M., Yamaguchi, H. and Lizuku, (1972) Toxic action of anti-HCG antibody to human trophoblast. *Int. J. Fertil.* 17, 65—71.

Morisada, M., Yamaguchi, H. and Lizuka, R. (1976) Immunobiological function of the syncytiotrophoblast: a new theory. *Amer. J. Obstet. Gynecol.* 125, 3—16.

Morris, N., Osborn, S. B. and Payling Wright, H. (1955) Effective circulation of the uterine wall in late pregnancy, measured with $^{24}NaCl$. *Lancet* 1, 323—325.

Morris, R. H., Vassalli, P., Beller, F. K. and McCluskey, R. I. (1964) Immunofluorescent studies of renal biopsies in the diagnosis of toxemia of pregnancy. *Obstet. Gynecol.* 24, 32—46.

Morse, J. H. (1968) Immunological studies of phytohaemagglutinin. I. Reactions between phytohaemagglutinin and normal sera. *Immunology* 14, 713—724.

Morse, J. H. (1976) The effect of human chorionic gonadotropin and placental lactogen on lymphocyte transformation in vitro. *Scand. J. Immunol.* 5, 779—787.

Morse, J. H., Stearns, G., Arden, J., Agosto, G. M. and Canfield, R. E. (1976) The effects of crude and purified human gonadotropin on in vitro stimulated human lymphocyte cultures. *Cell. Immunol.* 25, 178—188.

Moskalewski, S. Ptak, W. and Czarnik, Z. (1975) Demonstration of cells with IgG receptor in human placenta. *Biol. Neonate* 26, 268—273.

Mouton, R. P., Stoop, J. W., Ballieux, R. E. and Mul, N. A. J. (1970) Pneumococcal antibodies in IgA of serum and external secretions. *Clin. exp. Immunol.* 7, 201—210.

Munk-Anderson, G. (1958) Excess of group O-mothers in ABO-haemolytic disease. *Acta pathol. microbiol. scand.* 42, 43—50.

Murgita, R. A, and Tomasi, T. B. (1975) Suppression of the immune response by α-fetoprotein. I. The effect of mouse α-fetoprotein on the primary and secondary antibody response. *J. exp. Med.* 141, 269—286.

Murgita, R. A, and Wigzell, H. (1976) The effects of mouse alpha-fetoprotein on T-cell-dependent and T-cell-independent immune responses in vitro. *Scand. J. Immunol.* 5, 1215—1220.

Murgita, R. A., Goidl, E. A., Kontiainen, S. and Wigzell, H. (1977) α-fetoprotein induces suppressor T cells in vitro. *Nature (London)* 267, 257—259.

Murillo, G. J. and Goldman, A. S. (1970) The cells of human colostrum. II. Synthesis of IgA and β1C. *Pediat. Res.* 4, 71—75.

Murray, J. and Calman, R. M. (1953) Immunity of the newborn. A study of the transfer of anti-streptolysin from mother to foetus during pregnancy. *Brit. med. J.* 1, 13—15.

Murray, S. and Barron, S. L. (1971) Rhesus isoimmunisation after abortions. *Brit. med. J.* 3, 90—92.

Murray, S., Barron, S. L. and McNay, R. A. (1970) Transplacental haemorrhage after abortion. *Lancet* 1, 631—634.

Naeslund, J. (1951) Studies on placental permeability with radio-active isotopes of phosphorus and iron. *Acta obstet. gynaecol. scand.* 30, 231—246.

Naeslund, J. and Nylin, G. (1946) Investigation of permeability of placenta with aid of red blood corpuscles tagged with radio-active phosphorus. *Acta med. scand.*, Suppl. 170, 390—398.

Naiman, J. L., Punnett, H. H., Destiné, M. L. and Lischner, H. W. (1966) Yy chromosomal chimaerism. *Lancet* 2, 590.

Naiman, J. L., Punnett, H. H., Lischner, H. W., Destiné, M. L. and Arey, J. B. (1969) Possible graft-versus-host reaction after intrauterine transfusion for Rh erythroblastosis fetalis. *New Engl. J. Med.* 281, 697—701.

Naito, S., Mickey, M. R., Hirata, A. and Terasaki, P. I. (1971) Autolymphocytotoxins following immunisation by pregnancy, transplantation, and disease. *Tissue Antigens* 1, 219—228.

Nakajima, S., Baba, A. S. and Tamura, N. (1977) Complement system in human colostrum. Presence of nine complement components and factors of alternative pathway in human colostrum. *Int. Arch. Allergy appl. Immunol.* 54, 428—433.

Namba, T., Brown, S. B. and Grob, D. (1970) Neonatal myasthenia gravis: report of two cases and review of the literature. *Pediatrics* 45, 488—504.

Nathan, D. J. and Snapper, I. (1958) Simultaneous placental transfer of factors responsible for L-E cell formation and thrombocytopenia. *Amer. J. Med.* 25, 647—653.

Nathenson, G., Schorr, J. B. and Litwin, S. D. (1971) Gm factor fetomaternal gamma globulin incompatibility. *Pediat. Res.* 5, 2—9.

Naughton, M. A., Merrill, D. A., McManus, L. M., Fink, L. M., Berman, E., White, M. J. and Martinez-Hernandez, A. (1975) Localization of the β chain of human chorionic gonadotropin on human tumour cells and placental cells. *Cancer Res.* 35, 1887—1890.

Nature (1970) In pursuit of the Y chromosome. *Nature (London)* 226, 897.

Need, J. A. (1975) Pre-eclampsia in pregnancies by different fathers: immunological studies. *Brit. med. J.* 1, 548—549.

Need, J. A., Jenkins, D. M. and Scott, J. S. (1976) The response of lymphocytes to phytohaemagglutinin in women with pre-eclampsia. *Brit. J. Obstet. Gynaecol.* 83, 438—440.

Neill, J. M., Gaspari, E. L., Richardson, L. V. and Sugg, J. Y. (1932) Diptheria antibodies transmitted from mother to child. *J. Immunol.* 22, 117—124.

Nelson, J. H. and Hall, J. E. (1964) Studies on the thymolymphatic system in humans. I. Morphologic changes in lymph nodes in pregnancy at term. *Amer. J. Obstet. Gynecol.* 90, 482—484.

Nelson, J. H. and Hall, J. E. (1965) Studies on the thymolymphatic system in humans. II. Morphologic changes in lymph nodes in early pregnancy and during the puerperium. *Amer. J. Obstet. Gynecol.* 93, 1133—1136.

Nelson, J. H., Hall, J. E., Manuel-Limson, G., Freidberg, H. and O'Brien, F. J. (1967) Effect of pregnancy on the thymolymphatic system. I. Changes in the intact rat after exogenous HCG, estrogen and progesterone administration. *Amer. J. Obstet. Gynecol.* 98, 895—899.

Nelson, J. H., Jr., Lu, T., Hall, J. E., Krown, S., Nelson, J. H. and Fox, C. W. (1973) The effect of trophoblast on immune state of women. *Amer. J. Obstet. Gynecol.* 117, 689—699.

Nemirovsky, M. S. (1970) The induction of congenital abnormalities in mice by means of heterologous anti-mouse placenta serum. *Experientia* 26, 1138—1139.

Nemirovsky, T. and Trainin, N. (1973) Leukaemia induction in C_3H mice following their inoculation with normal AKR lymphoid cells. *Int. J. Cancer* 11, 172—177.

Newcomb, R. W., Normansell, D. and Stanworth, D. R. (1968) A structural study of human exocrine IgA globulin. *J. Immunol.* 101, 905—914.

Nisula, B. C. and Kohler, P. O. (1974) Effect of antiserum to human chorionic gonadotropin on growth and function of choriocarcinoma in vivo and in vitro. *Cancer Res.* 34, 512—515.

Nordbring, F. (1957a) The appearance of antistreptolysin and antistaphylolysin in human colostrum. *Acta paediat.* 46, 481—496.

Nordbring, F. (1957b) The failure of newborn premature infants to absorb antibodies from heterologous colostrum. *Acta paediat.* 46, 569—578.

Normington, E. A. M. and Jennison, R. F. (1969) Rhesus sensitisation and abortion. *Brit. med. J.* 4, 495—496.

Nutt, J., Clarke, F., Welch, R. G. and Hall, R. (1974) Neonatal hyperthyroidism and long-acting thyroid stimulator protector. *Brit. med. J.* 4, 695—696.

Ockleford, C. D. (1977) Antibody clearance by micropinocytosis: a possible role in foetal immunoprotection. *Lancet* 1, 310.

Ockleford, C. D. and Whyte, A. (1977) Differentiated regions of human placental cell surface associated with exchange of materials between maternal and foetal blood: coated vesicles. *J. cell. Sci.* 25, 293—312.

Ogra, P. L. and Ogra, S. S. (1973) Local antibody response to poliovaccine in the human female genital tract. *J. Immunol.* 110, 1307—1311.

Ogra, S. S., Ogra, P. L., Lippes, J. and Tomasi, T. B. (1971) Immunohistologic localization of immunoglobulins, secretory component, and lacteroferrin in the developing human fetus. *Proc. Soc. exp. Biol. Med.* 139, 570—574.

Ohama, K. and Kadotani, T. (1971) Lymphocyte reaction in mixed wife-husband leukocyte cultures in relation to infertility. *Amer. J. Obstet. Gynecol.* 109, 477—479.

Ohama, K. and Kajii, T. (1974) Mixed culture of fetal and adult lymphocytes. *Amer. J. Obstet. Gynecol.* 119, 552—556.

Okuda, T. and Grollman, A. (1966) Renal lesions in rats following injection of placental extracts. An experimental study of the pathogenesis of toxemia of pregnancy. *Arch. Pathol.* 82, 246—258.

Olding, L. (1972) The possibility of materno-foetal transfer of lymphocytes in man. *Acta paediat. scand.* 61, 73—75.

Olding, L. B. and Oldstone, M. B. A. (1974) Lymphocytes from human newborns abrogate mitosis of their mothers' lymphocytes. *Nature (London)* 249, 161—162.

Olding, L. B. and Oldstone, M. B. A. (1976) Thymus-derived peripheral lymphocytes from human newborns inhibit division of their mothers' lymphocytes. *J. Immunol.* 116, 682—686.

Olding, L. B., Murgita, R. A, and Wigzell, H. (1977) Mitogen-stimulated lymphoid cells from human newborns suppress the proliferation of maternal lymphocytes across a cell-impermeable membrane. *J. Immunol.* 119, 1109—1114.

Oldstone, M. B. A., Tishon, A. and Moretta, L. (1977) Active thymus derived suppressor lymphocytes in human cord blood. *Nature (London)* 269, 333—335.

Oliver, R. T. D. (1974) Are there Y-linked histocompatibility antigens in man? *Eur. J. Immunol.* 4, 519—520.

O'Reilly, R. J., Patterson, J. H., Bach, F. H., Bach, M. L. and Hong, R. (1973) Chimerism detected by HL-A typing. *Transplantation* 15, 505—507.

Osborn, J. J., Dancis, J. and Julia, J. F. (1952) Studies on the immunology of the newborn infant. II. Interference with active immunization by passive transplacental circulating antibody. *Pediatrics* 10, 328—334.

Overweg, J. and Engelfriet, P. C (1969) Cytotoxic leucocyte iso-antibodies formed during the first pregnancy. *Vox Sang.* 16, 97—104.

Owen, R. D., Wood, H., Foord, A. G., Sturgeon, P. and Baldwin, L. G. (1954) Evidence for actively acquired tolerance to Rh antigens. *Proc. nat. Acad. Sci.* 40, 420—424.

Pacsa, A. S. and Pejtsik, B. (1977) Impairment of immunity during pregnancy and antiviral effect of amniotic fluid. *Lancet* 1, 330—331.

Pahwa, S. G., Pahwa, R., Grimes, E. and Smithwick, E. (1977) Cellular and humoral components of monocyte and neutrophil chemotaxis in cord blood. *Pediat. Res.* 11, 677—680.

Papiernik, M. (1970) Correlation of lymphocyte transformation and morphology in the human fetal thymus. *Blood* 36, 470—479.

Parish, W. E., Carron-Brown, J. A. and Richards, C. B. (1967) The detection of antibodies to spermatozoa and to blood group antigens in cervical mucus. *J. Reprod. Fertil.* 13, 469—483.

Park, B. H., Holmes, B. and Good, R. A. (1970) Metabolic activities in leukocytes of newborn infants. *J. Pediat.* 76, 237—241.

Park, W. W. (1957) The occurrence of sex chromatin in chorioepitheliomas and hydatidiform moles. *J. Pathol. Bact.* 74, 197—206.

Park, W. W. (1971) *Choriocarcinoma. A Study of its Pathology.* William Heinemann, London.

Parker, R. H. and Beierwaltes, W. H. (1961) Thyroid antibodies during pregnancy and in the newborn. *J. clin. Endocrinol.* 21, 792—798.

Parkman, R., Mosier, D., Unmansky, I., Cochran, W., Carpenter, C. B. and

Rosen, F. S. (1974) Graft-versus-host disease after intrauterine and exchange transfusions for haemolytic disease of the newborn. *New Engl. J. Med.* 290 359—363.

Parmely, M. J., Beer, A. E. and Billingham, R. E. (1976) In vitro studies on the T-lymphocyte population of human milk. *J. exp. Med.* 144, 358—370.

Parmely, M. J., Reath, D. B., Beer, A. E. and Billingham, R. E. (1977) Cellular immune responses of human milk T lymphocytes to certain environmental antigens. *Transplant. Proc.* 9, 1477—1483.

Parmiani, G. and Della Porta, G. (1973) Effects of antitumour immunity on pregnancy in the mouse. *Nature (London) New Biol.* 241, 26—28.

Paterson, W. G. (1976) Letter commenting on: 'Advanced abdominal pregnancy with severe pre-eclampsia', by Anderton, Duncan and Lunt. *Brit. J. Obstet. Gynaecol.* 83, 336.

Pattillo, R. A. and Gey, G. O. (1968) The establishment of a cell line of human hormone-synthesizing trophoblastic cells in vitro. *Cancer Res.* 28, 2131—1234.

Pattillo, R. A., Gey, G. O., Delfs, E., Huang, W. Y., Hause, L., Garancis, J., Knoth, M., Amatruda, J., Bertino, J., Friesen, H. G. and Mattingly, R. F. (1971) The hormone-synthesizing trophoblastic cell in vitro: a model for cancer research and placental hormone synthesis. *Ann. N.Y. Acad. Sci.* 172, 288—298.

Pattillo, R. A., Hussa, R. O., Story, M. T., Ruckert, A. C. F., Shalaby, M. R. and Mattingly, R. F. (1977) Tumour antigen and human chorionic gonadotropin in CaSki cells: a new epidermoid cervical cancer cell line. *Science* 196, 1456—1458.

Payne, R. (1964) Neonatal neutropenia and leucoagglutinins. *Pediatrics* 33, 194—204.

Payne, R. and Rolfs, M. R. (1958) Fetomaternal leukocyte incompatibility. *J. clin. Invest.* 37, 1756—1763.

Pearse, W. H. and Kaiman, H. (1967) Human chorionic gonadotropin and skin homograft survival. *Amer. J. Obstet. Gynecol.* 98, 573—574.

Pearson, M. G. and Pinker, G. D. (1956) ABO blood groups and toxaemia of pregnancy. *Brit. med. J.* 1, 777—778.

Pearson, P. L., Bobrow, M. and Vosa, C. G. (1970) Technique for identifying Y chromosomes in human interphase nuclei. *Nature (London)* 226, 78—80.

Peer, L. A. (1958) Behaviour of skin grafts exchanged between parents and offsprings. *Ann. N.Y. Acad. Sci.* 73, 584—589.

Pegrum, G. D. (1971) Mixed cultures of human foetal and adult cells. *Immunology* 21, 159—164.

Pegrum, G. D., Ready, D. and Thompson, E. (1968) The effects of phytohaemagglutinin on human fetal cells grown in culture. *Brit. J. Haematol.* 15, 371—376.

Pellegrino, H. A., Pellegrino, A. and Kahan, B. D. (1970) Solubilization of fetal HL-A antigens. *Transplantation* 10, 425—430.

Pence, H., Petty, W. M. and Rocklin, R. E. (1975) Suppresssion of maternal responsiveness to paternal antigens by maternal plasma. *J. Immunol.* 114, 525—528.

Penrose, L. S. (1946) On the familial appearance of maternal and fetal incompatibility. *Ann. Eugen.* 13, 141—145.

Pentycross, C. R. (1969) Lymphocyte transformation in young people. *Clin. exp. Immunol.* 5, 213—216.

Perlman, P., Perlman, H. and Wigzell, H. (1972) Lymphocyte mediated cytotoxicity in-vitro. Induction and inhibition by humoral antibody and nature of effector cells. *Transplant Rev.* 13, 91—114.

Peters, D. K. (1975) The kidney in allergic disease. In: *Clinical Aspects of Immunology*. Eds.: Gell, Coombs and Lachmann. 3rd Ed. Blackwell, Oxford, pp. 1217—1239.

Peters, D. K. and Lachmann, P. J. (1974) Immunity deficiency in pathogenesis of glomerulonephritis. *Lancet 1* 58—60.

Petit, J. C., Galinha, A. and Salomon, J. C. (1973) Immunoglobulins in the intestinal content of the human fetus with special reference to IgA. *Eur. J. Immunol.* 3, 373—375.

Petrucco, O. M., Thomson, N. M., Lawrence, J. F. and Weldon, M. W. (1974) Immunofluorescent studies in renal biopsies in pre-eclampsia, *Brit. med. J.* 1, 473—476.

Petrucco, O. M., Seamark, R. F., Holmes, K., Forbes, I. J. and Symonds, R. G. (1976) Changes in lymphocyte function during pregnancy. *Brit. J. Obstet. Gynaecol.* 83, 245—250.

Pike, L. H. and Dickens, A. M. (1954) ABO blood groups and toxaemia of pregnancy. *Brit. med. J.* 2, 321—323.

Pinsker, M. C. and Mintz, B. (1973) Change in cell-surface glycoproteins of mouse embryos before implantation. *Proc. nat. Acad. Sci.* 70, 1645—1648.

Pitt, J. (1976) Breast milk leucocytes. *Pediatrics* 58, 769—770.

Platt, R., Steward, A. E. and Emery, E. W. (1958) The aetiology, incidence and heredity of pre-eclamptic toxaemia of pregnancy, *Lancet* 1, 552—556.

Playfair, J. H. L., Wolfendale, M. R. and Kay, H. E. M. (1963) The leucocytes of the peripheral blood in the human foetus. *Brit. J. Haematol.* 9, 336—344.

Polani, P. E. and Mutton, D. E. (1971) Y-fluorescence of interphase nuclei, especially circulating lymphocytes. *Brit. med. J.* 1, 138—142.

Poskitt, P. K. F., Kurt, E. A., Paul, B. B., Selvaraj, R. J., Sbarra, A. J. and Mitchell, G. W. (1977) Response to mitogen during pregnancy and the post partum period. *Obstet. Gynecol.* 50, 319—323.

Potter, J. F. and Schoeneman, M. (1970) Metastasis of maternal cancer to the placenta and fetus. *Cancer* 25, 380—388.

Powell, A. E. (1974) Maternal lymphocytes: suppression by human chorionic gonadotrophin. *Science* 184, 913—914.

Prall, R. H. and Kantor, F. S. (1966) Serum complement in eclamptogenic toxemia. *Amer. J. Obstet. Gynecol.* 95, 530—533.

Prehn, R. T. (1960) Specific homograft tolerance induced by successive matings and implications concerning choriocarcinoma. *J. nat. Cancer Inst.* 25, 883—886.

Preston, F. E., Malia, R. G., Tipton, R. H. and Smith, A. J. (1972) Intravascular coagulation and pre-eclamptic toxaemia. *Lancet* 1, 34—35.

Propp, R. and Alper, C. A. (1968) C′3 synthesis in the human fetus and lack of transplacental passage. *Science* 162, 672—673.

Pross, S. H., Hallock, J. A., Armstrong, R. and Fishel, C. W. (1977) Complement and Fc receptors on cord blood and adult neutrophils. *Pediat. Res.* 11, 135—137.

Purtilo, D. T., Hallgren, H. M. and Yunis, E. J. (1972) Depressed maternal lymphocyte response to phytohaemagglutinin in human pregnancy. *Lancet* 1, 769—771.

Queenan, J. T., Shah, S., Kubarych, S. F. and Holland, B. (1971) Role of induced abortion in rhesus immunisation. *Lancet* 1, 815—817.

Quie, P. G., Messner, R. P. and Williams, R. C. (1968) Phagocytosis in subacute bacterial endocarditis. *J. exp. Med.* 128, 553—570.

Rabson, A. S., Rosen, S. W., Tashjian, A. H. and Weintraub, B. D. (1973) Production of human chorionic gonadotrophin in vitro by a cell line derived from a carcinoma of the lung. *J. nat. Cancer Inst.* 50, 669—674.

Race, R. R. (1944) An 'incomplete' antibody in human serum. *Nature (London)* 153, 771—772.

Rachelefsky, G. S., McConnachie, P. R., Terasaki, P. I. and Steihm, E. R. (1973) Deficient killer function in newborn and young infant lymphocytes. *Pediat. Res.* 7, 371.

Rao, S. S. and Shahani, S. K. (1961) Antigenicity of HCG. *Immunology* 4, 1—12.

Raptopoulou, M. and Goulis, G. (1977) Physiological variations of T cells during the menstrual cycle. *Clin. exp. Immunol.* 28, 458—460.

Rather, L. J. (1971) Ambroise Paré, the Countess Margaret, multiple births, and hydatidiform mole. *Bull. N.Y. Acad. Med.* 47, 508—515.

Ratner, B. and Gruehl, H. L. (1929) Transmission of respiratory anaphylaxis (asthma) from mother to offspring. *J. exp. Med.* 49, 833—845.

Ratner, B., Jackson, H. C. and Gruehl, H. L. (1927a) Transmission of protein hypersensitiveness from mother to offspring. IV. Passive sensitization in utero. *J. Immunol.* 14, 291—302.

Ratner, B., Jackson, H. C. and Gruehl, H. L. (1927b) Transmission of protein hypersensitiveness from mother to offspring. V. Active sensitization in utero. *J. Immunol.* 14, 303—319.

Rebello, R. Green, F. H. Y. and Fox, H. (1975) A study of the secretory immune system of the female genital tract. *Brit. J. Obstet. Gynaecol.* 82, 812—816.

Reisfeld, R. A. and Hertz, R. (1960) Purification of chorionic gonadotropin from the urine of patients with trophoblastic tumours. *Biochim. biophys. Acta* 43. 540—543.

Remold, H. G. and David, J. R. (1971) Further studies on migration inhibitory factor (MIF): evidence for its glycoprotein nature. *J. Immunol.* 107, 1090—1098.

Renkonen, K. O. and Timonen, S. (1967) Factors influencing the immunization of Rh-negative mothers. *J. med. Genet.* 4, 166—168.

Renkonen, K. O., Mäkelä, O. and Lehtovaara, R. (1962) Factors affecting the human sex ratio. *Nature (London)* 194, 308—309.

Revillard, J. P., Robert, M., Betuel, H., Latour, M., Bonneau, M., Brochier, J. and Traeger, J. (1972) Inhibition of the mixed lymphocyte reaction by antibodies. *Transplant. Proc.* 4, 173—176.

Rhodes, P. (1965) Sex of the foetus in antipartum haemorrhage. *Lancet* 2, 718—719.

Riggio, R. R., Parrillo, J. E., Bull, F. G., Schwartz, G. H., Stenzel, K. H. and Rubin, A. L. (1971) Inhibition of lymphocyte transformation by a placental glycoprotein. *Transplantation* 12, 400—401.

Robert, M., Betuel, H. and Revillard, J. P. (1973) Inhibition of the mixed lymphocyte reaction by sera from multipara. *Tissue Antigens* 3, 39—56.

Robertson, W. B., Brosens, I. and Dixon, H. G. (1967) The pathological response of the vessels of the placental bed to hypertensive pregnancy. *J. Pathol. Bacteriol.* 93, 581—592.

Robinson, E., Shulman, J., Ben-Hur, H., Zuckerman, H. and Neuman, Z. (1963) Immunological studies and behaviour of husband and foreign homografts in patients with chorioepithelioma. *Lancet* 1, 300—302.

Robinson, E., Ben-Hur, N., Zuckerman, H. and Neuman, Z. (1967) Further immunologic studies in patients with choriocarcinoma and hydatidiform mole. *Cancer Res.* 27, 1202—1204.

Robinson, M. (1951) Infant morbidity and mortality. A study of 3266 infants. *Lancet* 1, 788—794.

Rocklin, R. E., Zuckerman, J. E., Alpert, E. and David, J. R. (1973) Effect of multiparity on human maternal hypersensitivity to foetal antigen. *Nature (London)* 241, 130—131.

Rodewald, R. (1976) Intestinal transport of peroxidase-conjugated IgG fragments in the neonatal rat. In: *Maternofoetal Transmission of Immunoglobulins.* Ed.: Hemmings. Cambridge University Press, Cambridge. pp. 137—153.

Roffman, B. Y. and Simons, M. (1969) Syncytial trophoblastic embolism associated with placenta increta and pre-eclampsia. *Amer. J. Obstet. Gynecol.* 104, 1218—1220.

Romano, E. L., Hughes-Jones, H. C. and Mollison, P. L. (1973) The direct antiglobulin reaction in ABO haemolytic disease of the newborn. *Brit. med. J.* 1, 524—526.

Rosen, F. S. (1974) Complement: ontogeny and phylogeny. *Transplant. Proc.* 6, 47—50.

Rosenberg, D., Grand, M. and Silbert, D. (1963) Neonatal hyperthyroidism. *New Engl. J. Med.* 268, 292—296.

Rosenfield, R. E. (1955) A-B haemolytic diseases of newborn. Analysis of 1480 cord blood specimens, with special reference to the direct anti-globulin test and to the group O mother. *Blood* 10, 17—28.

Rosenfield, R. E. and Ohno, G. (1955) A-B haemolytic disease of the newborn. *Rev. Hémat.* 10, 231—235.

Rosenthal, M. (1977) Enhanced phagocytosis of immune complexes in pregnancy. *Clin. exp. Immunol.* 28, 189—191.

Rowe, D. S., Crabbe, P. A. and Turner, M. W. (1968) Immunoglobulin D in serum, body fluids and lymphoid tissues. *Clin. exp. Immunol.* 3, 477—490.

Rowe, D. S., Hug,K., Faulk, W. P., McCormick, J. N. and Berker, H. N. (1973a) IgD on the surface of peripheral blood lymphocytes of the human newborn. *Nature (London) New Biol.*, 242, 155—157.

Rowe, D. S., Hug, K., Forni, L. and Pernis, B. (1973b) Immunoglobulin D as a lymphocyte receptor. *J. exp. Med.* 138, 965—972.

Ruddy, S., Klemperer, M. R., Rosen, F. S., Austen, K. F. and Kumate, J. (1970) Hereditary deficiency of the second component of complement (C2) in man: correlation of C2 haemolytic activity with immunochemical measurements of C2 protein. *Immunology* 18, 943—954.

Rudolf, R. H. and Thomas, E. D. (1970) Histocompatibility studies in patients with trophoblastic tumours. *Amer. J. Obstet. Gynecol.* 108, 1126—1129.

Ruoslahti, E., Tallberg, Th. and Seppälä, M. (1966) Origin of proteins in amniotic fluid. *Nature (London)* 212, 841.

Ruoslahti, E., Seppälä, M., Pihko, H. and Vuopio, P. (1971) Studies of carcino-fetal proteins. II. Biochemical comparison of α-fetoprotein from human fetuses and patients with hepatocellular cancer. *Int. J. Cancer 8*, 283—288.

Sabin, A. B., and Fieldsteel, A. H. (1962) Antipoliomyelitic activity of human and bovine colostrum and milk. *Pediatrics* 29, 105—115.

Sabin, A. B., Michaels, R. H., Krugman, S., Eiger, M. E., Berman, P. H. and Warren, J. (1963) Effect of oral poliovirus vaccine in newborn children. I. Excretion of virus after ingestion of large doses of type I or a mixture of all three types, in relation to level of placentally transmitted antibody. *Pediatrics* 31, 623—640.

Salvaggio, A. T., Nigogosyan, G. and Mack, H. C. (1960) Detection of trophoblast in cord blood and fetal circulation. *Amer. J. Obstet. Gynecol.* 80, 1013—1021.

Salzmann, K. D. (1955) Do transplacental hormones cause eclampsia? *Lancet* 2, 953—956.

Samuel, S., Pildes, R. S., Lewison, M. and Rosenthal, I. M. (1971) Neonatal hyperthyroidism in an infant born of an euthyroid mother. *Amer. J. Dis. Child.* 121, 440—443.

Sawyer, M. K., Forman, M. L. and Kuplic, L. S. (1971) Developmental aspects of the human complement system. *Biol. Neonate* 19, 148—162.

Saxena, B. B., Hasan, S. H., Haour, F. and Schmidt-Gollwitzer, M. (1974) Radioreceptor assay of human chorionic gonadotropin: detection of early pregnancy. *Science* 184, 793—795.

Scheinberg, H., Cook, C. D. and Murphy, J. A. (1954) The concentration of copper and ceruloplasmin in maternal and infant plasma at delivery. *J. clin. Invest.* 33, 963.

Schiff, R. I., Mercier, D. and Buckley, R. (1975) Inability of gestational hormones to account for the inhibitory effects of pregnancy plasmas on lymphocyte response in-vitro. *Cell. Immunol.* 20, 69—80.

Schindler, A-M., Graf, E. and Martin-Du-Pan, R. (1972) Prenatal diagnosis of fetal lymphocytes in the maternal blood, *Obstet. Gynecol.* 40, 340—346.

Schlesinger, J. J. and Covelli, H. D. (1977) Evidence for transmission of lymphocyte responses to tuberculin by breast-feeding. *Lancet* 2, 529—532.

Schlumberger, H. D. and Anderer, F. A. (1969) Infertility of mice induced by antibodies specific for human chorionic gonadotrophin. *Acta endocrinol.* 60, 681—688.

Schmidt, P. J., Hertz, R. and Leyshon, W. C. (1961) Blood group factors in women with choriocarcinoma as compared with those of their husbands. *Amer. J. Obstet. Gynecol.* 82, 651—653.

Schoen, I., Konwaler, B. E. and Novak, E. (1954) The sex incidence of the fetus or child in maternal choriocarcinoma. *Amer. J. Obstet. Gynecol.* 67, 1134—1138.

Schröder, J. (1974) Passage of leucocytes from mother to fetus. *Scand. J. Immunol,* 3, 369—373.

Schröder, J. (1975) Are fetal cells in maternal blood mainly B lymphocytes? *Scand. J. Immunol.* 4, 279—285.

Schröder, J. and De la Chapelle, A. (1972) Fetal lymphocytes in the maternal blood. *Blood* 39, 153—162.

Schröder, J., Tiilikainen, A. and De la Chapelle, A. (1974) Foetal leucocytes in the maternal circulation after delivery. I. Cytological aspects. *Transplantation* 17, 346—354.

Schulman, I., Smith, C. H. and Ando, R. E. (1954) Congenital thrombopenic purpura: observations on three infants born of a non-affected mother; demonstration of platelet agglutinins and evidence for platelet isoimmunization. *Amer. J. Dis. Child.* 88, 784—786.

Schwartz, E. S., Gang, N. F. and Gelfand, M. M. (1974) Studies on human placenta. I. Isolation and partial characterization of a glycoprotein from the chorionic villus. *Amer. J. Obstet. Gynecol.* 118, 857—863.

Schwartz, J., Kehaty, T. and Foldes, J. J. (1974) Phagocytosis of foetal erythrocytes by trophoblast cells. *IRCS Library Compendium* 2, 1002.

Schwartz, R. S. (1974) Trojan-Horse lymphocytes. *New Engl. J. Med.* 290, 397—398.

Sclare, G. (1960) Congenital hyperthyroidism. *Biol. Neonate* 2, 132—146.

Scott, J. R. and Beer, A. E. (1973) Immunological factors in first pregnancy Rh immunisation. *Lancet* 1, 717—718.

Scott, J. R. and Beer, A. E. (1976) Immunologic aspects of pre-eclampsia. *Amer. J. Obstet. Gynecol.* 125, 418—427.

Scott, J. R., Beer, A. E. and Stastny, P. (1976) Immunogenetic factors in pre-eclampsia and eclampsia. *J. Amer. med. Assoc.* 235, 402—404.

Scott, J. R., Beer, A. E., Guy, R., Liesch, M. and Elbert, G. (1977) Pathogenesis of Rh immunisation in primigravidas. Fetomaternal versus maternofetal bleeding. *Obstet. Gynecol.* 49, 9—14.

Scott, J. S. (1958) Pregnancy toxaemia associated with hydrops foetalis, hydatidiform mole and hydramnios. *J. Obstet. Gynaecol. Brit. Commonw.* 65, 689—701.

Scott, J. S. (1962) Choriocarcinoma. Observations on the etiology. *Amer. J. Obstet. Gynecol.* 83, 185—193.

Scott, J. S. and Jenkins, D. M. (1976) Immunogenetic factors in aetiology of pre-eclampsia/eclampsia (gestosis). *J. med. Genet.* 13, 200—207.

Searle, R. F., Jenkinson, E. J. and Johnson, M. H. (1975) Immunogenicity of mouse trophoblast and embryonic sac. *Nature (London)* 255, 719—720.

Seegal, B. C. and Loeb, E. N. (1940) Effect of anti-placenta serum on development of foetus in the pregnant rat. *Proc. Soc. exp. Biol. Med.* 45, 248—252.

Seegal, B. C. and Loeb, E. N. (1946) The production of chronic glomerulonephritis in rats by the injection of rabbit anti-rat-placental serum. *J. exp. Med.* 84, 211—221.

Seigler, H. G. and Metzgar, R. S. (1970) Embryonic development of human transplantation antigens. *Transplantation* 9, 478—486.

Seip, M. (1960) Systemic lupus erythematosus in pregnancy with haemolytic anaemia, leucopenia and thrombocytopenia in the mother and her newborn infant. *Arch. Dis. Childh.* 35, 364—366.

Sell, K. W., Mori, W., Rack, J. H., Gurner, B. W. and Coombs, R. R. A. (1969) Organ-specific membrane antigens. Attempts to produce specific antisera for mixed antiglobulin tests on disaggregated cells. *Brit. J. exp. Pathol.* 50, 413—426.

Seppälä, M. and Ruoslahti, E. (1972) α-fetoprotein in normal and pregnancy sera. *Lancet* 1, 375—376.

Seppälä, M. and Tolonen, M. (1970) Histocompatibility and human placentation. *Nature (London)* 225, 950—951.

Serr, D. M. and Ismajovich, B. (1963) Determination of the primary sex ratio from human abortions. *Amer. J. Obstet. Gynecol.* 87, 63—65.

Sever, J. L. and Terasaki, P. I. (1970) Maternal-fetal incompatibility. III. Central nervous system and cardiac anomalies. in: *Histocompatibility Testing*. Munksgaard, Copenhagen. pp. 495—500.

Shahani, S. and Southam, A. (1962) Immunofluorescent study of the ABO blood group antigens in human spermatozoa. *Amer. J. Obstet. Gynecol.* 84, 660—666.

Shek, P. N. and Dubiski, S. (1975) Maternal-foetal transfer of normal IgM in the rabbit. *Immunology* 29, 365—369.

Sherman, W. B., Hampton, S. F. and Cooke, R. A. (1940) The placental transmission of antibodies in the skin-sensitive type of human allergy. *J. exp. Med.* 72. 611—621.

Shim, B-S., Kang, Y-S., Kim, W-J., Cho, S-H. and Lee, D-B. (1969) Self-protective activity of colostral IgA against tryptic digestion. *Nature (London)* 222, 787—788.

Shulman, N. P., Aster, R. H., Pearson, H.A. and Hiller, M. C. (1962) Immunoreactions involving platelets. VI. Reactions of maternal isoantibodies responsible for neonatal purpura. Differentiation of a second platelet antigen system. *J. clin. Invest.* 41, 1059—1069.

Siegal, F. P. (1976) IgG on infant's B lymphocytes: enhanced binding of IgG by IgM-bearing lymphoid cells in early childhood. *Scand. J. Immunol.* 5, 721—729.

Silvers, W. K. and Poole, T. W. (1975) The influence of foster nursing on the survival and immunologic competence of mice and rats. *J. Immunol.* 115, 1117—1121.

Silverstein, A. M. (1972a) Immunological maturation in the foetus: modulation of the pathogenesis of congenital infectious diseases. In: *Ontogeny of Acquired Immunity*. CIBA Foundation Symposium. Eds.: Porter and Knight. Elsevier, North-Holland, Amsterdam. pp. 17—25.

Silverstein, A. M. (1972b) Fetal immune responses in congenital infection. *New Engl. J. Med.* 286, 1413—1414.

Simmons, R. L. and Russell, P. S. (1962) The antigenicity of mouse trophoblast. *Ann. N.Y. Acad. Sci.* 99, 717—732.

Simmons, R. L., Lipschultz, M. L., Rios, A. and Ray, P. K. (1971) Failure of neuraminidase to unmask histocompatibility antigens on trophoblast. *Nature (London) New Biol.* 231, 111—112.

Singal, D. P., Berry, R. and Naipaul, N. (1971) HL-A inhibiting activity in human seminal plasma. *Nature (London) New Biol.* 233, 61—62.

Sjögren, H. O., Hellström, I., Bansal, S. C. and Hellström, K. E. (1971) Suggestive evidence that the 'blocking antibodies' of tumour-bearing individuals may be antigen-antibody complexes. *Proc. nat. Acad. Sci.* 68, 1372—1375.

Sjöstedt, S., Grubb, R. and Linell, F. (1951) Blood group incompatibility in abortion and sterility. *Acta pathol. microbiol. scand.* 28, 375—387.

Slade, B. (1973) Antibodies to α-foetoprotein cause foetal mortality in rabbits. *Nature (London)* 246, 493—494.

Slater, L. M., Bostick, W. and Fletcher, L., (1977) Decreased mortality of murine graft-versus-host disease by human chorionic gonadotropin. *Transplantation* 23, 103—104.

Slotnick, V. and Brent, R. L. (1966) The production of congenital malformations using tissue antisera. V. Fluorescent localization of teratogenic antisera in the maternal fetal tissue of the rat. *J. Immunol.* 96, 606—610.

Smith, C. W. and Goldman, A. S. (1968) The cells of human colostrum. I. In vitro studies of morphology and function. *Pediat. Res.* 2, 103—109.

Smith, G. H. (1945) Iso-agglutinin titers in heterospecific pregnancy. *J. Pathol. Bacteriol.* 57, 113—121.

Smith, J. K., Caspary, E. A, and Field, E. J. (1972) Immune responses in pregnancy. *Lancet* 1, 96.

Smith, K., Duhring, J. L., Greene, J. W., Rochlin, D. B. and Blakemore, W. S. (1961) Transfer of maternal erythrocytes across the human placenta. *Obstet. Gynecol.* 18, 673—676.

Smith, M. A., Evans, J. and Steel, C. M. (1974) Age-related variation in proportion of circulating T-cells. *Lancet* 2, 922—924.

Snary, D., Woods, F. R. and Crumpton, M. J. (1976). Disruption of solid tissue for plasma membrane preparation. *Anal. Biochem.* 74, 457—465.

Soliman, M. D. E., Fadel, H. E. and El-Mehairy, M. M. (1971) Serum complement activity during normal pregnancy. *Int. J. Gynecol. Obstet.* 9, 181—184.

Solish, G. I., Gershowitz, H. and Behrman, S. J. (1961) Occurrence and titre of isohemagglutinins in secretions of the human uterine cervix. *Proc. Soc. exp. Biol. Med.* 108, 645—649.

Solnick, C., Gleichmann, H., Kavanah, M. and Schwartz, R. S. (1973) Immunosuppression and malignant lymphomas in graft-versus-host reactions. *Cancer Res.* 33, 2068—2077.

Srivannaboon, S. (1971) Antigenicity of human choriocarcinoma. *Int. J. Fertil.* 16, 36—41.

Stanbridge, E. J. (1976) Suppression of malignancy in human cells. *Nature (London)* 260, 17—20.

Stastny, P. (1965) Accelerated graft rejection in the offspring of immunised mothers. *J. Immunol.* 95, 929—936.

Stastny, P. (1972) Tissue typing antisera from immunization by pregnancy. *Tissue Antigens* 2, 123—127.

Steblay, R. W. (1962) Localisation in human kidney of antibodies formed in sheep against human placenta. *J. Immunol.* 88, 434—442.

Stefanini, M., Mele, R. H. and Skinner, D. (1958) Transitory congenital neutropenia: a new syndrome. *Amer. J. Med.* 25, 749—758.

Steigman, A. J. and Lipton, M. M. (1958) Neonatal immunity. II. Poliocidal effects of human amniotic fluids. *Proc. Soc. exp. Biol. Med.* 99, 576—579.

Steinberg, A. G. and Wilson, J. A. (1963) Hereditary globulin factors and immune tolerance in man. *Science* 140, 303—304.

Stern, K., Davidsohn, I. and Masaitis, L. (1956) Experimental studies on Rh immunisation. *Amer. J. clin. Pathol.* 26, 833—843.

Stern, K., Goodman, H. S. and Berger, M. (1961) Experimental iso-immunization to hemo-antigens in man. *J. Immunol.* 87, 189—198.

Steven, D. (1975) Anatomy of the placental barrier. In: *Comparative Placentation. Essays in Structure and Function.* Ed.: Steven. Academic Press, London, pp. 25—57.

Stevens, V. C. (1973) Immunisation of female baboons with hapten coupled gonadotrophins. *Obstet. Gynecol.* 42, 496—506.

Stevens, V. C. (1974) Fertility control through active immunization using placenta proteins. In: *Immunological Approaches to Fertility Control.* Karolinska Symposia on Research Methods in Reproductive Endocrinology. Ed.: Diczfalusy. Karolinska Institute, Stockholm. pp. 357—375.

Stevens, V. C. (1976) Antifertility effects from immunizations with intact, subunits and fragments of HCG. In: *Physiological Effects of Immunity against Reproductive Hormones.* Eds.: Edwards and Johnson. Cambridge University Press, Cambridge. pp. 249—274.

Stevens, V. C. and Crystle, C. D. (1973) Effects of immunisation with hapten coupled HCG on the human menstrual cycle. *Obstet. Gynecol.* 42, 485—495.

Stevenson, A. C., Davison, B. C. C., Say, B., Ustuopler, S., Durmas, L., Abdul-Einen, M., and Toppozada, H. K. (1971) Contribution of feto-maternal incompatibility to aetiology of pre-eclamptic toxaemia. *Lancet* 2, 1286—1289.

Stevenson, A. C., Say, B., Ustaoglu, S. and Durmus, A. (1976) Aspects of pre-eclamptic toxaemia of pregnancy, consanguinity, and twinning in Ankara. *J. med. Genet.* 13, 1—8.

Stiehm, E. R. (1975) Fetal defense mechanisms. *Amer. J. Dis. Child.* 129, 438—443.

Stiehm, E. R. and Fudenberg, H. H. (1966) Serum levels of immune globulins in health and disease: a survey. *Pediatrics* 37, 715—727.

Stiehm, E. R., Ammann, A. J. and Cherry, J. D. (1966) Elevated cord macroglobulins in the diagnosis of intrauterine infections. *New Engl. J. Med.* 275, 971—977.

Stimson, W. H. (1976) Studies on the immunosuppressive properties of a pregnancy-associated α-macroglobulin. *Clin. exp. Immunol.* 25, 199—206.

Stimson, W. H. (1977) Identifications of pregnancy-associated α-macroglobulin on the surface of peripheral blood leucocyte populations. *Clin. exp. Immunol.* 28, 445—452.

Stimson, W. H. and Blackstock, J. C. (1975) Synthesis of a pregnancy-associated α-macroglobulin by human leucocytes. *Experientia* 31, 371—373.

Stites, D. P., Wybran, J., Carr, M. C. and Fudenberg, H. H. (1972) Development of cellular immunocompetence in man. In: *Ontogeny of Acquired Immunity.* Eds.: Porter and Knight. Associated Scientific Publishers, Amsterdam. pp. 113—129.

Stites, D. P., Carr, M. C. and Fudenberg, H. H. (1974) Ontogeny of cellular immunity in the human fetus. Development of responses to phytohaemagglutinin and to allogeneic cells. *Cell. Immunol.* 11, 257—271.

Stolbach, L. L., Krant, M. J. and Fishman, W. H. (1969) Ectopic production of an alkaline phosphatase isoenzyme in patients with cancer. *New Engl. J. Med.* 281, 757—762.

Stoliar, O. A., Pelley, R. P., Kaniecki-Green, E. Klaus, M. H. and Carpenter, C. C. J. (1976) Secretory IgA against enterotoxins in breast milk. *Lancet* 1, 1258—1261.

Stossel, T. P., Alper, C. A. and Rosen, F. S. (1973) Opsonic activity in the newborn: role of properdin. *Pediatrics* 52, 134—137.

Straus, E. K. (1961) Occurrence of antibody in human vaginal mucus. *Proc. Soc. exp. Biol. Med.* 106, 617—621.

Strauss, L. and Driscoll, S. G. (1964) Congenital neuroblastoma involving the placenta. Report of two cases. *Pediatrics* 34, 23—31.

Streilein, J. W. and Grebe, S. (1976) 'Graft-versus-host reaction: a review'. *Adv. Immunol.* 22, 119—221.

Strelkauskas, A. J., Wilson, B. S. and Dray, S. (1975) Inversion of levels of human T & B cells in early pregnancy. *Nature (London)* 258, 331—332.

Sullivan, J. F. and Jennings, E. R. (1966) Transplacental fetal-maternal haemorrhage. *Amer. J. clin. Pathol.* 46, 36—42.

Sundqvist, K., Bergström, S. and Håkansson, S. (1977) Surface antigens of human trophoblasts. *Dev. compar. Immunol.* 1, 241—253.

Sussman, S. (1961) The passive transfer of antibodies to Escherichia coli O111:B4 from mother to offspring. *Pediatrics* 27, 308—313.

Sutherland, J. M., Esselborn, V. M., Burket, R. L., Skillman, T. B. and Benson, J. T. (1960) Familial nongoitrous cretinism apparently due to maternal antithyroid antibody: report of family. *New Engl. J. Med.* 263, 336—341.

Sweet, L. K. and Connerty, H. V. (1941) Congenital melanoma. Report of a case in which antenatal metastasis had occurred. *Amer. J. Dis. Child.* 1029—1040.

Swinburne, L. M. (1970) Leucocyte antigens and placental sponge. *Lancet* 2, 592—594.

Szulman, A. E. (1964) The histological distribution of blood group substances A & B in man as disclosed by immunofluorescence. III. The A, B and H antigens in embryo and fetuses from 18 mm in length. *J. exp. Med.* 119, 503—515.

Szulman, A. E. (1972) The A, B and H blood-group antigens in human placenta. *New Engl. J. Med.* 286, 1028—1031.

Tait, B. D., d'Apice, A. J. F. and Morris, P. J. (1974) Maternal cell mediated immunity to foetal transplantation antigens. *Tissue Antigens* 4, 586—594.

Takano, K. and Miller, J. R. (1972) ABO incompatibility as a cause of spontaneous abortion: evidence from abortuses. *J. med. Genet.* 9, 144—150.

Tamerius, J., Hellström, I. and Hellström, K. E. (1975) Evidence that blocking factors in the sera of multiparous mice are associated with immunoglobulins. *Int. J. Cancer* 16, 456, 464.

Tashjian, A. H., Weintraub, B. D., Barowsky, N. J., Rabson, A. S. and Rosen, S. W. (1973) Sub-units of human chorionic gonadotropin: unbalanced synthesis and secretion by clonal cell strains derived from a bronchogenic carcinoma. *Proc. nat. Acad. Sci.* 70, 1419—1422.

Taylor, A. I. and Polani, P. E. (1965) XX/XY mosaicism in man. *Lancet* 1, 1226.

Taylor, J. F. (1967) Sensitisation of Rh negative daughters by their Rh positive mothers. *New Engl. J. Med.* 276. 547—551.

Taylor, P. V. and Hancock, K. W. (1973) Viability of human trophoblast in vitro. *J. Obstet. Gynaecol. Brit. Commonw.* 80, 834—838.

Taylor, P. V. and Hancock, K. W. (1975) Antigenicity of trophoblast and possible antigen-masking effects during pregnancy. *Immunology* 28, 973—982.

Taylor, P. V., Gowland, G., Hancock, K. W. and Scott, J. S. (1975) Effect of length of gestation on maternal cellular immunity to human trophoblast antigens. *Amer. J. Obstet. Gynecol.* 125, 528—531.

Taylor, W. C. and Kullman, G. (1961) The detection of foetal erythrocytes in blood smears. *J. Obstet. Gynaecol. Brit. Commonw.* 68, 261—263.

Ten Broeck, C. and Bauer, J. H. (1923) The transmission of tetanus antitoxin through the placenta. *Proc. Soc. exp. Biol. Med.* 20, 399—400.

Teoh, E. S. (1967) Chorionic gonadotrophin in the serum and urine of Asian women in normal pregnancy. *J. Obstet. Gynaecol. Brit. Commonw.* 74, 74—79.

Terasaki, P. I., Mickey, M. R., Yamazaki, J. N. and Vredevoe, D. (1970) Maternal-fetal incompatibility. I. Incidence of HL-A antibodies and possible association with congenital anomalies. *Transplantation* 9, 538—543.

Terry, W. D., Henkart, P. A., Coligan, J. E. and Todd, C. W. (1975) Carcinoembryonic antigen: characterisation and clinical applications. *Transplant. Rev.* 20, 100—129.

Than, G. N., Csaba, I. F., Karg, N. J., Szabo, D. G., Ambrus, M. and Bajtai, G. (1975) Immunosuppressive effect of pregnancy-associated alpha$_2$-glycoprotein. *Lancet* 1, 515.

Thiede, H. A., Choate, J. W., Gardner, H. H. and Santay, H. (1965) Immunofluorescent examination of the human chorionic villus for blood group A and B substance. *J. exp. Med.* 121, 1039—1049.

Thiede, H. A., Choate, J. W. and Dyre, S. (1968) Pregnancy and the lymphocyte. *Amer. J. Obstet. Gynecol.* 102, 642—653.

Thom, H. and McKay, E. (1971) Observations on infants of mothers with antibodies to γ-globulin. *Biol. Neonate* 19, 397—408.

Thomaidis, T., Agathopoulos, A. and Matsaniotis, N. (1969) Natural isohaemagglutinin production by the fetus. *J. Pediat.* 74, 39—48.

Thomas, J. H., MacArthur, R. I. and Humprey, L. J. (1976) Fc receptors on the human placenta. *Obstet. Gynecol* 48, 170—171.

Thompson, K. D. and Linna, T. J. (1973) Bursa-dependent and thymus-dependent 'surveillance' of a virus-induced tumour in the chicken. *Nature (London) New Biol.* 245, 10—12.

Thomson, D., Paterson, W. G., Smart, G. E., MacDonald, H. K. and Robson, J. S. (1972) The renal lesions of toxaemic and abruptio placentae studied by light and electronmicroscopy. *J. Obstet. Gynaecol. Brit. Commonw.* 79, 311—320.

Thomson, J. A. and Riley, I. D. (1966) Neonatal thyrotoxicosis associated with maternal hypothyroidism. *Lancet* 1, 635—636.

Thomson, J. A, Dirmikis, S. M., Munro, D. S., Smith, B. R., Hall, R. and Mukhtan, D. E. (1975) Neonatal hyperthyroidism and long-acting thyroid stimulator protector. *Brit. med. J.* 2, 36.

Thomson, N. C., Stevenson, R. D., Behan, W. M., Sloan, D. P., and Horne, C. H. W. (1976) Immunological studies in pre-eclamptic toxaemia. *Brit. med. J.* 1, 1307—1309.

Thomson, S., Arnott, W. M. and Matthew, G. D. (1939) Blood complement in acute glomerulonephritis. *Lancet* 2. 734—735.

Thong, Y. H., Steele, R. W., Monroe, M. V., Hensen, S. A. and Bellanti, J. A. (1973) Impaired in-vitro cell-mediated immunity to rubella virus during pregnancy. *New Engl. J. Med.* 289, 604—606.

Tighe, J. R., Garrod, P. R. and Curran, R. C. (1967) The trophoblast of the human chorionic villus. *J. Pathol. Bacteriol.* 93, 559—567.

Tiilikainen, A. and Kauranen, H. (1969) Anti-lymphocyte antibodies and toxaemia of pregnancy. *Acta pathol. microbiol. scand.* 77, 346.

Tiilikainen, A., Schröder, J. and De la Chapelle, A. (1974) Foetal leucocytes in the maternal circulation after delivery. II. Masking of HL-A antigens. *Transplantation* 17, 355—360.

Timmerman, W. A. (1931) Zur Frage der Uebertragung des Typhus 'H' und 'O'-Agglutinin von Mutter auf Kind. *Z. Immun.-Forsch.* 70, 388—399.

Toivanen, P. and Hirvonen, T. (1970a) Placental weight in human foeto-maternal incompatibility. *Clin. exp. Immunol.* 7, 533—539.

Toivanen, P. and Hirvonen, T. (1970b) Sex ratio of newborns: preponderance of males in toxemia of pregnancy. *Science* 170, 187—188.

Tomasi, T. B. and Zigelbaum, S. (1963) The selective occurrence of γ1A globulins in certain body fluids. *J. clin. Invest.* 42, 1552—1560.

Tominaga, T. and Page, E. W. (1966) Sex chromatin of trophoblastic tumours. *Amer. J. Obstet. Gynecol.* 96, 305—309.

Tomkins, G. A. (1968) Chromosome studies on cultured lymphoblast cell lines from cases of New Guinea Burkitt lymphoma, myeloblastic and lymphoblastic leukaemia and infectious mononucleosis. *Int. J. Cancer* 3, 644—653.

Tomoda, Y., Fuma, M., Saiki, N., Ishizuka, N. and Akaza, T. (1976) Immunologic studies in patients with trophoblastic neoplasia. *Amer. J. Obstet. Gynecol.* 126, 661—667.

Tønder, O., Morse, P. A. and Humphrey, L. J. (1974) Similarities of Fc receptors in human malignant tissue and normal lymphoid tissue. *J. Immunol.* 113, 1162—1169.

Tongio, M. M. and Mayer, S. (1977) Narrowing of feto-maternal immunization at time of delivery. *Tissue Antigens* 9, 174—176.

Tongio, M. M., Berrebi, A., Pfeiffer, B. and Mayer, S. (1971) Serological studies on lymphocytotoxic antibodies in primiparous women. *Tissue Antigens* 1, 243—257.

Tongio, M. M., Berrebi, A. and Mayer, S. (1972) A study of lymphocytotoxic antibodies in multiparous women having had at least four pregnancies. *Tissue Antigens* 2, 378—388.

Tongio, M. M., Mayer, S. and Lebec, A (1975) Transfer of HLA antibodies from the mother to the child. *Transplantation* 20, 163—166.

Tourville, D. R., Ogra, S. S., Lippes, J. and Tomasi, T. B. (1970) The human female reproductive tract: immunohistological localisation of γA, γG, γM, secretory 'piece', and lactoferrin. *Amer. J. Obstet. Gynecol.* 108. 1102—1108.

Tovey, G. H. (1945) Study of protective factors in heterospecific blood group pregnancy and their role in prevention of haemolytic disease of newborn. *J. Pathol. Bacteriol.* 57, 295—305.

Tovey, L. A. D. and Maroni, E. S. (1976) Rhesus isoimmunisation. In: *Immunology of Human Reproduction.* Eds.: Scott and Jones. Academic Press, London. pp. 187—227.

Tovey, L. A. D. and Robinson, A. E. (1975) Reduced severity of Rh haemolytic disesase after anti-D immunoglobulin. *Brit. med. J.* 4, 320—322.

Tribe, C. R., Smart, G. E. and MacKenzie, J. C. (1974) Pre-eclampsia and the kidney. *Brit. med. J.* 2, 335.

Tuffrey, M., Barnes, R. D., Lund, P., Catty, D. and King T. D. (1976) Manipulation of mouse embryos to study the role of maternal antibody upon the IgG_{2a} levels in the progeny of immunised maternal recipients using allotypic markers. In: *Maternofoetal Transmission of Immunoglobulins.* Ed.: Hemmings. Cambridge University Press, Cambridge. pp. 253—260.

Tunicliff, R. (1910) Observations on the anti-infectious power of the blood of infants. *J. infect. Dis.* 7, 698—707.

Turk, J. L. (1972) *Immunology in Clinical Medicine.* Heinemann, London, pp. 217—221.

Turner, J. H., Wald, N. and Quinlivan, W. (1966) Cytogenetic evidence concerning possible transplacental transfer of leukocytes in pregnant women. *Amer. J. Obstet. Gynecol.* 95, 831—833.

Turner, J. H., Hutchinson, D. L., Hayashi, T. T., Petricciani, J. C. and Germanowski, J. (1975) Fetal and maternal risks associated with intrauterine transfusion procedures. *Amer. J. Obstet. Gynecol.* 123, 251—256.

Usategui-Gomez, M. and Morgan, D. F. (1966) Maternal origin of the group specific (Gc) proteins in amniotic fluid. *Nature (London)* 212, 1600—1601.

Usategui-Gomez, M. and Stearns, S. (1969) Comparative study of the Rh-D antibody titres of amniotic fluids and corresponding maternal sera in Rh-D sensitised pregnancies. *Nature (London)* 221, 82—83.

Usategui-Gomez, M., Morgan, D. F. and Toolan, H. W. (1966) A comparative study of amniotic fluid, maternal sera and cord sera by disc electrophoresis. *Proc. Soc. exp. Biol. Med.* 123, 547—551.

Vaerman, J-P. and Férin, J. (1974) Local immunological response in the vagina, cervix and endometrium. In: *Immunological Approaches to Fertility Control.* Karolinska Symposia on Research Methods in Reproductive Endocrinology. Ed.: Diczfalusy. Karolinska Inst., Stockholm. pp. 281—305.

Vahlquist, B. and Högstedt, C. (1949) Minute absorption of diphtheric antibodies from the gastrointestinal tract in infants. *Pediatrics* 4, 401—405.

Vahlquist, B., Lagercrantz, R. and Nordbring, F. (1950) Maternal and foetal titres of antistreptolysin and antistaphylolysin at different stages of gestation. *Lancet* 2, 851—853.

Vaitukaitis, J. L. (1974) Human chorionic gonadotropin as a tumor marker. *Ann. clin. Lab. Sci.* 4, 276—280.

Valentine, G. H. (1958) ABO incompatibility and haemolytic disease of the newborn. *Arch. Dis. Childh.* 33, 185—190.

Van Beek, W. P., Smets, L. A. and Emmelot, P. (1973) Increased sialic acid density in surface glycoprotein of transformed and malignant cells — a general phenomenon? *Cancer Res.* 33, 2913—2922.

Van Beek, W. P., Smets, L. A. and Emmelot, P. (1975) Changed surface glycoprotein as a marker of malignancy in human leukaemic cells. *Nature* 253, 457—460.

Vandenbroucke, J. and Verstraete, M. (1955) Thrombocytopenia due to platelet agglutinins in the newborn. *Lancet* 1, 593—594.

Van der Werf, A. J. M. (1971) Are lymphocytotoxic iso-antibodies induced by the early human trophoblast? *Lancet* 1, 595.

Van Furth, R., Schuit, R. E. and Hijmans, W. (1965) The immunological development of the human fetus. *J. exp. Med.* 122, 1173—1188.

Van Rood, J. J., Eernisse, J. G., Van Leeuwen, A. (1958) Leucocyte antibodies in sera from pregnant women. *Nature (London)* 181, 1735—1736.

Van Rood, J. J., Van Leeuwen, A., Van Santen, M. C. T. (1970) Anti HL-A2 inhibitor in normal serum. *Nature (London)* 226, 366—367.

Vassalli, P. and McCluskey, R. T. (1965) The coagulation process and glomerular disease. *Amer. J. Med.* 39, 179—183.

Vassalli, P., Morris, R. H. and McCluskey, R. T. (1963a) The pathogenic role of fibrin deposition in the glomerular lesions of toxemia of pregnancy. *J. exp. Med.* 118, 467—477.

Vassalli, P., Simon, G. and Rouiller, C. (1963b) Production of ultra-structural glomerular lesions resembling those of toxaemia of pregnancy by thromboplastin infusion in rabbits. *Nature (London)* 199, 1105—1106.

Virélla, G., Amélia Silveira Nunes, M. and Tamaguini, G. (1972) Placental transfer of human IgG subclasses. *Clin. exp. Immunol.* 10, 475—478.

Vitums, V. C. and Sites, J. G. (1968) Leukaemia in pregnancy. Data on 9 cases with an important new finding. *Med. Ann. D.C.* 37, 588—593.

Vives, J., Gelabert, A. and Castillo R. (1976) HL-A antibodies and period of gestation: decline in frequency of positive sera during last trimester. *Tissue Antigens* 7, 209—212.

Voigt, J. C. and Britt, R. P. (1969) Feto-maternal haemorrhage in therapeutic abortion. *Brit. med. J.* 4, 395—396.

Von Schoultz, B. (1974) A quantitative study of the pregnancy zone protein in the serum of pregnant and puerperal women. *Amer. J. Obstet. Gynecol.* 119, 792—797.

Vos, G. H. (1965) A comparative observation of the presence of anti-Tj^a-like hemolysins in relation to obstetric history, distribution of the various blood groups and the occurrence of immune anti-A or anti-B hemolysins among aborters and nonaborters. *Transfusion* 5, 327—335.

Vossen, J. M. and Hijmans, W. (1975) Membrane-associated immunoglobulin determinants on bone-marrow and blood lymphocytes in pediatric age group and on fetal tissues. *Ann. N.Y. Acad. Sci.* 254, 262—279.

Vyas, G. N. and Fudenberg, H. H. (1970) Immunobiology of human anti-IgA. A serological and immunogenetic study of immunization of IgA in transfusion and pregnancy. *Clin. Genet.* 1, 45—64.

Vyas, G. N., Levin, A. S. and Fudenberg, H. H. (1970) Intrauterine isoimmunization caused by maternal IgA crossing the placenta. *Nature (London)* 226, 275—276.

Walden, P. A. M., Pentycross, C. R., Leyton, R., Browne, P., Dent, J. and Vernon, P. (1976) Leucocyte migration in response to PPD in patients with trophoblastic tumours. *Eur. J. Cancer* 12, 277—282.

Waldman, R. H., Cruz, J. M. and Rowe, D. S. (1972a) Immunoglobulin levels and antibody to Candida albicans in human cervicovaginal secretions. *Clin. exp. Immunol.* 10, 427—434.

Waldman, R. H., Cruz, J. M. and Rowe, D. S. (1972b) Intravaginal immunization of humans with Candida albicans. *J. Immunol.* 109, 662—664.

Waldmann, T. A. and McIntire, K. R. (1972) Serum-alpha-fetoprotein levels in patients with ataxia-telangiectasia. *Lancet* 2, 1112—1115.

Walford, R. (1966) Increased incidence of lymphoma after injection of mice with cells differing at weak histocompatibility loci. *Science* 152, 78—80.

Walkanowska, J., Conte, F. A. and Grumbach, M. M. (1969) Practical and theoretical implications of fetal/maternal lymphocyte transfer. *Lancet* 1, 1119—1122.

Walker, J. S., Freeman, C. B. and Harris, R. (1972) Lymphocyte reactivity in pregnancy. *Brit. med. J.* 3, 469.

Wallach, E. E., Brody, J. I. and Oski, F. A. (1969) Fetal immunization as a consequence of bacilluria during pregnancy. *Obstet. Gynecol.* 33, 100—105.

Walsh, J. J. and Lewis, B. V. (1970) Transplacental haemorrhage due to termination of pregnancy. *J. Obstet. Gynaecol. Brit. Commonw.* 77, 133—136.

Wands, J. R., Alpert, E. and Isselbacher, K. J. (1975) Serial studies and partial characterization of a serum inhibitor of cellular immunity in acute hepatitis-B and chronic active hepatitis. *Gastroenterology* 69, 878.

Wang, A. C., Faulk, W. P., Stuckey, M. A. and Fudenberg, H. H. (1970)

Chemical differences of adult, fetal and hypogammaglobulinemic IgG immunoglobulins. *Immunochemistry* 7, 703—708.

Warburton, D. and Naylor, A. F. (1971) The effect of parity on placental weight and birth weight. An immunological phenomenon? A report of the collaborative study of cerebral palsy. *Amer. J. hum. Genet.* 23, 41—54.

Ward, H. K., Walsh, R. J. and Kooptzoof, O. (1957) Rh antigens and immunological tolerance. *Nature (London)* 179, 1352—1353.

Wardle, E. M. and Mennon, I. S. (1969) Fibrinolysis in pre-eclamptic toxaemia of pregnancy. *Brit. med. J.* 2, 625—627.

Warren, R. J., Lepow, M. L., Bartsch, G. E. and Robbins, F. C. (1964) The relationship of maternal antibody, breast feeding, and age to the susceptibility of newborn infants to infection with attenuated polioviruses. *Pediatrics* 34, 4—13.

Wass, M., Rawlings, G. T., Pentrycross, C. R. and Bagshawe, K. D. (1977) Response of lymphocytes from cancer patients to human chorionic gonadotrophin. *Lancet* 1, 171—172.

Wasz-Höckert, O., Wager, O., Hautala, T. and Widholm, O. (1956) Transmission of antibodies from mother to foetus. A study of the diphtheria level in the newborn with oesophageal atresia. *Ann. Med. exp. Biol. Fenn.* 34, 444—446.

Waterhouse, J. A. H. and Hogben, L. (1947) Incompatibility of mother and foetus with respect to iso-agglutinogen A and its antibody. *Brit. J. soc. Med.* 1, 1—17.

Watkins, S. M. (1972) Lymphocyte response to phytohaemagglutinin in pregnancy. *J. Obstet. Gynaecol. Brit. Commonw.* 79, 990—993.

Wei, P. Y. and Chiang, W. T.(1967) Tissue culture study of abnormal trophoblast. Growth pattern and nuclear sex. *Amer. J. Obstet. Gynecol.* 98, 1144—1147.

Weiner, W., Child, R. M., Garvie, J. M. and Peck, W. H. (1958) Foetal cells in maternal circulation during pregnancy. *Brit. med. J.* 2, 770—771.

Weintraub, B. D. and Rosen, S. W. (1971) Ectopic production of human chorionic somatomammotropin by non-trophoblast cancers. *J. clin. Endocrinol. Metab.* 32, 94—101.

Weintraub, B. D. and Rosen, S. W. (1973) Ectopic production of the isolated beta subunit of human chorionic gonadotropin. *J. clin. Invest.* 52, 3135—3142.

Whang-Peng, J., Leikin, S., Harris, C., Lee, E. and Stites, J. (1973) The transplacental passage of fetal leucocytes into the maternal blood. *Proc. Soc. exp. Biol. Med.* 142, 50—53.

White, L. P., Linden, G., Breslow, I. and Harzfeld, L. (1961) Studies of melanoma, the effect of pregnancy on survival in human melanoma. *J. Amer. med. Assoc.* 177, 235—238.

Whyte, A., Loke, Y. W. and Stoddart, R. W. (In press) Saccharide distribution in human trophoblast demonstrated using fluorescein-labeled lectins. *Histochem. J.*

Wide, L. (1969) Early diagnosis of pregnancy. *Lancet* 2, 863—864.

Wiener, A. S. (1944) A new test (blocking test) for Rh sensitisation. *Proc. Soc. exp. Biol. Med.* 56, 173—176.

Wiener, A. S., Freda, V. J., Wexler, I. B. and Brancato, G. J. (1960) Pathogenesis of ABO hemolytic disease. *Amer. J. Obstet. Gynecol.* 79, 567—592.

Wild, A. E. (1960) Proteins of the liquor amnii. *Brit. med. J.* 1, 802.

Wild, A. E. (1961) The association between protein and bilirubin in liquor amnii. *Clin. Sci.* 21, 221—231.

Wild, A. E. (1976) Mechanism of protein transport across the rabbit yolk sac endoderm. In: *Maternofoetal Transmission of Immunoglobulins.* Ed.: Hemmings. Cambridge University Press, Cambridge. pp. 155—167.

Wiley, L. D. (1974) Presence of a gonadotrophin on the surface of pre-implanted mouse embryos. *Nature (London)* 252, 715—716.

Winchester, R. J., Fu, S. M., Wernet, P., Kunkel, H. G., Dupont, B. and Jersild, C. (1975) Recognition by pregnancy serum of non-HL-A alloantigens selectively expressed on B lymphocytes. *J. exp. Med.* 141, 924—929.

Winter, G. C. B., Byles, A. B. and Yoffey, J. M. (1965) Blood lymphocytes in new-born and adult. *Lancet* 2, 932—933.

Wislocki, G. B. and Bennett, H. S. (1943) The histology and cytology of the human and monkey placenta, with special reference to the trophoblast. *Amer. J. Anat.* 73, 335—350.

Wolf, R. L., Lomnitzer, R. and Rabson, A. R. (1977) An inhibitor of lymphocyte proliferation and lymphokine production released by unstimulated foetal monocytes. *Clin. exp. Immunol.* 27, 464—468.

Woodrow, J. C. and Donohoe, W. T. A. (1968) Rh immunisation by pregnancy. Results of a survey and their relevance to prophylactic therapy. *Brit. med. J.* 4, 139—144.

Woodrow, J. C., Clarke, C. A., Donohoe, W. T. A., Finn, F., McConnell, R. B., Sheppard, P. M., Lehane, D., Russell, S. H., Kulke, W. and Durkin, C. M., (1965) Prevention of Rh-haemolytic disease: a third report. *Brit. med. J.* 1, 279—283.

Woodrow, J. C., Clarke, C. A., Donohoe, W. T. A., Finn, R., McConnell, R. B., Sheppard, P. M., Lehane, D., Roberts, F. M. and Gimlette, T. M. D. (1975) Mechanism of Rh prophylaxis: an experimental study on specificity of immunosuppression. *Brit. med. J.* 2, 57—59.

Woodruff, M. F. A. and Lennox, B. (1959) Reciprocal skin grafts in a pair of twins showing blood chimaerism. *Lancet* 2, 476—478.

World Health Organisation Technical Report Series (1968) Immunology of malaria. *WHO Tech. Rep. Ser.* 396, 1—50.

Wray, V. P. and Walborg, E. F. (1971) Isolation of tumour cell surface binding sites for concanavalin A and wheat germ agglutinin. *Cancer Res.* 31, 2072—2079.

Wren, B. G. and Vos, G. H. (1961) Blood group incompatibility as a cause of spontaneous abortion. *J. Obstet. Gynaecol. Brit. Commonw.* 68, 637—647.

Wrezlewicz, W., Rashkoff, E., Lucas, T., Ramasamy, N. and Sawyer, P. N. (1977) Effect of human chorionic gonadotropin and antithymocyte-globulin on the electrophoretic mobility of human lymphocytes. *Transplant. Proc.* 9, 1441—1445.

Wybran, J., Carr, M. C. and Fudenberg, H. H. (1972) The human rosette-forming cell as a marker of a population of thymus-derived cells. *J. clin. Invest.* 51, 2537—2542.

Wynn, R. M. (1967) Fetomaternal cellular relations in the human basal plate: An ultrastructural study of the placenta. *Amer. J. Obstet. Gynecol.* 97, 832—850.

Yachnin, S. (1972) Inhibition of phytohaemagglutinin-induced lymphocyte transformation by α globulins: Lack of correlation with phytohaemagglutinin precipitation by serum proteins. *J. Immunol.* 108, 845—847.

Yachnin, S. (1975) Fetuin, an inhibitor of lymphocyte transformation. The interaction of fetuin with phytomitogens, and a possible role for fetuin in fetal development. *J. exp. Med.* 141, 242—256.

Yachnin, S. (1976) Demonstration of the inhibitory effect of human alphafetoprotein on in-vitro human lymphocyte transformation. *Proc. nat. Acad. Sci.* 73, 2857—2861.

Yachnin, S. and Lester, E. (1976) Inhibition of human lymphocyte transformation by human alphafoetoprotein (HAFP); comparison of foetal and hepatoma HAFP and kinetic studies of in-vitro immunosuppression. *Clin. exp. Immunol.* 26, 484—490.

Yachnin, S. and Lester, E. P. (1977) Inhibition of human lymphocyte transformation by human α-fetoprotein (HAFP): HAFP monomers and multimers and a resistant lymphocyte subpopulation. *J. Immunol.* 119, 555—557.

Yamini, G., Chard, T. and Blake, M. E. (1972) Some biological effects of antisera to human placental lactogen in rodents. *J. Endocrinol.* 55, 29—30.

Yang, S. L., Kleinman, A. M. and Wei, P. Y. (1975) Immunologic aspects of term pregnancy toxemia — study of immunoglobulins and complement. *Amer. J. Obstet. Gynecol.* 122, 727—731.

Younger, J. B., St. Pierre, R. L. and Zmijewski, C. M. (1969) Effect of human chorionic gonadotropin on antibody production. *Amer. J. Obstet. Gynecol.* 105, 9—13.

Youtanannkorn, V. and Matangkasombut, P. (1972) Human maternal cell mediated immune reaction to placental antigens. *Clin. exp. Immunol* 11, 549—555.

Youtanannkorn, V. and Matangkasombut, P. (1973) Specific plasma factors blocking human maternal cell-mediated immune reaction to placental antigens. *Nature (London) New Biol.* 242, 110—111.

Youtanannkorn, V., Matangkasombut, P. and Osathanondh, V. (1974) Onset of human maternal cell-mediated immune reaction to placental antigens during the first pregnancy. *Clin. exp. Immunol.* 16, 1—6.

Yu, V. Y. H., Waller, C. A., MacLennan, I. C. M. and Baum, J. D. (1975) Lymphocyte reactivity in pregnant women and newborn infants. *Brit. med. J.* 1, 428—430.

Zak, S. J. and Good, R. A. (1959) Immunochemical studies of human serum gamma-globulin. *J. clin. Invest.* 38, 579—586.

Zarou, D. M., Lichtman, H. C. and Hillman, L. M. (1964) The transmission of chromium-51 tagged maternal erythrocytes from mother to fetus. *Amer. J. Obstet. Gynecol.* 88, 565—571.

Zeek, P. and Assali, N. (1950) Vascular changes in the decidua associated with eclamptogenic toxemia of pregnancy. *Amer. J. clin. Pathol.* 20, 1099—1109.

Zilliacus, R., De la Chapelle, A., Schröder, J., Tiilikainen, A., Kohne, E. and Kleihauer, E. (1975) Transplacental passage of foetal blood cells. *Scand. J. Haematol.* 15, 333—338.

Zimmerman, A. and Schmickel, R. (1971) Fluorescent bodies in maternal circulation. *Lancet* 1, 1305.

Zimmerman, E. F., Voorting-Hawking, M. and Michael, J. G. (1977) Immunosuppression by mouse sialylated α-foetoprotein. *Nature (London)* 265, 354—356.

Zipurksy, A., Hull, A., White, F. D. and Israels, L. G. (1959) Foetal erythrocytes in maternal circulation. *Lancet* 1, 451—452.

Zipurksy, A, Pollock, J., Neelands, P., Chown, B. and Israels, L. G. (1963) The transplacental passage of fetal red blood cells and the pathogenesis of Rh immunisation during pregnancy. *Lancet* 2, 489—493.

Zipursky, A., Brown, E. J. and Bienenstock, J. (1973) Lack of opsonization potential of 11S human secretory γA. *Proc. Soc. exp. Biol. Med.* 142, 181—184.

Zmijewski, C. M., Zmijewski, H. E. and Huneycutt, H. C. (1967) The relationship of the frequencies of white cell antibodies and red cell antibodies in the sera of multiparous women. *Int. Arch. Allergy appl. Immunol.* 32, 574—582.

Zuelzer, W. W. and Kaplan, E. (1954a) ABO heterospecific pregnancy and hemolytic disease. I. Patterns of maternal A and B isoantibodies in unselected pregnancies. *Amer. J. Dis. Child.* 88, 158—178.

Zuelzer, W. W. and Kaplan, E. (1954b) ABO heterospecific pregnancy and hemolytic disease. II. Patterns of A and B isoantibodies in the cord blood of normal infants. *Amer. J. Dis. Child.* 88, 179—192.

Zuelzer, W. W. and Rutzky, J. (1953) Megaloblastic anemia of infancy. *Adv. Pediat.* 6, 243—306.

Author index

Subject index

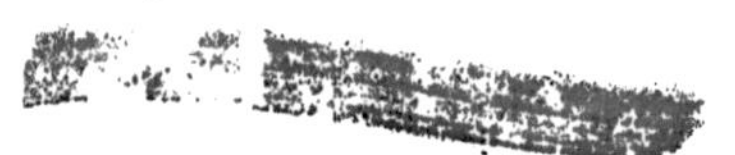